D1707275

Pulmonary Function Testing

Principles and Practice

Pulmonary Function Testing
Principles and Practice

Edited by

Steven A. Conrad, M.D.

Instructor
Department of Medicine
Clinical Assistant Professor
Department of Physiology and Biophysics
Louisiana State University Medical Center
Shreveport, Louisiana

Gary T. Kinasewitz, M.D.

Associate Professor
Pulmonary Diseases Section
Department of Medicine
Associate Professor
Department of Physiology and Biophysics
Louisiana State University Medical Center
Shreveport, Louisiana

Ronald B. George, M.D.

Professor and Chief
Pulmonary Diseases Section
Department of Medicine
Medical Director
Department of Respiratory Therapy
Louisiana State University Medical Center
Shreveport, Louisiana

Churchill Livingstone
New York, Edinburgh, London, and Melbourne 1984

Acquisitions Editor: *William R. Schmitt*
Copy Editor: *Donna C. Balopole*
Production Editor: *Karen Goldsmith Montanez*
Production Supervisor: *Kerry Ann O'Rourke*
Compositor: *Progressive Typographers, Inc.*
Printer/Binder: *The Maple-Vail Book Manufacturing Group*

© **Churchill Livingstone Inc. 1984**

Distributed in the United Kingdom by Churchill Livingstone,
Robert Stevenson House, 1–3 Baxter's Place, Leith Walk,
Edinburgh EH1 3AF and by associated companies, branches
and representatives throughout the world.

First published in 1984

Printed in U.S.A.

ISBN 0-443-08182-4

9 8 7 6 5 4 3 2 1

Library of Congress Cataloging in Publication Data
Main entry under title:

Pulmonary function testing.

Includes bibliographies and index.
1. Pulmonary function tests.   I. Conrad, Steven A.
II. Kinasewitz, Gary T.   III. George, Ronald B.
[DNLM: 1. Respiratory Function Tests. WF 141 P982]
RC734.P84P84   1984   616.2′4   84-11395

ISBN 0-443-08182-4

Manufactured in the United States of America

Contributors

Andrew L. Chesson, Jr., M.D.
Associate Professor, Department of Neurology, Louisiana State University Medical Center, Shreveport, Louisiana

Steven A. Conrad, M.D.
Instructor, Department of Medicine, and Clinical Professor, Department of Physiology and Biophysics, Louisiana State University Medical Center, Shreveport, Louisiana

Howard Eigen, M.D.
Director, Section of Pediatric Pulmonology, and Professor of Pediatrics and Respiratory Therapy, Indiana University School of Medicine; Director, Pediatric Pulmonary Function Laboratory, James Whitcomb Riley Hospital for Children, Indianapolis, Indiana

Ronald B. George, M.D.
Professor and Chief, Pulmonary Diseases Section, Department of Medicine, and Medical Director, Department of Respiratory Therapy, Louisiana State University Medical Center, Shreveport, Louisiana

Stephen G. Jenkinson, M.D.
Associate Professor, Department of Medicine, University of Texas Health Science Center at San Antonio; Chief, Pulmonary Diseases Section, Audie L. Murphy Memorial Veterans Hospital, San Antonio, Texas

Gary T. Kinasewitz, M.D.
Associate Professor, Pulmonary Diseases Section, Department of Medicine, and Associate Professor, Department of Physiology and Biophysics, Louisiana State University Medical Center, Shreveport, Louisiana

Foreword

Assessment of lung function is technically intricate and requires a solid competence in pulmonary medicine and a journeyman knowledge of physics, physical chemistry, mathematics, and computer science. However, the real art lies in presenting the results in a conceptualized manner to the practitioner charged with care of his patient. His ability to use this information will depend entirely upon the breadth, depth, and correctness of his concepts of the function of the lungs. The authors of this book have dealt elegantly with performance of these tests, and with the manner in which the results should be interpreted. In this foreword, I want to say a little about the historical development of pulmonary function testing.

Concepts are the stuff of knowledge, the tools of effective thought. The ancients did not lack for "knowledge." They had an immense amount of it! In the two centuries before Christ, the library at the Museum in Alexandria grew to contain 700,000 rolls. We know that most of that "knowledge" was erroneous, but some of it was not. The earth was round, its diameter had been estimated with surprising accuracy, the planets moved in heavenly paths different from the paths of the stars, the circle had been squared, and so on. However, the modern concepts of respiration were slow to evolve, and ancient ideas were hard to dispel. It was not until the seventeenth century that the process of ventilation was recognized.

Robert Hooke (1635 – 1702), as Curator to the Royal Society, had a duty to perform an experiment at each meeting of the society. On October 24, 1677, he presented a demonstration of artificial respiration. First he showed, with an open-chest dog and a bellows pump, that motion of the chest wall was not necessary to life of the animal, so long as the lungs were ventilated. Then he made multiple small perforations in the exposed pleural surfaces, thus allowing the entering air to escape by this route, and, exerting a steady pressure, he showed that motion of the lungs played no part in this vital process either. As long as fresh air continually entered the lungs, it made no difference whether the lungs moved or not. Thereby, he proved the purpose of the lungs is to expose the blood to fresh air, and that the motions of the chest and of the lungs are merely the normal means whereby this "ventilation of the blood" comes to pass.

Sir Humphrey Davy (1778 – 1829) was the first to address the matter of the volume of the lung. He had apprenticed to a surgeon-apothecary at Penzance and, early in his career, was director of the laboratory of the Pneumatic Institution at Clifton. He recognized that all the air could not be expelled from the lung by voluntary effort. In the last decade of the eighteenth century, he used hydrogen as a tracer to measure the total lung capacity, including the residual volume. At the same time, he demonstrated that the intrapulmonary mixing process is essentially complex exponential in character. However, Davy's work was not followed by immediately fruitful medical application.

On the inauguration of spirometry, Bartels has this to say: "Spirometry, as the name implies, is the 'measurement of breathing.' Both the name and the general principles of the methodology derive from Hutchinson, who also fathered the concept of the vital capacity." A great deal of "fruitful medical application" followed Hutchinson's spirometric work, but it followed it at a very respectful distance, about three-quarters of a century!

It was well into the present century before pulmonary function testing served any general clinical use. The Cardiopulmonary Laboratory of the University of Rochester School of Medicine and Dentistry, where I originally trained, came into being in the third decade and was, perhaps, the second or third such laboratory in North America. When I established the Lung Station of Charity Hospital of New Orleans in 1942, it was the fifth or sixth one this side of the Atlantic. Today, any general medical and surgical hospital offers these tests on a routine basis.

Concepts can only become useful in an environment where they are needed, and where they fulfill that need. The incentive to form the laboratory in which I trained had been a virtual epidemic of silicosis in the northern tier of counties of New York State. Almost every means known for the induction of silicosis was rampant in the manufactories of that area. Castings were sandblasted with silica sand. Welding was performed with silica-coated rods, often inside tanks without the proper use of suckers. Gun painting with silica-containing enamels was widespread. Silica-abrasive grinding wheels were everywhere. Men worked about the cupolas of furnaces without respirators. Only mining and stone cutting were missing. Preventive measures were generally ignored, and silicosis was not recognized under workman's compensation laws of the state. Lawsuits brought under common law began to succeed, then swelled to a tide. Juries made large awards without regard to functional impairment. The incentive to evaluate functional impairment suddenly became very strong!

By the time I joined that laboratory in 1938, proper industrial hygienic measures had been instituted, and silicosis had disappeared from that region except for a handful of old-time cases. We were hard put to find a few patients to complete studies inaugurated by Alberto Hurtado and Nolan Kaltreider. By then, however, a new force was felt. Thoracic surgery had been advancing at a fast pace, a pace that sometimes outran the functional capacity of the lungs of patients.

Soon, a consciousness of air pollution grew, not only the kind attributed to industry and soft-coal-burning home fires, but also the personal variety, cigarette smoking. The British taught us that chronic bronchitis was a serious disease, clearly related to air pollution, both public and personal. Whereas for long it had been taught that soft coal dust was harmless, perhaps even protective against silicosis, the truly disastrous effect of black lung upon pulmonary function was finally recognized. Jethro Gough led us to a new understanding of the tissue pathology of the emphysematous and fibrotic pulmonary disorders. New therapeutic measures to ameliorate the effects of impaired lung function came to hand.

More recently, our Social Security laws have generated a need for objective appraisal of viability. Most of these needs and more are still with us. This text, *Pulmonary Function Testing: Principles and Practice,* is a new help to fulfill these needs.

George R. Meneely, M.D., M.A.C.P.

Preface

Like most areas of medicine, the field of pulmonary function testing has undergone tremendous change in the past 20 years. Expanding knowledge of the pathophysiology of disease is redefining the role of the pulmonary function laboratory in clinical practice. The growth of critical care medicine has moved the traditional pulmonary function tests, such as spirometry and blood gas analysis, from the laboratory to the bedside and the emergency room, an important advance in the practice of pulmonary medicine. New tests and new adaptations, such as sleep analysis and exercise testing, have expanded the role of the cardiopulmonary technologist in the diagnosis and treatment of diseases affecting the lungs and other organs.

With the move to the bedside, to the physician's office, and even into the home, more medical and nonmedical people, including physicians, nurses, respiratory therapists, technologists, and even patients and their families, are now performing serial testing of ventilatory function. Neurologists and electroencephalographers are active in the sleep laboratory, and cardiologists, pulmonologists, nurse specialists, and EKG technicians are involved in the exercise laboratory. This book is designed to meet the needs of this heterogenous group of specialists.

We have attempted to write this book in a simple and direct manner, for use as an introduction by medical and allied health students and at the same time to provide a reference for the practicing respiratory therapist, cardiopulmonary technologist, and physician. The contributors include not only adult pulmonary disease specialists, but a neurologist, a pediatric pulmonologist, and an engineer.

The preparation of this book has involved the support of many people, to whom we extend our sincere gratitude. We are indebted to Cathy Couvillion and Carol Potter for manuscript preparation, Jay Chawla, C.C.P.T., for technical assistance, and to Mr. William Schmitt at Churchill Livingstone for his assistance and encouragement. Special thanks go to George R. Meneely, M.D., M.A.C.P., for his erudite contributions and for his review of the manuscript, and to Mona Conrad, C.R.T.T., for her technical assistance and her encouragement throughout the endeavor. Finally, we thank the faculty, house staff, and allied health specialists with whom we work, who provided us with both the inspiration and the time to write this book.

Steven A. Conrad, M.D.
Gary T. Kinasewitz, M.D.
Ronald B. George, M.D.

Contents

Section I
PHYSIOLOGICAL BASIS

1

Structure and Control of the Respiratory System

Ronald B. George, M.D.

The process of respiration includes gas exchange between the atmosphere and alveoli and between the alveoli and the blood in the pulmonary capillaries. This chapter describes the various components of the respiratory system in relation to their contributions to gas exchange. These components, as outlined in Table 1-1, include the structures involved in the control of respiration, the ventilatory pump mechanism, the airways, pulmonary circulation, and the terminal respiratory unit.

CONTROL OF RESPIRATION

Ventilation is controlled so as to maintain Po_2 and Pco_2 relatively constant over a wide range of physical activity with large variations in the rate of oxygen consumption and CO_2 production. Information from chemoreceptors in the brain and major arteries and input from mechanoreceptors in the lung and chest wall are integrated in the respiratory center located in the central nervous system (CNS) so that alveolar ventilation is adjusted to the appropriate level; tidal volume and respiratory rate are altered in such a way that energy expenditure is minimized. Output from the respiratory center is the product of an interaction between the automatic control center in the brain stem, which provides the basic respiratory drive, and an anatomically distinct cortical control system that may modulate or even override the lower centers, as outlined in Figure 1-1. Recently, sophisticated techniques using microelectrodes have enabled the stimulation of nerve groups to provide more precise identification of the structures involved in the control of respiration.

Table 1-1 Functions of Various Components of the Respiratory System

Function	Component
Control of respiration	Respiratory center; peripheral chemoreceptors; afferent and efferent nerves
Ventilatory pump	Respiratory muscles; chest wall and pleura
Distribution of air	Upper and lower respiratory tracts out to the terminal bronchioles
Circulatory pump	Right ventricle
Distribution of blood	Pulmonary arteries and veins
Gas exchange	Terminal respiratory units
Lung clearance and defense	Mucociliary escalator; alveolar fluid; macrophages; lymphatics

Autonomic Regulation of Respiration

The respiratory muscles have no intrinsic automaticity of their own and cease to function if the spinal cord is sectioned caudal to the medulla. The brain stem provides the rhythmic stimulus to breathing. A group of neurons has been identified in the region of the nucleus parabrachialis medialis in the rostral pons (Fig. 1-2). This neuronal group, the *pneumotaxic center,* apparently generates the

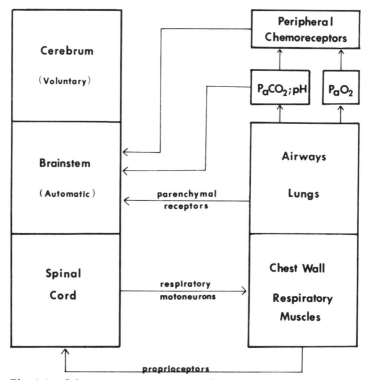

Fig. 1-1. Schematic respresentation of the respiratory control system.

Fig. 1-2. A schematic representation of the dorsal surface of the lower brain stem. APC, apneustic center; CP, cerebellar peduncle; DRG, dorsal respiratory group; IC, inferior colliculus; PNC, pneumotaxic center; VRG, ventral respiratory group. (Modified from Berger AJ, et al: N Engl J Med 297:138, 1977)

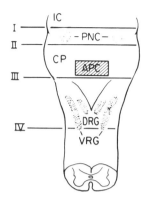

pattern of rhythmic respiratory activity; electrical stimulation of this area results in premature switching from inspiration to expiration. Destruction or separation of this pneumotaxic center at the level of the area vestibularis produces a series of inspiratory gasps interrupted by weak expiratory efforts called apneustic breathing.[1] This pattern is accentuated in vagotomized cats, leading investigators to postulate the presence of an *apneustic center* in the caudal pons.[2]

In addition, two distinct aggregations of respiratory neurons have been identified within the substance of the medulla, the *dorsal respiratory group* in the nucleus of the tractus solitarius and the *ventral respiratory group* located near the nucleus ambiguus and nucleus retroambigualis.[3] The dorsal group stimulates the ventral group, and fibers from the ventral respiratory group control the intercostal, abdominal, and auxiliary muscles of respiration. The reticular formation of the brain yields stimuli that produce a "wakefulness" drive and modify the automatic respiratory response.

Cortical Modulation of Respiration

The voluntary control of respiration originates in cortical neurons that project to the motoneurons of the respiratory muscles. Thus, a conscious individual may voluntarily stop breathing completely or may hyperventilate to an extremely low level of arterial Pco_2. The vital capacity maneuver, which is performed frequently in the pulmonary function laboratory, is an example of a voluntary respiratory act. Cortical input appears to be inhibitory on the brain stem's respiratory center; thus, removal of this inhibitory effect produces an increased sensitivity to CO_2.[4]

Spinal Pathways and Integration

The efferent fibers from the cortical centers descend through the spinal cord via the corticospinal tracts, whereas the involuntary fibers project down the ventrolateral cord. Impulses from both these control systems are integrated at the anterior horn cell of the respiratory motoneuron. Inhibition of expiratory neurons occurs during inspiration and vice versa, so reflex contraction of antagonist muscles is prevented.[5] In addition, pain, temperature, touch, and proprioceptive receptors from the body travel via the lateral columns to the control centers in the CNS where they may alter respiration.

Mechanoreceptors

There are at least three different types of pulmonary parenchymal receptors, all of which are capable of altering the depth and frequency of respiration when stimulated by mechanical deformation of tissue. The *stretch receptors* are located in the smooth muscle of the airways. Lung inflation excites these stretch receptors, provoking inhibition of inspiratory and stimulation of expiratory activity (Hering-Breuer reflex). *Irritant receptors,* located between the epithelial cells of the airways, respond to mechanical or chemical stimuli, such as inhalation of noxious fumes, producing bronchoconstriction and hyperpnea. Stimulation of these receptors also seems to enhance the ventilatory response to CO_2. The *juxtacapillary receptors* (J receptors) in the interstitium of the lung near the alveolar-capillary membrane are thought to respond to distortion of the interstitial space with an increase in afferent activity.[6] These J receptors may be responsible for the rapid shallow breathing pattern characteristic of pulmonary edema or interstitial fibrosis.

There are also chest wall mechanoreceptors, which sense and modulate the forces generated by the respiratory muscles during inspiration.[7] *Tendon receptors* have been identified in the diaphragm and chest wall that may prevent injury caused by excessive or potentially injurious tension in the respiratory muscles. *Muscle spindles* sense the expansion of the chest wall during inspiration and augment inspiration motoneuron output if movement of the chest wall and consequent tidal volume is restricted (Fig. 1-3). The muscle spindles serve as an immediate feedback system to maintan adequate ventilation in the presence of increased respiratory loads.

Chemoreceptors

Changes in P_{O_2}, P_{CO_2}, or pH in arterial blood evoke a compensatory change in ventilation that tends to restore these parameters to near normal levels. The most important of these stimuli in healthy individuals is P_{CO_2}, because over a wide range of metabolic activity and CO_2 production there is normally little variation in Pa_{CO_2}.

In normal individuals, an increase in Pa_{CO_2} elicits a proportional increase in minute ventilation. Most (80 percent) of this increase results from the change in concentration of hydrogen ions in the cerebrospinal fluid (CSF) that bathe the

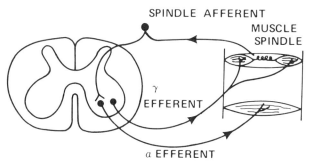

Fig. 1-3. Muscle spindles contain stretch receptors and also muscle fibers supplied by gamma efferents. This system can control contraction of the main muscle. (Reprinted by permission from West JB: Respiratory Physiology— The Essentials. © 1974 The Williams & Wilkins Co., Baltimore.)

central chemoreceptors located near the ventrolateral surface of the medulla.[8] The change in hydrogen ions is the result of CO_2, which rapidly diffuses across the blood-brain barrier, altering the ratio of CO_2 to bicarbonate in the CSF and thereby increasing hydrogen ion concentration. Normally, there is little protein present to buffer changes in pH; however, active transport of bicarbonate across the blood-brain barrier, buffering by neuronal cells, and alteration of cerebral blood flow blunt the effects of changes in pH.[8]

About one-fifth of the increased ventilation evoked by hypercapnia is caused by stimulation of peripheral chemoreceptors located in the carotid and aortic bodies.[9] Hypoxia, on the other hand, increases ventilation solely by stimulating the peripheral chemoreceptors in the major arteries.[10] In contrast to the central stimulatory effect of CO_2, hypoxia is a depressant to central respiratory neurons. In normal individuals at sea level, approximately 10 percent of the normal resting respiratory drive is a result of hypoxic stimulation from the carotid and aortic bodies.[11] Hypoxia, however, stimulates ventilation in a hyperbolic manner after Po_2 falls below a level of about 75 torr.[10] Because of the hyperbolic shape of the response to hypoxia, the decrease in Po_2 from 50 to 40 torr will cause a marked increase in minute ventilation. This was thought to be caused by the shape of the hemoglobin dissociation curve, since rapid desaturation of hemoglobin occurs at these lower levels of Po_2. However, recent information suggests that it is Po_2 rather than oxygen saturation that stimulates the chemoreceptors. There is an interaction between hypoxia and hypercapnia at the peripheral chemoreceptors, so that the ventilatory response to hypoxia is increased in the presence of hypercapnia and vice versa.[10]

Hydrogen ions per se stimulate both the central chemoreceptors of the medulla and the peripheral receptors in the aortic and carotid bodies.[12] It has been shown experimentally that a low pH at a constant Pco_2 results in an increase in minute ventilation.[13] The ventilatory response to hypercapnia may either be augmented by acidosis or attenuated by alkalosis.

Measurement of Chemosensitivity

Sensitivity of the chemoreceptors was measured in the past by asking the subject to inhale gases containing different mixtures of oxygen and CO_2 and comparing changes in arterial Po_2 or Pco_2 with the resultant increase in minute ventilation. In the traditional steady-state technique, a particular gas mixture containing low oxygen or high CO_2 was inhaled for at least 10 min prior to the measurement of ventilation. Serial measurements were required with different concentrations of CO_2 and oxygen, making this a cumbersome and time-consuming procedure.

Measurement of chemosensitivity was simplified by the introduction of a nonsteady-state rebreathing method for determining ventilatory response to carbon dioxide.[14] When a subject breathes a gas mixture containing 7 percent CO_2, rapid equilibration of alveolar gas with arterial blood and CNS are achieved. Pco_2 at all three sites will increase at the same rate (4 to 6 torr/min) so that if alveolar Pco_2 is determined with a rapid gas analyzer and is compared to

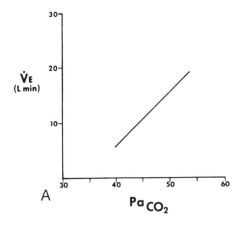

A

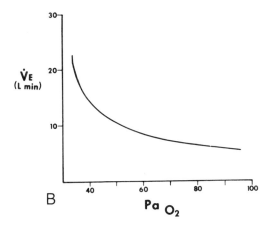

B

Fig. 1-4. (A) The normal relationship between arterial Pco_2 and minute ventilation at a Pa_{O_2} of 100 mmHg. During hypoxia the ventilatory response to an increase in Pa_{CO_2} is increased. (B) The normal relationship between Po_2 and minute ventilation at a Pa_{CO_2} of 40 mmHg. The ventilatory response to a hypoxic stimulus is increased by hypercapnea.

the minute ventilation, the ventilatory response to CO_2 can be determined within 4 min. The slope of the line relating ventilation to alveolar Pco_2 ($\Delta\dot{V}/\Delta Pco_2$) is the ventilatory response to CO_2, and normal values range from 0.5 to 8.0 liter/min/torr Pco_2 (Fig. 1-4A). Responses are generally lower in women, possibly because of their smaller vital capacity.

The ventilatory response to hypoxia can be determined by a similar technique in which the patient inspires 7 percent CO_2 in air. Since the hypoxic ventilatory response is influenced by Pco_2, a portion of the expired air is diverted through a CO_2 absorber. This allows maintenance of a constant arterial Pco_2 while Po_2 progressively falls as oxygen is removed from the rebreathing circuit (Fig. 1-4B). Alveolar Po_2 can be measured, or alternatively, arterial oxygen saturation may be measured using an ear oximeter. In patients with an increased alveolar-arterial oxygen gradient, arterial Po_2 must be measured directly.

THE VENTILATORY PUMP

The ventilatory pump is a bellows comprised of the ribs, bony thorax, and respiratory muscles. Contraction of the diaphragm during inspiration causes an enlargement of the thoracic cage, producing relatively negative pressures at the alveolar level. This causes atmospheric air to be drawn into the alveoli. With expiration the diaphragm relaxes, the thorax becomes smaller, and air flows from the alveoli back out into the atmosphere through the same system of conducting airways. Ventilation is therefore a to-and-fro movement of air. This is called *tidal flow,* that is, like the tides of the ocean.

The Thorax and Diaphragm

The bony thorax consists of the spine, ribs, and sternum. These bony structures are connected by ligaments and cartilage in such a way that the ribs move upward and outward during inspiration and downward and inward during expiration. The basic shape of the thorax is that of a truncated cone (Fig. 1-5). Both the superior and inferior ends of this cone are inclined anteriorly so that the posterior portion of the cone, the spine, is longer than the anterior portion, the sternum.

The diaphragm is the principal muscle of respiration and during rest it performs the majority of the work of ventilation. During inspiration the diaphragmatic muscles contract and the diaphragm moves down toward the abdomen like a piston. The movement of this wide-bore piston over a relatively small distance moves large volumes of gas with a minimal amount of musclar work. Movement of the chest wall is coupled to the lungs by the negative pressure in the pleural cavity, so that when the chest wall expands the lungs expand with it. When the lungs expand, the gas within the lungs falls to a subatmospheric pressure and creates a flow of air into the lungs. Fresh air will continue to flow

Superior Sulcus
(Domes of Pleura)

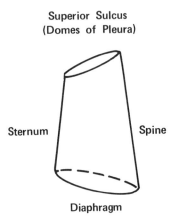

Sternum   Spine

Diaphragm

Fig. 1-5. Simplified diagram of the cone-shaped thorax (lateral view). There is anterior-posterior compression so that the thorax is widened laterally; the anterior wall (sternum) is shorter than the posterior wall (spine) and the superior and inferior planes are inclined anteriorly.

into the lungs until the intrapulmonary gas pressure equals atmospheric pressure. Expiration begins with the elastic recoil of the chest wall and lung, compressing the air contained within the lungs and resulting in a pressure greater than atmospheric pressure. This causes gas to flow out of the lungs until atmospheric pressure is reached once again.

Motor innervation to the diaphram occurs via the phrenic nerve, which is derived from the third through fifth cervical nerves and descends with the diaphragm during fetal growth. Sensory nerves leading to the center of the diaphragm also are carried in the phrenic nerve; thus, irritation of the central portion of the diaphragm may cause pain that is referred to the neck or shoulder areas, areas also innervated by the third, fourth, and fifth cervical segments. Sensory innervation of the periphery of the diaphragm and the chest wall itself occurs via the intercostal nerves.

The Pleura

As the lungs grow laterally from the mediastinum during fetal development, they grow into a part of the coelomic cavity. This cavity is lined with undifferentiated mesenchyme. As the lungs extend into the cavity they are invested with the mesenchymal lining, which becomes the visceral and parietal layers of the pleura. The visceral pleura is adherent to the lungs and the parietal pleura lines the chest wall and mediastinum. The visceral and parietal pleura join one another at the lung hila. The parietal pleura contains abundant pain fibers derived from the intercostal nerves; irritation of this membrane produces a characteristic, well-localized type of chest pain that is exacerbated by chest wall movement (pleuritic pain). The visceral pleura does not contain pain fibers.

The pleural space is airtight and the two pleural surfaces, parietal and visceral, are separated by only a thin film of lubricating fluid. In the intact system at rest, the lung has a natural tendency to become smaller and the chest wall a natural tendency to become larger. The two surfaces thus pull against each other across the pleural space, and since no air can enter, a negative pressure is produced. It is this negative pleural pressure that links the lung to the chest wall and transmits movements of the chest wall to the lung. At rest, average intrapleural pressure is about -4 cm H_2O. In the upright position, the pressure in the pleural cavity is more negative at the top of the lungs than at the lung bases because of the effect of gravity on the lungs themselves.

Fluid is constantly flowing through the pleural space, forming the lubricating film. Pleural fluid is formed from the systemic capillaries in the parietal pleura and is absorbed into the plexus of capillaries under the visceral pleura. The visceral pleural capillaries drain via the pulmonary veins into the left atrium.

DISTRIBUTION OF AIR

The Upper Respiratory Tract

Before atmospheric air reaches the alveolar-capillary membrane the air must be conditioned so that it does not injure the delicate surface area. The upper respiratory tract is primarily designed to purify, warm, and humidify the air; it consists of the nose, paranasal sinuses, pharynx, and larynx. In addition to conditioning inspired gas, these structures perform other important functions, such as smell, swallowing, and speech.

The *nose* contains baffles that are bathed by thin, watery secretions designed to trap foreign particles and add moisture to the inspired air. With normal, quiet breathing, inspired air is heated to body temperature and its relative humidity is increased to over 90 percent during passage through the nose. Resistance to airflow is higher in the nose than in the mouth because of this intricate system of baffles. This explains mouth breathing during vigorous exercise. In this case, the valuable air conditioning function of the nose is lost, and dry, cold air may enter the lower airways. In patients with abnormal irritability of the bronchi, inspiration of cold air through the mouth during exercise may initiate bronchospasm. Patients with tracheostomy and those being ventilated via endotracheal tubes also lose the function of the nose, and inspired gas must be artificially humidified and warmed to prevent drying and irritation of the lower airways.

The *paranasal sinuses* are lined by ciliated columnar epithelium and communicate with the nasal passages by narrow openings that may become occluded when inflamed. Their function is not completely clear, but they add resonance to voice sounds and may insulate the cranial vault. They also provide lightness to the skull without unduly compromising its protective function. The sinuses may become inflamed and cause drainage of material into the pharynx (postnasal drip). This material may be aspirated into the lower respiratory tract, especially during sleep, and become a source of chronic bronchial irritation.

The *pharynx* is divided by the soft palate into the nasopharynx and the oropharynx. The adenoids, tonsils, and eustachian tubes are located in the nasopharynx. At the base of the tongue is the epiglottis, which protects the laryngeal opening during swallowing. In unconscious patients the base of the tongue may fall posteriorly and obstruct the laryngeal opening. In order to avoid this, the head should be hyperextended and the lower jaw pulled forward. Alternatively, the patient may be placed in a position in which gravity causes the tongue to fall forward, such as on his side.

The *larynx* contains the vocal cords, a vital part of the defenses of the respiratory system because they participate in coughing. Coughing is a major clearance mechanism for material that collects in the larger airways and is initiated by irritation of nerves in the walls of the trachea and large bronchi. Coughing is produced by closure of the vocal cords combined with contraction of the respiratory and abdominal muscles so that high pressure is created in the lower airways. Sudden opening of the vocal cords then allows a rush of air to be expelled, carrying larger particles of mucus with it. Normally, the respiratory tract is free of bacteria below the level of the larynx; however, when lung clearance mechanisms are compromised, the trachea often becomes colonized with bacteria.

One or both vocal cords may become paralyzed by surgery or injury to the nerves in the neck or thorax. The left recurrent laryngeal nerve descends into the mediastinum and around the arch of the aorta before returning to the larynx. This nerve may become disrupted by cancer involving lymph nodes adjacent to the left hilum; hoarseness is an ominous sign in patients with carcinoma of the lung. Other diseases, such as granulomas, lymphomas, and aortic aneurysms, may also interrupt the left recurrent laryngeal nerve in the mediastinum.

If both vocal cords are paralyzed, they become flaccid near the midline and breathing may be hindered. Large airway obstruction produces a characteristic combination of symptoms, signs, and pulmonary function abnormalities.[15] Bilateral vocal cord paralysis causes a variable extrathoracic airway obstruction, which produces inspiratory stridor associated with hoarseness, dyspnea, and anxiety. Tests of ventilatory function, such as a flow-volume curve, may be relatively normal on expiration; however, during inspiration there is a decrease in peak airflow.

Carcinoma of the larynx also produces the combination of hoarseness and stridor. Since this is a fixed obstruction, stridor usually occurs during inspiration and expiration, and pulmonary function tests show both inspiratory and expiratory flow limitation.

The Lower Respiratory Tract

The lower respiratory tract begins at the junction of the larynx with the trachea, and includes the trachea, bronchi, bronchioles, and alveoli. The air conduction system of the lungs is a series of dichotomously branching bronchi and bronchioles ending blindly in some 300 million alveoli, which collectively form the gas exchange surface (Fig. 1-6). Normally, there are about 23 generations of airways, of which the first 16 or so are conducting airways where no gas

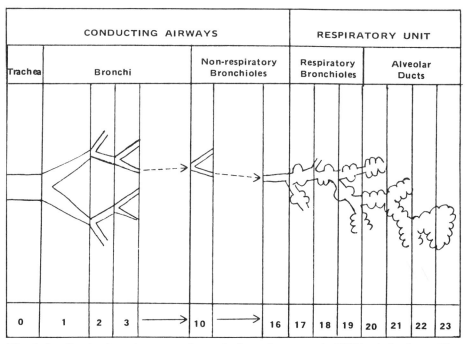

CONDUCTING AIRWAYS			RESPIRATORY UNIT	
Trachea	Bronchi	Non-respiratory Bronchioles	Respiratory Bronchioles	Alveolar Ducts

| 0 | 1 | 2 | 3 | →10 | →16 | 17 | 18 | 19 | 20 | 21 | 22 | 23 |

Fig. 1-6. Conducting airways and terminal respiratory unit (TRU) of the lung. The relative size of the respiratory unit is greatly enlarged. Figures at the bottom indicate the approximate number of generations from trachea to alveoli. (Modified with permission from Weibel ER: Morphometry of the Lung. Academic Press, New York, 1963. Copyright by Academic Press, Inc. (London) Ltd.)

exchange occurs and the last 7 or so are respiratory airways where alveoli appear in progressively larger numbers.[16] The average diameter of a daughter branch is smaller than that of its parent branch, but the total cross-sectional area of each successive generation *increases* from trachea to alveoli; thus, the total area of the respiratory bronchioles is much greater than that of the trachea (Fig. 1-7).

The Trachea

The trachea begins at the base of the neck and extends about 10 to 12 cm to its bifurcation into the right and left main bronchi. It lies immediately anterior to the esophagus and behind the aorta, and often lies slightly to the right of the midline after entering the thorax. Its transverse diameter is greater than its anterior-posterior diameter, and it is held open by a series of horseshoe-shaped cartilaginous rings bound posteriorly by fibrous bands. The lining of the trachea is composed of ciliated columnar epithelium and contains mucous glands. Carina position varies according to the position of the neck and the level of inspiration, but it is normally at about the level of the second anterior rib, just below the aortic

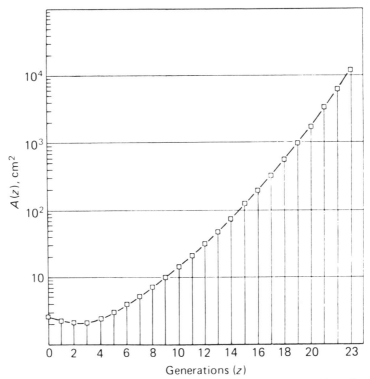

Fig. 1-7. Total cross-section of the airways in the human lung by generation. Although each generation of airways is smaller than its parent, the *total* cross-sectional area of each generation is greater than the *total* area of the previous generation. With permission from Weibel ER: Morphometry of the Lung. Academic Press, New York, 1963. Copyright by Academic Press Inc. (London) Ltd.

arch. The angle between the right and left main bronchi is normally acute, varying from 50 to 100 degrees.

The Bronchi and Bronchioles

The two main bronchi begin at the tracheal carina. The right main bronchus divides almost immediately into the right upper lobe bronchus and the intermediate bronchus. The left main bronchus is considerably longer, extending across the midline approximately 5 cm before it divides into the left upper and left lower lobe bronchi. The major bronchi contain large numbers of mucous glands and their surface is innervated by branches of both the parasympathetic and sympathetic nervous systems. The parasympathetic nerves are connected to the brain via the vagus nerves. Irritant receptors in large airways initiate the cough reflex, and resultant motor stimuli cause bronchoconstriction and mucus secretion.

The right main bronchus is larger and less deviated from the axis of the trachea than the left; thus, it may be considered an extension of the trachea itself. This is a possible explanation for the more frequent aspiration of foreign material into the right lung. The main bronchi divide into five lobar bronchi — the upper, middle, and lower on the right, and the upper and lower on the left. The lobes are separated from each other by fissures that are lined by two layers of visceral pleura.

The lobar bronchi divide into segmental bronchi, 10 on the right and 9 on the left (Fig. 1-8). Segments are usually separated by delicate connective tissue planes but not fissures. There is some disagreement concerning nomenclature of the bronchopulmonary segments; however, the classification of the Thoracic Society of Great Britain, shown in Figure 1-8, is the one most commonly used. A thorough knowledge of the lung segments has become necessary in recent years because of the high incidence of bronchogenic carcinoma, one of the most common neoplasms. These neoplasms commonly occur in lobar and segmental bronchi and produce characteristic patterns on chest x-ray film based on their anatomic location.

The segmental bronchi bifurcate further until the terminal bronchiole is reached. Bronchial mucosa is lined with pseudostratified ciliated columnar epithelium with interspersed goblet cells. The height of the cells gradually diminishes in the smaller bronchi to become cuboid. Bronchial mucous glands lie in the submucosa with their ducts penetrating the mucosa to empty into the lumen. These glands are especially prevalent in the medium-sized bronchi and sparse in the smaller bronchi. The *Reid index,* which measures the average depth of penetration of glands into the bronchial wall, is a measure of the relative hypertrophy of these mucous glands in persons with chronic bronchitis. Normally, the mucous glands should not extend more than halfway through the bronchial wall. Hypertrophy of these glands is associated with an increase in mucus production and with a chronic productive cough in patients with bronchitis.

The wall of a large bronchus is shown in Figure 1-9. The mucosa contains several types of cells, each with specialized functions. The ciliated cell contains motile cilia that beat in a coordinated manner to move the mucous layer toward the mouth. The goblet cells interspersed among the ciliated epithelial cells secrete mucus. There are also nonciliated, nonsecretory cells interspersed in the mucosa. These brush cells contain microvilli similar to those in the gut, and may function to control fluid balance in the airway lumen. Basal cells have no special function but serve as precursors, differentiating into whichever cell type is needed to replace the population of lost cells. Chronic irritation, as in cigarette smoking, causes these basal cells to differentiate into epidermoid cells rather than ciliated columnar cells.

Kulchitsky cells occur most commonly in newborns. These cells appear to be innervated and may produce kinins during the newborn period.[17] These cells are the precursors of bronchial carcinoid tumors and probably of oat cell carcinomas. Clumps of argyrophilic cells have been discovered in bronchial, bronchiolar, and

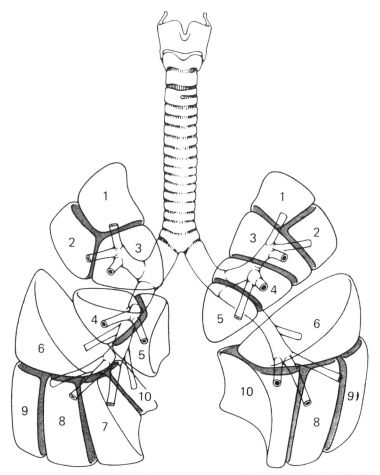

Fig. 1-8. The bronchopulmonary segments. *Upper lobes:* (1) apical, (2) posterior, (3) anterior, (4) superior lingular, and (5) inferior lingular segments. *Middle lobe:* (4) lateral and (5) medial segments. *Lower lobes:* (6) apical (superior), (7) medial basal, (8) anterior basal, (9) lateral basal, and (10) posterior basal segments. The medial basal segment (7) is absent in the left lung. [From Weibel ER: Design and structure of the human lung. Ch. 15. In Fishman AP (ed): Pulmonary Diseases and Disorders. Copyright © 1980, The McGraw-Hill Book Company. Used with the permission of the McGraw-Hill Book Company.

alveolar epithelium; these innervated neuroepithelial bodies are strategically located in such a manner that they may serve to "sniff" the air flowing by them and regulate the caliber of the airways. This would provide a sensitive autoregulatory mechanism for the distribution of inspired air.[18]

The mucosa of smaller bronchioles contains cuboidal epithelium that gradually loses cilia as the terminal bronchiole is approached. The walls of the terminal

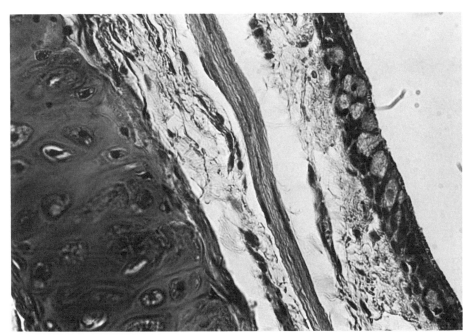

Fig. 1-9. Section through the wall of a large bronchus (×400). The lumen (right) is lined with pseudostratified columnar epithelial cells containing tiny cilia, which propel mucus toward the trachea. The submucosa is surrounded by a thin layer of smooth muscle. To the left is a part of the cartilage that lends support to the bronchial wall. (Courtesy of Warren D. Grafton, M.D.)

bronchiole are quite different from those of the larger airways (Fig. 1-10). Ciliated cells become less numerous and no glands or goblet cells are present. Nonciliated Clara cells become evident. The role of Clara cells is not settled; however, they may secrete surfactant into the small peripheral airways to promote airway stability and add to the mucous lining of the lung periphery. Each terminal bronchiole has a diameter of about 1 mm, but the aggregate cross-sectional area of all terminal bronchioles is greater than that of any previous generation (see Fig. 1-7).

The Alveoli

Beyond the terminal bronchiole the airways contain progressively larger numbers of alveoli. As shown in Figure 1-6, after approximately three generations of respiratory bronchioles, alveolar ducts are found. These are completely lined by alveoli. The bronchial arteries do not extend beyond the terminal bronchioles, and the blood supply to the alveoli is derived totally from the pulmonary circulation. The walls of alveoli contain a rich network of pulmonary capillaries and it is here that the exchange of carbon dioxide for oxygen occurs.

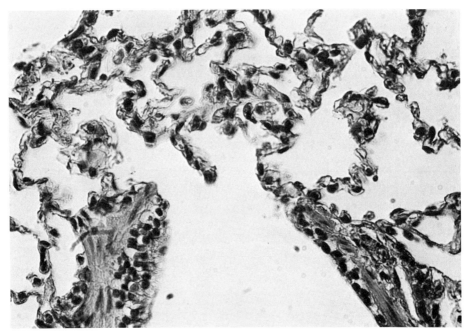

Fig. 1-10.   Section through a terminal bronchiole ($\times 400$). At the center of the picture the terminal bronchiole is dividing into two respiratory bronchioles, whose walls contain alveoli. The respiratory bronchioles end in alveolar sacs. (Courtesy of Warren D. Grafton, M.D.)

Ventilation of the conducting airways ceases to be bulk flow at the level of the alveolar ducts. Further distally, movement of gases is by gaseous diffusion. Ventilation of the gas exchange surfaces, therefore, depends on how far the gases must travel from the alveolar duct to the alveolar wall. If the small peripheral airways become partly or completely occluded, collateral ventilation of alveoli may occur via the pores of Kohn, holes in the alveolar walls that connect alveoli directly, or via the canals of Lambert, tiny passages from distal airways to adjacent alveoli. This collateral ventilation increases the physiological dead space and adds to the ventilation/perfusion mismatching seen in diseases that affect the small airways.[19] However, it prevents lung segments distal to the obstructed airways from becoming atelectatic.

THE CIRCULATORY PUMP

The circulatory pump is the right ventricle, powered by the contraction of the myocardium. The pulmonic valve prevents regurgitation of blood into the right ventricle during diastole and assures a constant flow through the pulmonary artery to the capillaries. The capillaries cover the surface of the alveolar wall in a latticework pattern, allowing optimum contact of the red blood cells with the alveolar capillary surface. The capillaries coalesce to form the pulmonary veins, which bring oxygenated blood into the left atrium.

The pulmonary circulation is a low-pressure system, and mean pulmonary artery pressure is normally around 15 torr at rest. Low hydrostatic pressure keeps the flow of fluids relatively small from the pulmonary capillaries into the interstitial space. Fluid is rapidly removed from the interstitium by the abundant lymphatics of the lungs; this efficient system keeps the alveoli free of fluid so gas exchange may occur.

The entire cardiac output flows through this low-pressure system, although at any given time the capillaries contain only about 100 ml blood at rest. This blood moves into the capillaries in a pulsatile manner with each heart beat, so that each 100 ml of blood remains in the capillaries for about 0.8 sec (with a normal heart rate of 80 beats/min). This is more than adequate for gas exchange to occur. Blood flow through the capillaries increases markedly during exercise, and this decreases the time available for gas exchange; but this is usually not a problem, as gas exchange is essentially complete within about 0.25 sec.

DISTRIBUTION OF BLOOD

The lungs have a dual blood supply consisting of the bronchial arteries, which contain oxygenated blood, and the pulmonary arteries, which contain mixed venous blood. The bronchial arteries usually arise from the aorta just beyond its arch, although they may arise from intercostal, subclavian, or internal mammary arteries. They supply the bronchi and surrounding tissues down to the level of the terminal bronchiole. Distal to this, the terminal respiratory units (TRU) are supplied solely by the pulmonary artery. Bronchial arteries surround the bronchi and divide with them, forming a fine capillary plexus on the submucosa of the bronchi. Venous capillaries arise from this network and form a plexus in the adventitia that drains into the bronchial veins. The bronchial veins empty into the pulmonary veins, and therefore into the systemic circulation, near the pulmonary hila.

The pulmonary artery emerges from the right ventricle and divides into right and left main pulmonary arteries anterior to the tracheal carina (Fig. 1-11A). The left pulmonary artery is slightly higher than the right in most cases, and the right crosses the midline before dividing into the upper and lower branches. The pulmonary arteries divide into branches corresponding to the divisions of the bronchial tree and end in the terminal arterioles, which enter the center of the TRUs adjacent to the terminal bronchioles. These in turn break up into pulmonary capillaries, which form networks in the interalveolar septa. Pulmonary veins form at the periphery of the TRUs and converge separate from the arteries and bronchi, eventually forming the main pulmonary veins, which end in the left atrium (Fig. 1-11B). In addition to the alveolar capillaries, the pulmonary veins also drain the larger bronchi via the bronchial veins, which enter the pulmonary

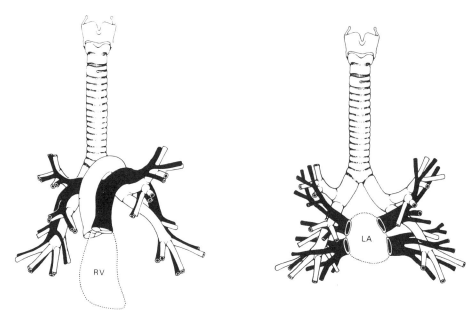

Fig. 1-11.   The pulmonary hila, showing the arteries (left) and veins (right). Note the relationships of the major vessels to the trachea, bronchi, and aorta. [Reprinted from Weibel ER: Design and structure of the human lung. Ch. 15. In Fishman AP (ed): Pulmonary Diseases and Disorders. Copyright © 1980, McGraw-Hill. Used with the permission of the McGraw-Hill Book Company.]

veins near the hilum. The bronchial venous blood accounts for a significant portion of the right-to-left shunt that occurs normally in the lungs (up to 5 percent of cardiac output).

THE GAS EXCHANGE AREA

In the past, different authors have used various names for the smaller divisions of the lung architecture. To prevent confusion, the *terminal respiratory unit* (TRU) is herein defined as that portion of the lung distal to the terminal nonrespiratory bronchiole.[20,21] The TRU has been called the acinus by Lauweryns[22] and the primary lobule by Miller.[23] A TRU measures less than 1 cm in diameter and is visible on the chest radiograph if it is filled with fluid, as in some cases of early alveolar filling. Three to five TRUs combine to form a pulmonary lobule,[24] which is separated from its neighboring lobules by an interlobular septum containing lymphatic channels. The interlobular septa may become visible as Kerley's "B" lines on chest films if they are distended by fluid or fibrosis.

A stylized version of a TRU is illustrated in Figure 1-12. The unit is designed to perform its basic function of gas exchange in an efficient manner. The terminal

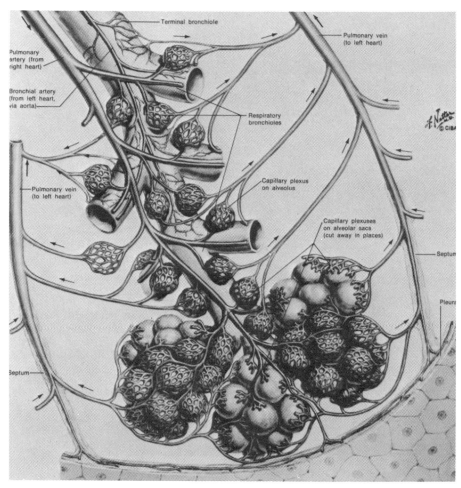

Fig. 1-12.   A terminal respiratory unit (TRU), the basic gas-exchanging unit of the lungs.
The pulmonary arterial branch enters the center of the TRU along with the terminal
bronchiole. It anastomoses with the pulmonary venule in the alveolar walls, forming a
dense capillary network for gas exchange. Venous drainage is to the periphery of the TRU,
where the venous branches lie. They coalesce to form the major pulmonary veins, which
carry oxygenated blood. (© 1979, 1980 CIBA Pharmaceutical Company, Division of
CIBA-GEIGY Corporation. Reprinted with permission from the CIBA Collection of
Medical Illustrations by Frank H. Netter, M.D. Vol 7. All rights reserved.)

bronchiole enters the center of the TRU accompanied by a branch of the
pulmonary artery carrying unoxygenated blood from the body tissues. The
arteriole divides into a rich network of pulmonary capillaries that covers the
alveolar walls and drains into the pulmonary venules, which lie in the periphery
of the TRU. These venules converge into larger branches situated in the interlobular septa. This arrangement results in the organized perfusion of a lobule
from the center to the periphery.

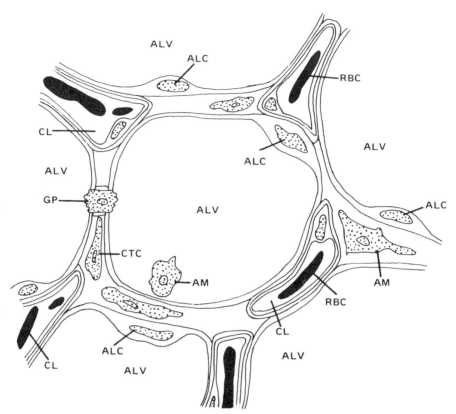

Fig. 1-13. Cells of the alveoli. ALV, alveolus; AM, alveolar macrophage; CL, capillary lumen; CTC, connective tissue cell; RBC, red blood cell; ALC, alveolar lining cells; GP, granular pneumocytes.

The alveoli themselves are lined with a thin layer of epithelial cells. Ninety-five percent of these cells are thin type I alveolar lining cells (Fig. 1-13). These have large, thin cytoplasmic extensions that may extend into two or more alveoli. They provide a minimal barrier to gas exchange. Interspersed among these lining cells are the type II granular pneumocytes, which contain lamellar bodies and are the source of the surfactant lining layer of the alveoli. The alveolar-capillary membrane itself is 4 to 8 μm thick and is composed of the alveolar epithelium, the interstitium containing the basement membrane, and the pulmonary capillary endothelium. The alveolar walls are lined with a thin layer of surfactant that is continuous with the mucous layer in the bronchi.

LUNG CLEARANCE AND DEFENSES

The lung is unique among internal organs in its continuous direct contact with the environment. Major irritants that invade the respiratory tract are such organic agents as bacteria, fungal spores, and viruses, and such inorganic agents as industrial exhaust, dusts, and cigarette smoke. In general, organic agents cause acute illnesses whereas inorganic agents cause chronic debilitating diseases. This is not always true, however, and infectious and noninfectious agents may act together to produce disease. Complicated and effective defense mechanisms have been developed by the body to protect the respiratory tract from these inhaled substances.[25]

Particle Deposition in the Respiratory Tract

The deposition of particles in the lungs depends on their size and density, the distance over which they must travel, and the relative humidity. The method of breathing (i.e., mouth breathing versus nose breathing), the rate of airflow, the minute ventilation, and the depth of breathing also influence the method of deposition of the aerosol. Defense mechanisms vary, depending on where in the respiratory tract particles are deposited as well as their size and composition. In general, particles larger than 10 μm in diameter are deposited in the upper respiratory passages, those between 2 and 10 μm in the bronchial tree, and those between 0.5 and 3 μm in the gas exchange areas of the lungs (TRUs). Modern nebulizers are capable of generating aerosols containing small particles in high concentrations and thus are an efficient means of depositing particles in the distal parts of the respiratory tract.

Transport Systems of the Lungs

Three transport systems are available in the lungs to remove inhaled particles, as shown in Table 1-2. These systems work together, although they operate through different pathways and at different rates.[25] The fastest is the "mucociliary escalator," which functions to transport deposited particles from the level of the terminal bronchioles to the major airways where they are coughed up, or to the glottis where they are expectorated or swallowed. The transport rate of this system is about 3 mm/min and becomes more rapid proximally where the streams converge. Approximately 90 percent of the particles directly deposited on the mucous layer are cleared within 2 hr. In the main bronchi the mucociliary apparatus is formed by the ciliated epithelial cells, the goblet cells, and the mucous glands, which open directly into the mucosa. In the smaller bronchi and bronchioles, mucus is formed from goblet cell secretions. In the respiratory

Table 1-2 Pulmonary Transport Systems

System	Transport Time
Mucociliary escalator	Minutes
Alveolobronchiolar fluid flow	Hours, days, weeks
Lymphohematogenous drainage	Variable

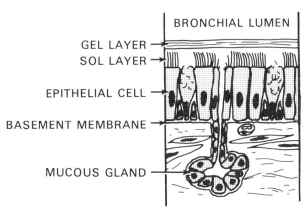

Fig. 1-14. The mucociliary escalator. The gel layer of mucus is propelled toward the trachea by the movement of the cilia on the surface of the cells.

bronchioles mucous glands are not normally seen and the epithelium is lined by a thin layer of material, probably surfactant, which flows proximally.

The mucus, which is the transport medium, is a complex mucopolysaccharide arranged in a double layer on the surface of the epithelium (Fig. 1-14). The external layer is a viscous gel that acts as a trap to catch and transport deposited particles. The internal sol layer is a thin liquid in which the villi are able to move easily. The cilia themselves move with a characteristic biphasic rhythm. Beating within the liquid layer and striking the gel layer with their tips they exhibit a periodic movement, forming wave bands that move the mucus up the bronchial tree toward the larynx.

Many factors, such as toxic fumes and cigarette smoke, affect the wave pattern of the cilia and may cause them to stop beating completely, causing the movement of mucus to slow. Dehydration may change the composition of the liquid layer and thus interfere with ciliary action. Slowing of the movement of mucus allows inhaled particles to stay in the lungs longer, permitting multiplication of infectious organisms.

From the alveoli, deposited material is transported out into the mucociliary transport system by the slow but constant flow of alveolar fluid into the bronchioles. This second transport system takes 24 hr to several days and particles may be carried free in this fluid or within phagocytic cells (Table 1-2). The principal phagocytic cell is the *alveolar macrophage,* a monocytic cell from the bone marrow that is able to adapt to the high oxygen environment within the alveoli. This is the major cell processor for inhaled particles and is responsible for detoxification, destruction, and transport of particles that reach the alveoli. The alveolar macrophage migrates or is carried from the alveolus to the mucous layer by the flow of alveolar fluid. Following phagocytosis, bacteria are killed and inert particles are digested by powerful enzymes in the cellular lysosomes. If the alveolar macrophages are unable to handle the agent because of inflammation, toxic effects on the cells, or overwhelming numbers of particles, neutrophils may invade the alveoli as a second line of defense. The bactericidal mechanisms of the phagocytes are enhanced by the flow of specific immunoglobulins onto the alveolar surface.

The third transport system is lymphohematogenous drainage of the lungs (Table 1-2). The alveolar septum contains connective tissue and is a potential space that may act as a vehicle for the exit of macrophages from the alveoli. From there, macrophages may enter pulmonary capillaries or the lymphatics of the lung. Inhaled particles probably do not enter lymphatics directly unless inflammation is present, but are carried within phagocytic cells. Foreign particles may be stored for long periods in the lung lymphatics. The speed of transport via the lymphatic system is variable and may take months or years. Since lymph flow is augmented by the movement of respiration, decreased movement of some parts of the lung, as in kyphoscoliosis, may slow clearance of particles via lymphatics in these areas.

Particles larger than 3 μm are deposited largely in the tracheobronchial tree and are therefore subject mainly to transport by the mucociliary escalator. Smaller particles are deposited in the gas exchange areas of the lung where there is no mucociliary activity and transport mechanisms are slower. In these areas, detoxification becomes more important. In animals, after an aerosol bacterial challenge, detoxification mechanisms far outweigh transport mechanisms in the early and decisive postexposure period.

The Pulmonary Lymphatics

The lungs and pleura are richly supplied with lymphatics. The purpose of the large flow of lymph from the lungs is twofold. First, it forms a natural mechanism for the removal of excess fluid that moves into the interstitial spaces from the pulmonary capillaries, thus keeping the alveoli relatively free of fluid. Second, it forms an important part of the alveolar defense mechanism by transporting macrophages containing inhaled particles from distal areas of the lungs. It is largely because of this lymphatic system that bronchogenic carcinoma travels out of the lungs readily. The lymphatics from the TRUs converge in the interlobular septa; when they are distended, these septa may become visible as an early sign of increased lung water (Kerley "B" lines). Movement of lymph is caused by respiratory movements combined with a series of valves in the lymphatic vessels that assures proximal flow. The lymphatics line the pulmonary arteries and veins, as well as the bronchi themselves, and converge at the pulmonary hila where the lymph glands are found. From here the lymph is carried via the thoracic duct on the left and the right lymphatic duct on the right. These vessels enter the systemic venous circulation at the junctions of the subclavian and internal jugular veins (Fig. 1-15).

The bronchopulmonary lymph nodes surround the divisions of the lobar bronchi; thus, hilar glands are clustered at the lung roots. The hilar lymph nodes

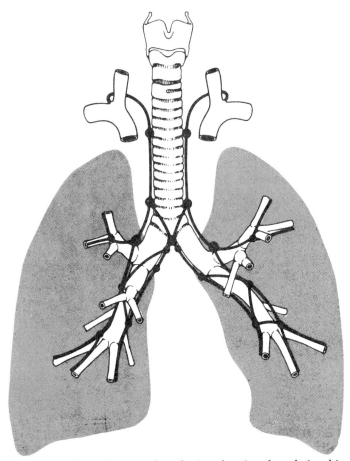

Fig. 1-15. The pulmonary lymphatics, showing the relationship of main lymphatic channels and lymph nodes to the bronchial tree. [From Weibel ER: Design and structure of the human lung. Ch. 15. In Fishman AP (ed): Pulmonary Diseases and Disorders. Copyright © 1980, The McGraw-Hill Book Company. Used with the permission of the McGraw-Hill Book Company.]

occur around the upper and lower lobe bronchi and communicate richly via the subcarinal nodes with the opposite side. Paratracheal nodes are found on either side of the trachea and are most prominent on the right. The "azygos" node is found adjacent to the azygos vein at the junction of the right upper lobe bronchus and right main bronchus. The pulmonary lymphatic system communicates with the lower deep cervical nodes above and with the abdominal lymphatics below.

In addition to the hilar and mediastinal lymph nodes, there are also lymphatics along the distribution of the internal mammary arteries, near the intercostal arteries adjacent to the posterior ribs, and in the anterior and posterior mediastinum. There is some disagreement as to the drainage of the various lobes of the lung, and indeed, drainage channels may vary among individuals. In general, the lower lobes drain into the hilar and subcarinal nodes, whereas the upper lobes more often drain directly to the paratracheal nodes. Thus, cancers arising in lower lobe bronchi must traverse an extra set of lymph nodes, the hilar group, before reaching the paratracheal chain. The rich system of anastamoses among lymph node groups may account at least in part for the variation in lymphatic drainage of the lobes.

REFERENCES

1. Gautier H, Bertrand F: Respiratory effects of pneumo-taxic center lesions and subsequent vagotomy in chronic cats. Resp Physiol 23:71, 1975
2. Krieger AJ, Christensen HD, Sapru HN, Wang SC: Changes in ventilatory patterns after ablation of various respiratory feedback mechanisms. J Appl Physiol 33:431, 1972
3. Mitchell RA, Berger, AJ: Neural regulation of respiration. Am Rev Resp Dis 3:206, 1975
4. Plum F, Posner JB: The diagnosis of stupor and coma. p. 197. In Howell JBL, Campbell EJM (eds): Breathlessness. F.A. Davis, Philadelphia, 1966
5. Newsom DJ: Control of the muscles of breathing. p. 221. In Widdicombe JG (ed): Respiratory Physiology: MTP International Review of Science. Series 1, Vol. 2. Butterworth, London, 1974
6. Paintal AS: Vagal sensory receptors and their reflex effects. Physiol Rev 53:159, 1973
7. Euler C Von: On the role of proprioceptors in perception and execution of motor acts with special reference to breathing. p. 139. In Pengelly LD, Rebuck AS, Campbell EJM (eds): Loaded Breathing. Longmans Canada, Don Mills, Ontario, 1974
8. Leusen I: Regulation of cerebrospinal fluid composition with reference to breathing. Physiol Rev 52:1, 1972
9. Mitchell RA, Loeschcke HH, Massion WH, Severinghaus JW: Respiratory responses mediated through superficial chemosensitive areas on the medulla. J Appl Physiol 18:523, 1963
10. Biscoe TJ: Carotid body: Structure and function. Physiol Rev 42:335, 1962
11. Stockley RA: The estimation of the resting reflex hypoxic drive to respiration in normal man. Resp Physiol 31:217, 1977
12. Kellogg RH: Central chemical regulation in respiration. p. 507. In Fenn WO, Rahn H (eds): Handbook of Physiology, Vol. 1, Respiration. American Physiological Society, Washington, DC, 1964
13. Biscoe TJ, Purnes MJ, Sampson SR: The frequency of nerve impulses in single carotid body chemoreceptor afferent fibers recorded in vivo with intact circulation. J Physiol (Lond) 208:121, 1970
14. Read DJC: A clinical method for assessing the ventilatory response to CO_2. Aust Ann Med 16:20, 1967
15. Light RW, George RB: Upper airway obstruction (editorial). Arch Intern Med 137:281, 1977
16. Weibel ER: Morphometry of the Lung. Academic Press, New York, 1963
17. Lauweryns JM, Peuskens JC, Cokelacre M: Argyrophil, fluorescent and granulated (peptide and amine producing?) AFG cells in human infant bronchial epithelium. Light and electron microscopic studies. Life Sci 9:1417, 1970
18. Lauweryns JM, Peuskens JC: Neuroepithelial bodies (neuroreceptor or secretory organs?) in human infant bronchial bronchiolar epithelium. Anat Rec 172:471, 1972
19. Terry PB, Traystman RJ, Newell HH, et al: Collateral ventilation in man. N Engl J Med 298:10, 1978
20. Von Hayek H: The Human Lung. Krohl VE (trans). Hafner Publishing, New York, 1960.

21. Staub NC: The interdependence of pulmonary structure and function. Anesthesiology 24:831, 1963
22. Lauweryns JM: The blood and lymphatic microcirculation of the lung. In Sommers SC (ed): Pathology Annual 1971. Appleton-Century-Crofts, New York, 1971
23. Miller WS: The Lung. Charles C Thomas, Baltimore, Md, 1937
24. Reid L, Simon G: The peripheral pattern in the normal bronchogram and its relation to peripheral pulmonary anatomy. Thorax 13:103, 1958
25. Green GM: In defense of the lung. Am Rev Resp Dis 102:691,1970

ADDITIONAL READING

Gee JBL, Smith GJW: Lung cells and disease. Basics RD. 9 (5):1, May 1981
Macklem PT: Respiratory muscles: The vital pump. Chest 78:753, 1980
Murray JF: The Normal Lung. Chapters 1–7. WB Saunders, Philadelphia, 1976
Weibel ER: Design and Structure of the Human Lung. p. 224. Chapter 15. In Fishman FP (ed): Pulmonary Diseases and Disorders. McGraw-Hill, New York, 1980

2

Respiratory Mechanics

Gary T. Kinasewitz, M.D.

The lungs and chest wall, acting in concert, comprise the ventilatory pump of the respiratory system. The chest wall includes not only the rib cage and diaphragm surrounding the lungs, but also the abdominal and accessory muscles of respiration, which are important during vigorous respiratory efforts. As with any mechanical pump, the ventilatory apparatus can be characterized by its elastic, flow resistive, and inertial properties. In the lung, inertia is negligible and can be ignored.[1]

ELASTIC PROPERTIES OF THE VENTILATORY PUMP

The elastic properties of the lung are due to the elastic tissue and collagen that surround the pulmonary vessels and bronchi and provide structural support within the alveolar walls.[2] As the lung expands, an elastic recoil pressure is generated not by the simple elongation of the elastic fibers, but rather by a geometrical rearrangement of the elastic fibers within the parenchyma. This rearrangement is analogous to a nylon stocking that, because of its knitted composition, can be stretched even though the individual fibers undergo very little elongation. In contrast, the collagen fibers are poorly extensible and act primarily to limit expansion at high lung volumes.[3]

Lung Pressures

At the end of a normal expiration, when the respiratory muscles are at rest, the elastic recoil of the lung (its tendency to collapse) is counterbalanced by the elastic recoil of the chest wall (its tendency to expand).[4] These opposing forces generate a subatmospheric pressure in the potential space between the parietal and visceral pleura. When the inspiratory muscles contract, the pleural pressure becomes more subatmospheric, decreasing gas pressure within the alveoli. Air at the mouth, which is at atmospheric pressure, flows into the lung and increases the alveolar volume until, at the end of inspiration, alveolar pressure is once again equal to atmospheric pressure. The transpulmonary pressure (PL), that is, the difference between alveolar pressure (PA) and pleural pressure (Ppl), is increased at this higher lung volume. Since alveolar pressure is zero under these conditions, the pleural pressure which maintains this lung volume is equal in magnitude (but opposite in direction) to the elastic recoil pressure of the lung [Pst(L)]. *Static compliance* (Cst), or distensibility of the lung, is a function of its elastic properties and may be measured as

$$Cst = \Delta V / \Delta P_L \qquad \text{(Eq. 2-1)}$$

where ΔV is the change in lung volume produced by a change in transpulmonary pressure (ΔP_L) in the absence of airflow. A static compliance curve for the lung can be constructed by relating lung volume to transpulmonary pressure over the entire vital capacity (Fig. 2-1). Since pleural pressure cannot be measured directly in humans, changes in esophageal pressure are used to estimate alterations in pleural pressure.[5] Lung compliance is influenced by the lung volume at which it is measured and the previous volume history of the lung, that is, whether the measurement is made during inspiration or expiration.

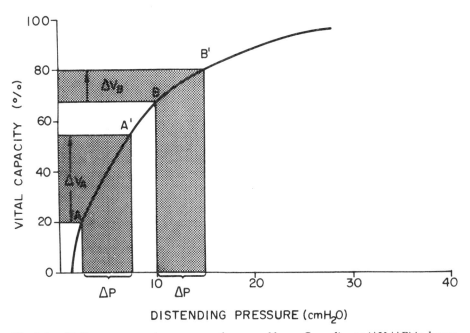

Fig. 2-1.   Static pressure-volume curve of a normal lung. Compliance ($\Delta V / \Delta P$) is dependent on the lung volume at which it is measured; an equal increase in distending pressure produces a greater increase in volume at low lung volumes (A-A[1]) than at high lung volumes (B-B[1]). [Reprinted with permission from Light RW: Mechanics of respiration, I. Statics of the respiratory system. p. 41. In George RB, Light RW, Matthay RA (eds): Chest Medicine. Churchill Livingstone, New York, 1983]

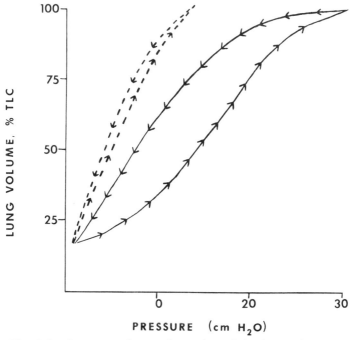

Fig. 2-2. Pressure-volume relationship of the lung when it is inflated and deflated with air (solid lines) and saline (dashed lines). The saline curve reflects the pressure required to overcome the tissue forces of the lung, and the difference between the two curves is the pressure required to overcome the surface forces within the lung.

The pressure-volume characteristics of the lung are nonlinear and a given increase in distending pressure will produce less of a volume increment at high lung volumes. More pressure is required to achieve a given increment in lung volume during inspiration than during expiration (Fig. 2-2). This *hysteresis* or difference between the inspiratory and expiratory pressure-volume curves is primarily caused by the extra pressure that must be generated during inspiration to overcome the surface tension of the liquid film lining the alveoli.[6] At any air-liquid interface a surface tension (T) is generated because the attraction between molecules in the liquid is much stronger than that between the liquid and the gas. These strong attractive forces within the liquid cause the surface area of the fluid to be as small as possible, just as a soap bubble blown at the end of a tube will contract to form a sphere (the smallest surface area for a given volume). The surface tension in the wall of the bubble tends to contract the bubble, whereas the pressure (P) of the gas within the bubble acts to expand it. At equilibrium the relationship within the "alveolar bubble" is described by Laplace's law,

$$P = 2T/r$$

(Eq. 2-2)

where *r* is the radius of curvature of the alveolus. If surface tension were constant throughout the lung, then as the alveolar radius decreased, the pressure of the gas within the smaller alveoli would rise and they would empty into larger communicating ones. Fortunately, the lining film of the lung contains a surface-active material secreted by type II pneumocytes. This *surfactant,* which is composed of phospholipid, primarily dipalmitoyl lecithin, serves two main functions. Its presence, particularly at low lung volumes, decreases alveolar surface tension, thereby increasing compliance and facilitating lung expansion. Furthermore, because alveolar surface tension decreases as its volume decreases, the pressures within all patent alveoli are equal and atelectasis from the emptying of small alveoli into larger ones is averted. The importance of surfactant is exemplified in the neonate. Premature infants frequently have a deficiency in surfactant production and manifest both alveolar instability and a decreased lung compliance. In neonatal acute respiratory distress syndrome, alveolar instability progresses to atelectasis with the development of large right-to-left shunts and extreme hypoxemia, whereas reduced lung compliance leads to alveolar hypoventilation. Injury to type II pneumocytes and loss of surfactant is also felt to play an important role in the pathogenesis of diffuse microatelectasis and decreased lung compliance characteristic of adult respiratory distress syndrome.

Static compliance is measured during breathholding at various lung volumes in the absence of airflow. Compliance can also be measured during the breathing cycle, in which case the pressure required to generate airflow is included in the measurement of transpulmonary pressure. In a normal individual, *dynamic compliance* (Cdyn) approximates static compliance (Cst) since the resistance of the airways is small. However, in a patient with airway disease Cdyn may be significantly less than Cst.[7] The pathological destruction of elastic fibers characteristic of emphysema, and to a lesser extent, the physiological loss of elastic tissue that occurs with increasing age are both associated with a decrease in the elastic recoil pressure of the lung and an increase in lung compliance.[8,9] Conversely, the increased collagen content of the lung seen in interstitial fibrosis is associated with an increased elastic recoil pressure and a fall in lung compliance. Lung compliance will also be reduced by airspace consolidation and edema, which interfere with lung expansion.

The chest wall, just like the lung, has elastic recoil; if the contact between the visceral and parietal pleural surfaces is disrupted by a pneumothorax so that pleural pressure is atmospheric, the chest will expand to about 70 percent of its total capacity (Fig. 2-3). At this equilibrium position the pressure across the chest wall (Pw) is zero. This may be expressed as

$$Pw = Ppl - Pbs \qquad \text{(Eq. 2-3)}$$

where Ppl is pleural pressure and Pbs is pressure at the body surface. When the volume of gas within the chest is increased above 70 percent of total lung capacity, energy must be expended to expand both the chest and lungs. Conversely, at volumes below the resting position of the chest wall, the recoil pressure of the chest is directed outward and tends to expand the lungs.

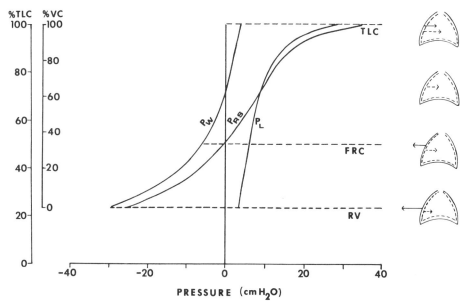

Fig. 2-3. Pressure-volume relationships of the lung (PL), chest wall (Pw), and total respiratory system (Prs) expressed as the percentage of total lung capacity and vital capacity. The direction and magnitude of the recoil pressure of the lung (dashed arrow) and chest wall (solid arrow) are indicated on the right. (Modified from Knowles JH, Hong SK, Rahn H: Possible errors using esophageal balloon in determination of pressure-volume characteristics of the lung and thoracic cage. J Appl Physiol 14:528, 1959, with permission)

Mechanically, the components of the ventilatory pump, lung, and chest wall are in series with each other so that the recoil pressure of the respiratory system (Prs) is the sum of its components:

$$Prs = Pw + P_L \qquad \text{(Eq. 2-4)}$$

When the respiratory muscles are completely at rest and the pressure at the surface of the lung is atmospheric, the pressure of the respiratory system equals alveolar pressure under static conditions. It is difficult to determine Prs accurately in the pulmonary function laboratory because complete relaxation of the respiratory muscles is difficult to achieve.

Lung Volumes

The quantity of gas contained within the lungs is subdivided into four primary lung volumes (Fig. 2-4). Combinations of two or more of these primary lung volumes make up the four lung capacities.

Tidal volume (TV) is the volume of air that enters and leaves the lungs during normal breathing. *Inspiratory capacity* (IC) is the maximal volume of air that may

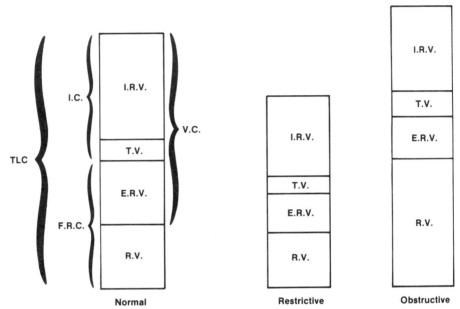

Fig. 2-4. The four primary lung volumes. The four capacities are composed of combinations of two or more lung volumes. In restrictive lung disease, both vital capacity and total lung capacity are reduced. In obstructive lung disease, FRC and TLC may be increased because of increased RV; vital capacity will be reduced if air trapping is severe. (Reproduced with permission from Kinasewitz GT: The laboratory in pulmonary diseases. p. 119. In Mandell HN (ed): Laboratory Medicine in Clinical Practice, John Wright-PSG Inc., Boston, 1983)

be inhaled from a normal resting level. The IC is composed of two lung volumes, TV and *inspiratory reserve volume* (IRV).

The volume of gas within the lung at the end of a normal expiration is *functional residual capacity* (FRC). Since the respiratory muscles are at rest at the end of a normal expiration, FRC is determined by the opposing recoil forces of the lung and chest wall. FRC is the lung volume at which the tendency of the lung to collapse is counterbalanced by the tendency of the chest wall to expand. FRC is composed of two primary lung volumes, *expiratory reserve volume* (ERV) and *residual volume* (RV). ERV is the maximal amount of gas that can be exhaled beginning from the end of a quiet expiration when the lung is at FRC. RV is the volume of gas remaining in the lung following a maximal expiratory effort. *Total lung capacity* (TLC) is the volume of air in the lungs following a maximal inspiration, that is, the sum of all four primary lung volumes. *Vital capacity* (VC) is the maximal amount of air that can be exhaled following a maximal inspiration. Although the VC and its subdivisions, TV, IRV, and ERV can be measured directly with a spirometer, RV and those lung capacities that include RV, that is, FRC and TLC, must be determined indirectly. In most pulmonary function laboratories, FRC is measured indirectly and RV is calculated by subtracting ERV from FRC.

Three techniques are commonly employed to determine FRC. Two, the *closed-circuit helium dilution* technique and *open-circuit nitrogen washout* method, rely on the use of a tracer to measure FRC. In principle, a known volume of gas with a known concentration of tracer gas is placed in communication with an unknown lung volume. After equilibration between the two compartments the final tracer concentration is measured, and by simple proportional calculation the final volume (V_f), which is the sum of both the known and unknown volumes, may be calculated as

$$V_f = V_i(C_i/C_f) \qquad \text{(Eq. 2-5)}$$

where V_i is the initial volume and C_i and C_f are the initial and final concentrations of the tracer, respectively. In the closed-circuit helium dilution technique, beginning at end-expiration (FRC) the subject breathes from a spirometer with a known volume of gas containing 10 percent helium.[10] Because helium is inert and doesn't cross the alveolar-capillary membrane, the volume of helium within the system remains constant. After equilibration has occurred, the total volume of the closed-circuit, that is, the lungs and spirometer, is calculated from Equation 2-5, and FRC is determined by subtracting the initial volume of the spirometer from that of the entire closed circuit. The open-circuit nitrogen washout technique utilizes the nitrogen present in the lung at FRC as the tracer substance.[11]

An alternative to the two tracer techniques for determining FRC is to measure the volume of gas present in the thorax by means of a *body plethysmograph*.[12] By measuring the changes in plethysmograph pressure and mouth pressure that occur during panting after a normal expiration, the amount of gas present within the thorax, for example, FRC, can be determined. (See Chapter 6 for a more detailed discussion of the technique.) It is important to note that FRC determined via one of the tracer dilution techniques may be less than the volume of thoracic gas measured via plethysmography. The dilution techniques measure the gas in the communicating spaces of the lung, whereas some lung diseases, for example, bullous emphysema, are characterized by the presence of large airspaces that are so poorly ventilated they are essentially noncommunicating spaces. Because the gas in these noncommunicating spaces is still compressible, it will be measured by the body plethysmograph. Indeed, the difference between the two determinations of FRC will indicate the volume of the poorly communicating compartment.

Total lung capacity is determined by the ability of the inspiratory muscles to expand the lungs and chest wall.[13] Similarly, in an individual free of airway disease, residual volume of the lungs is determined by the force exerted by the expiratory muscles in compressing the chest wall, "squeezing" air from the lungs.[14] A reduction in both vital capacity and total lung capacity is the hallmark of those disorders that produce a restrictive impairment. Infiltrative pulmonary diseases, for example, pulmonary fibrosis, reduce the distensibility of the lung; TLC and VC are therefore decreased in these disorders, primarily because of a reduction in inspiratory capacity. In the massively obese individual, the compliance of the chest wall is reduced and the diaphragm is displaced high into the thorax by the abdominal contents. Both TLC and VC are reduced in massive obesity, primarily because of a reduction in expiratory reserve volume. Other nonpulmonary conditions that may produce a pattern of restrictive impairment include skeletal deformities, ascites, pleural effusions, and pregnancy. Finally, disorders that decrease the strength of the respiratory muscles, for example, myasthenia gravis, will also reduce the amount of air that can be inspired (IC) and expired (ERV) from functional residual capacity, creating a restrictive pulmonary impairment.

In chronic obstructive lung disease the airways are narrowed and lose some of the peribronchial support that maintains their patency. During expiration premature airway closure may occur, trapping air behind the occluded bronchioles and increasing the residual volume of the lung.[14] This loss of elastic structural tissue, if widespread, may increase the distensibility of the lung and both FRC and TLC may actually become elevated.[13] Nonetheless, vital capacity is normal or even reduced when air trapping increases residual volume at the expense of vital capacity.

FLOW-RESISTIVE PROPERTIES OF THE LUNG

The transpulmonary pressure measured during expansion of the lungs includes the pressure generated to overcome the *flow resistance* of the airways and the frictional resistance to the displacement of lung tissue during inspiration, *tissue resistance.* Normally, tissue resistance caused by viscous forces within the lung is less than 20 percent of total (lung plus airway) pulmonary resistance, though it may increase significantly in severe interstitial lung diseases.

Airway Resistance

The driving pressure for airflow P(A-ao) is the difference between alveolar pressure (PA) and pressure of the airway opening (Pao). Airway resistance by definition can be calculated as

$$Raw = \frac{P(A\text{-}ao)}{\dot{V}} \qquad \text{(Eq. 2-6)}$$

where $\dot{V}$ is the rate of airflow. The driving pressure required to overcome a given resistance depends on whether airflow is *laminar* or *turbulent* (Fig. 2-5). The pressure-flow characteristics of laminar or streamlined flow in a tube of length *l* and radius *r* can be described by Poiseuille's equation,

$$\frac{\Delta P}{\dot{V}} = \frac{8nl}{r^4} \qquad \text{(Eq. 2-7)}$$

where n is the viscosity of the gas and ΔP and $\dot{V}$ are the driving pressure and flow rate, respectively. Note the critical importance of tube radius in determining

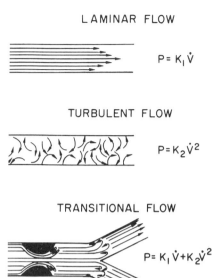

LAMINAR FLOW

$P = K_1 \dot{V}$

TURBULENT FLOW

$P = K_2 \dot{V}^2$

TRANSITIONAL FLOW

$P = K_1 \dot{V} + K_2 \dot{V}^2$

airway resistance ($\Delta P/\dot{V}$); if r is halved, the driving pressure must be increased 16-fold to maintain the same flow rate.

At high flow rates airflow becomes turbulent and there is a complete disorganization of the streamlined characteristic of laminar flow. During turbulent flow the driving pressure required to produce a given rate of airflow becomes proportional to the square of airflow,

$$\Delta P = K(\dot{V}^2) \qquad \text{(Eq. 2-8)}$$

where K is a constant that is proportional to the density of the gas. Note that during turbulent flow airway resistance ($\Delta P/\dot{V}$) is proportional to the rate of airflow.

The pattern of airflow, laminar or turbulent, in a tube is determined from the Reynolds number (Re), a dimensionless number calculated as

$$Re = \frac{2rvd}{n} \qquad \text{(Eq. 2-9)}$$

where v is average velocity, d the gas density, n the viscosity, and r the radius of the tube. In rigid, smooth tubes turbulence occurs when the Reynolds number exceeds 2,000. In the tracheobronchial tree, where irregularities in the airway wall and repeated branching of the airways occur, eddy currents frequently develop and flow assumes a transitional pattern that is a combination of both laminar and turbulent flow. The driving pressure required to produce a given flow under these conditions is dependent on both the density of the gas and its flow rate. Normally, flow is transitional through most of the tracheobronchial tree, with laminar patterns only in the small peripheral airways. At high flow rates, such as those achieved during exercise, flow may be turbulent in the trachea; irregularities in the bronchial wall caused by excessive mucus production, strictures, or tumors can produce turbulent flow in the segmental bronchi and beyond, even at low flow rates.

The upper respiratory tract is the site of a significant proportion of the resistance to airflow. The resistance of the nasal passages is extremely high; up to 50 percent of total airway resistance may be in the nose during nasal breathing.[15] This is the reason that mouth breathing predominates when minute ventilation is high, for example, during exercise. The mouth, pharynx, and larynx account for one-quarter of airway resistance during quiet breathing, but as much as one-half of Raw during exercise. Most of the remaining airway resistance is located in the large conducting airways. It will be recalled from Chapter 1 that the total cross-sectional area of the airways increases with each successive branching. The small peripheral airways less than 2 mm in diameter, that is, the terminal bronchioles and beyond, contribute only a small fraction, 10 to 20 percent, of total airway resistance.[16]

The major sites of increased airway resistance can be identified by comparing expiratory flow-volume curves of breathing air and a *helium-oxygen mixture* that is less dense than air. In normal individuals, the major sites of airway resistance are in the large central airways where airflow is turbulent and density-dependent. Breathing a helium-oxygen mixture will increase expiratory airflow at all but the lowest lung volumes. Those patients who have a significant portion of their airway resistance in the small peripheral airways of the lung, where flow is laminar and independent of density, will have a much smaller change in airflow at 50 percent of vital capacity ($\Delta \dot{V}max_{50\%}$) while breathing the helium-oxygen mixture.[17] This test may become particularly valuable if selective pharmacological manipulation of the large and small airways becomes practical.

Airway resistance varies inversely with lung volume because the diameter of the airways increases as the lungs expand. Depending on the transmural pressure, that is, the difference between pressure within the airways and the surrounding tissue, the airways can be compressed or distended. The airways (and extraalveolar blood vessels) are attached to the elastic elements of the lung, and as the lung expands, the rising elastic recoil pressure of the lung increases traction on the airway wall while pressure within the peribronchial space becomes more negative. The caliber of the airways therefore increases and airway resistance falls at high lung volumes (Fig. 2-6). At low lung volumes airway resistance increases as transmural pressure declines and the small airways at the lung bases may even close. The resistance of the airways can also be increased by contraction of the bronchial smooth muscle. An increment in bronchomotor tone not only narrows the airway, but also makes them less compliant so they distend less at any given transmural airway pressure. If the elastic recoil pressure of the lung is reduced, for example, from emphysema, at any given lung volume transmural airway pressure will be decreased and the airways made narrower. Similarly, the mucosal hypertrophy and excess mucus production characteristic of chronic bronchitis encroaches on the airway lumen and increases its resistance.

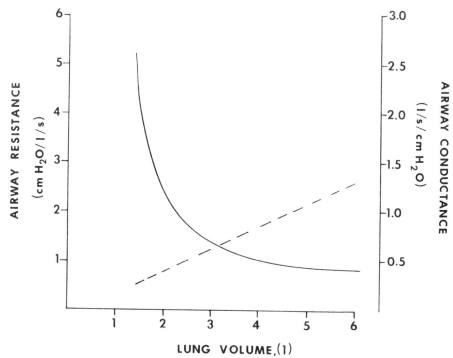

Fig. 2-6.   The relationship between airway resistance (Raw) and lung volume is hyperbolic, whereas that between airway conductance (the inverse of Raw) and lung volume is linear.

It is therefore important in assessing the measurement of Raw to take into account the effect of lung volume. Airway resistance is usually determined at a known lung volume, generally FRC.[18] Because the relationship between lung volume and airway resistance is hyperbolic, the relationship between lung volume and the inverse of Raw is linear. The inverse of airway resistance is *airway conductance* (Gaw), the flow per unit pressure change. This linear relationship between conductance and lung volume means the conductance per unit lung volume or *specific airway conductance* (Gaw/VL) will be independent of the lung volume at which it is measured.

Measurement of airflow during forced expiration is a common method of assessing the flow-resistive properties of the lung. To understand the determinants of expiratory airflow, it is useful to analyze the relationship between expiratory airflow and lung volume during a series of forced expirations made with varying degrees of expiratory effort, *expiratory flow-volume curves* (Fig. 2-7A). As previously discussed, because airway resistance is inversely proportional to lung volume, it is not surprising that maximal rate of airflow progressively declines as lung volume decreases. At high lung volumes, successively more forceful efforts produce progressive increases in expiratory flow rate. At low and intermediate lung volumes, however, modest expiratory efforts are sufficient

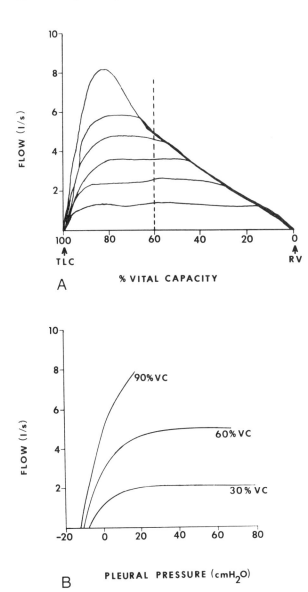

Fig. 2-7. Expiratory flow volume curves (A) with progressively more forceful efforts produce increments in flow at high lung volumes but not at low lung volumes. Measuring pleural pressure and expiratory flow at a constant lung volume, indicated by the vertical dashed line in part A, enables one to conduct an isovolume pressure flow curve at 60 percent of vital capacity, which is shown in part B. At high lung volumes the isovolume pressure flow curve does not plateau and expiration is effort-dependent.

to produce a maximal expiratory flow rate. This phenomena is more readily apparent when one examines the relationship between expiratory airflow and pleural pressure at a constant lung volume, the *isovolume pressure-flow curve.*[19] At any lung volume, as expiratory effort is progressively increased, pleural pressure increases and will exceed atmospheric pressure during a forceful expiration (Fig. 2-7B). Initially, the rate of airflow increases as pleural pressure rises, but at lung volumes below 75 percent of vital capacity, the flow plateaus and becomes fixed at a maximal level. Further increases in pleural pressure produce no additional increment in expiratory airflow, that is, airflow is effort-independent beyond this point. In contrast, at lung volumes above 75 percent of vital capacity airflow increases with progressive increments in pleural pressure and is effort-dependent. Previously, we have indicated that the driving pressure for expiratory airflow is the difference between alveolar pressure and pressure at the airway opening. Inasmuch as

$$P_A = Pst(L) + Ppl \qquad \text{(Eq. 2-10)}$$

and elastic recoil pressure at a given lung volume is constant, alveolar pressure must be increased as pleural pressure rises during increased expiratory efforts. If airflow remains constant in the presence of increasing driving pressure, then resistance to airflow must be increasing proportionally. This occurs because of the *dynamic compression* of the airways during a maximal forced expiration.

During expiration intrabronchial pressure progressively decreases from the alveolus to the mouth as driving pressure is dissipated from having to generate airflow. During a forced expiration when pleural pressure exceeds pressure at the airway opening, at some point along the airway the decrease in intrabronchial pressure equals the elastic recoil pressure of the lung (Fig. 2-8). At this *equal pressure point* (EPP) the pressure within the airway equals peribronchial (pleural) pressure and transmural pressure is zero.[20] The equal pressure point therefore divides the airways into two segments arranged in series. The upstream segment extends from the alveolus to the EPP and the downstream segment extends from the EPP to the airway opening. It is this latter segment that is subject to dynamic compression.

At the end of inspiration pleural pressure is subatmospheric and there is no equal pressure point. During forced expiration, as pleural pressure begins to rise and becomes less subatmospheric, pleural pressure will equal airway pressure at some point along the intrathoracic trachea. This equal pressure point is effected despite the increase in alveolar pressure produced by positive pleural pressure [$P_A = Pst(L) + Ppl$]. If the force of the expiratory muscles increases and pleural pressure rises still further, the EPP will occur at a more peripheral location in the tracheobronchial tree until, at some point in the lobar or segmental bronchi, a pleural pressure is reached beyond which further increases only increase compression of the airway and a maximal rate of expiratory airflow ($\dot{V}$max) for that lung volume is attained. Because the driving pressure for flow from the alveolus to the EPP is the elastic recoil pressure of the lung, the resistance of the upstream segment can be calculated as

$$Rs = \frac{Pst(L)}{\dot{V}max} \qquad \text{(Eq. 2-11)}$$

Thus far we have considered the site of airway compression or closure to be located at the EPP where transmural pressure (Ptm) is zero. Depending on the structure of the airway, its tethering to surrounding lung parenchyma, and the degree of bronchomotor tone, airway collapse may occur at a critical transmural pressure (Ptm_{crit}) other than zero.[21] Critical closing pressure is the distending

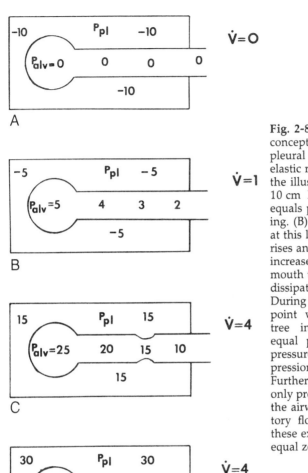

Fig. 2-8. The equal pressure point concept. (A) At the end of inspiration pleural pressure counterbalances the elastic recoil pressure of the lung [at the illustrated lung volume Pst(L) = 10 cm H_2O] and alveolar pressure equals pressure of the airway opening. (B) During a passive expiration at this lung volume pleural pressure rises and therefore alveolar pressure increases; as air moves toward the mouth the intrabronchial pressure is dissipated, generating the flow. (C) During a forceful expiration at some point within the tracheobronchial tree intrabronchial pressure will equal pleural pressure, the equal pressure point, and dynamic compression of the airway can occur. (D) Further increases in expiratory effort only produce greater compression of the airway while the rate of expiratory flow remains constant. In all these examples Ptm_{crit} is assumed to equal zero. (See text for dicusssion.)

pressure required to maintain airway patency. Whenever transmural pressure falls below Ptm_{crit}, airway collapse may occur. Airway pressure within the potentially collapsible airway is the difference between alveolar pressure and the pressure used to generate airflow, so that at any given flow rate transmural pressure (Ptm) across the bronchus is

$$Ptm = [P_A - \dot{V}(Rs)] - Ppl \qquad \text{(Eq. 2-12)}$$

Because alveolar pressure is the sum of elastic recoil pressure and pleural pressure,

$$Ptm = Pst(L) - \dot{V}(Rs) \qquad \text{(Eq. 2-13)}$$

As flow increases, Ptm falls until a level of airflow is attained at which Ptm drops below Ptm_{crit} and airway closure occurs. Once the airway is completely collapsed there is no flow. In the absence of airflow intrabronchial pressure increases; as soon as Ptm exceeds Ptm_{crit} airflow resumes. The collapsible segment of the airways therefore behaves as a variable resistor. Once pleural pressure sufficient to produce dynamic compression of the airways is reached, partial collapse of the bronchial segment occurs and resistance across this portion of the airway increases until Ptm equals Ptm_{crit}. Further increases in pleural pressure only increase the resistance of the collapsible segment, limiting airflow to a maximal level. Flow limitation occurs when Ptm = Ptm_{crit} so that

$$\dot{V}max = \frac{Pst(L) - Ptm_{crit}}{Rs} \tag{Eq. 2-14}$$

Note that when Ptm_{crit} equals zero, Equations 2-11 and 2-14 are identical.

It is apparent from this relationship that the maximal rate of expiratory airflow is dependent on three factors: (1) the elastic recoil pressure of the lung, (2) the critical closing pressure of the airway, and (3) the resistance of the airway upstream from the compressible segment. Elastic recoil pressure of the lung increases as lung volume increases. Diseases that alter the compliance of the lung will either increase or decrease $\dot{V}max$ at a given lung volume, depending on whether the elastic recoil pressure is increased, for example, pulmonary fibrosis, or reduced, for example, emphysema. An increase in bronchomotor tone or destruction of the supporting structures of the airway will decrease $\dot{V}max$ by increasing the critical closing pressure of the airway. Finally, a reduction in total cross-sectional area of the airways because of excessive mucus production, for example, chronic bronchitis, bronchospasm, or stricture, will reduce maximal expiratory flow.

The dynamic collapse of the airway is important in generating an effective cough. Because of airway compression that occurs during coughing, linear velocity of the expired air is increased across the narrowed segments. This increased linear velocity augments the shear forces that help to remove mucus and other particles from the bronchial wall.

Measuring Airflow

The dynamic aspects of pulmonary function are measured by monitoring the rate of airflow from the lungs during forceful expiration from total lung capacity to residual volume. The volume of air expelled during this *forced vital capacity* (FVC) maneuver should be similar to that expired during a slow vital capacity maneuver. However, some patients with obstructive lung disease increase their residual volume because of premature airway closure and air trapping during forced expiration; therefore, FVC may be less than slow VC in these individuals.

The forced expiratory spirogram is produced by having the patient inhale to

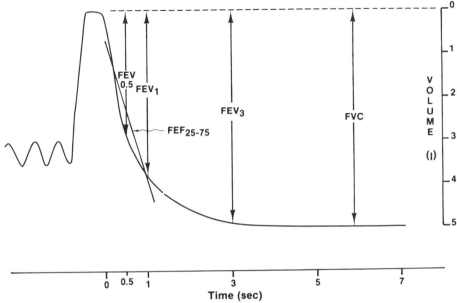

Fig. 2-9.   Normal forced expiratory spirogram with $FEV_{0.5}$, FEV_1, FEV_3, and $FEF_{25-75\%}$ indicated. Expiration is almost complete after 3 sec. (Reproduced with permission from Kinasewitz GT: The laboratory in pulmonary diseases. p. 119. In Mandell HN (ed): Laboratory Medicine in Clinical Practice, John Wright-PSG Inc., Boston, 1983)

total lung capacity, and then, as forcefully as possible, exhale to residual volume while the results are graphically recorded as a function of time (Fig. 2-9). Airflow (change in volume per unit time) is usually reported as the volume exhaled over particular time intervals or over particular segments of forced vital capacity. *Forced expired volumes* are measured at ½ ($FEV_{0.5}$), 1 (FEV_1) and 3 (FEV_3) sec after the start of expiration; these timed volumes are usually expressed as absolute volumes and a percentage of forced vital capacity, for example, $FEV_1/FVC\%$. In addition, *forced midexpiratory flow rate* ($FEF_{25-75\%}$) is the mean flow rate between 25 and 75 percent of forced vital capacity. The mean forced expiratory flow between 200 and 1,200 ml of expired volume ($FEF_{0.2-1.2}$) is a measure of airflow at large lung volumes.

The influence of lung volume on airflow can be more easily appreciated if expiratory airflow during the FVC maneuver is plotted as a function of the volume of gas within the lungs, a maximal expiratory *flow-volume curve* (Fig. 2-10). In the normal individual, after the initial rapid increase in airflow at onset of expiration, there is a gradual decline in airflow as both airway diameter and elastic recoil pressure of the lungs decrease with falling lung volumes. Obstructive airway disease is characterized by narrowing of the airways, and frequently, a decrease in the elastic recoil pressure of the lung. Increased total lung capacity, frequently observed in obstructive disease, has the compensatory effect of increasing both airway size and elastic recoil of the lung. Nonetheless, at any

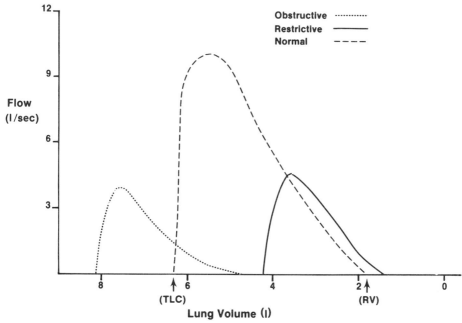

Fig. 2-10. Maximal expiratory flow as a function of lung volume. Even though the volume of air in the lungs is greater than normal in obstructive disease, expiratory airflow is clearly reduced. In restrictive lung disease, the low level of expiratory airflow is caused by the reduced lung volume. (Reproduced with permission from Kinasewitz GT: The laboratory in pulmonary diseases. p. 119. In Mandell HN (ed): Laboratory Medicine in Clinical Practice, John Wright-PSG Inc., Boston, 1983)

given lung volume expiratory airflow is subnormal. In restrictive lung disease, even though absolute values for expiratory airflow may be decreased, airflow is labeled normal or even supranormal when lung volume is considered.

Because airflow during the initial phase of a forced vital capacity maneuver is dependent on expiratory effort, the $FEF_{0.2-1.2}$, which is measured early during expiration, may be disproportionately reduced in comparison with other flow rates in the poorly motivated patient. On the other hand, FEV_1, FEV_3, and $FEF_{25-75\%}$ are all measured over large lung volumes, and therefore they will be relatively less influenced by a suboptimal effort. These latter tests are reliable indexes of airflow obstruction.

Diseases that produce airway obstruction, for example, asthma and chronic bronchitis, will reduce expiratory airflow in proportion to the severity of the disorder. Early or mild obstructive disease may reduce only FEV_3 and $FEF_{25-75\%}$, since these measurements include airflow at low lung volumes where airway narrowing will have a greater effect. However, all indexes of expiratory airflow will fall below normal with progressively worsening obstruction. In restrictive lung disorders, such as pulmonary fibrosis, FEV_1 and FEV_3 may be correspondingly decreased because vital capacity is reduced. Yet, when FEV_1 and FEV_3 are expressed as a percentage of forced vital capacity, for example, $FEV_1/FVC\%$, normal or increased values will be obtained.

Inspiratory flow rates are mainly determined by the inspiratory force generated by the respiratory muscles. Because pleural pressure is lower than intrabronchial pressure throughout inspiration, compression of the intrathoracic airways does not occur. Inspiratory flow rates are usually not helpful in evaluating patients with pulmonary disease because inspiratory flow in most individuals is principally effort-dependent. The most common cause of a reduced maximal inspiratory flow rate is poor patient effort. Reduced inspiratory flow is also seen in patients with weakness because of neuromuscular disease, for example, myasthenia gravis, or extrathoracic airway obstruction, for example, tracheomalacia. In the latter condition, as the pressure within the trachea becomes subatmospheric during inspiration the airway is compressed by surrounding (atmospheric) pressure, thereby reducing inspiratory flow. The *flow-volume loop* (in which inspiratory and expiratory airflow are plotted as a function of lung volume) is an important diagnostic aid. Expiratory flow may be completely normal with extrathoracic obstruction, whereas inspiratory flow will plateau at a low rate.[22]

Maximal voluntary ventilation (MVV), formerly termed maximal breathing capacity (MBC), is another test of dynamic lung function that is highly effort-dependent. Although abnormal results are common in patients with obstructive lung disease, individuals with poor strength, coordination, or motivation frequently have an abnormal MVV as well. In contrast, the MVV is fairly well preserved in patients with pure restrictive lung disease unless their impairment is severe.

DISTRIBUTION OF VENTILATION

The pleural pressure around the top of the lung is more negative than that at the lung base.[23] This vertical gradient of pleural pressure, 0.25 cm H_2O per centimeter distance, is generated by the effects of gravity on the lung. Because of this pleural-pressure gradient the transpulmonary pressure at the apex of the lung is greater than at the base, and consequently, the alveoli are larger at the apex than at the base of the lung at end-expiration (Fig. 2-11). Despite their smaller resting volume, during a tidal breath from FRC a greater proportion of inspired air goes to the alveoli at the base of the lung.[24] This preferential distribution of ventilation exists because the pressure-volume curves of the alveoli at the base are such that a given decrease in pleural pressure produces a greater increase in lung volume in that area. Note that at low lung volumes the intrapleural pressure at the base may exceed airway pressure and compression of alveoli, and collapse of the airways at the bottom of the lung may occur. Under these conditions, ventilation of this region is impossible until the pleural pressure at the bottom of the lung becomes subatmospheric; therefore, the initial portion of the air inspired from residual volume goes to the apexes.[24]

The distribution of ventilation will be altered in the presence of diseases that

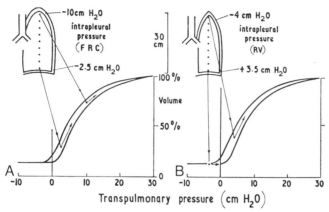

Fig. 2-11. Alveoli at the top and bottom of the lung operate on different portions of their compliance curve because of the vertical gradient of intrapleural pressure. A tidal breath from FRC will produce a greater increase in alveolar volume at the base of the lung (A) but the apex will be better ventilated if the tidal breath begins from RV (B). (Reproduced with permission from West JB: Ventilation/Blood Flow and Gas Exchange. Blackwell, Oxford, 1970)

affect the compliance and/or resistance of the lung in a nonuniform manner,[25] as shown in Figure 2-12. Consider the simple case of two lungs with identical compliances but a marked increase in the airway resistance of one lung (Fig. 2-12B). A decrease in pleural pressure of 2 cm H_2O will produce an equal driving pressure for inspiratory flow in both lungs, but, because of the increased airway resistance, airflow into lung A will be slower and it will take longer to reach the same volume as lung B. If inspiration is terminated because of a rapid respiratory rate while airflow into lung A is still occurring, then the volume of lung A will be less than that of lung B. If the resistance of both lungs were equal but the compliance of lung A were increased (Fig. 2-12C), then at a given decrease in pleural pressure air would enter both lungs at the same rate; however, because lung B is less compliant it will fill to capacity more quickly than lung A.

Under either of these circumstances, an increase in resistance or compliance, lung A fills asynchronously with lung B. If sufficient time is available both lungs will fill to capacity, whereas at rapid respiratory rates insufficient time would be available for lung A to fill completely and dynamic compliance would fall at rapid respiratory rates. In a normal individual, dynamic compliance decreases minimally at respiratory rates up to 100 breaths/min. However, in the presence of early disease of the small (less than 2 mm diameter) airways, compliance may become *frequency-dependent,* that is, it may fall with increasing respiratory frequency, even when the expiratory spirogram is normal.[7]

Regional inhomogeneity in the distribution of ventilation is decreased because of the interdependence of contiguous respiratory units.[26] Because the alveoli share common walls, the expansion of a respiratory unit exerts traction on the adjoining units and promotes synchronous ventilation within the lung. There

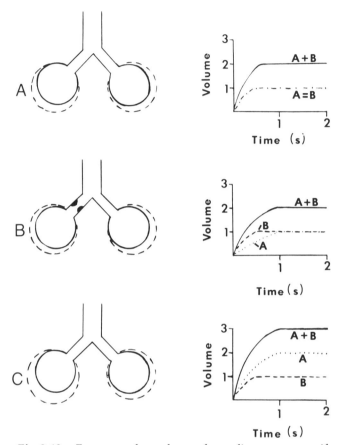

Fig. 2-12. Frequency dependence of compliance can occur if
either the compliance or resistance of the lung is increased in a
nonuniform manner. (A) Two lungs with equal compliances
and resistances fill synchronously (curve A = B), and as long
as the time of inspiration is 0.5 sec or greater the volume
within the lungs (curve A + B) and dynamic compliance
($\Delta V/\Delta P$) will be constant. (B) The resistance of the lung on the
left is increased so that the time it takes to fill, indicated by the
dotted curve A, is prolonged; when the duration of inspiration
is less than 1.0 sec, the volume of the lungs (curve A + B) and
dynamic compliance of A + B will fall. (C) The compliance of
the lung on the left is increased so that a greater volume of air
must flow into that unit before it is filled to capacity (dotted
curve A); therefore, it takes longer to fill. The dynamic compliance of A + B will also fall when the duration of inspiration
is less than 1.0 sec.

is also interdependence between the lung and chest wall; when the chest expands during inspiration a lag in regional filling will distort the chest wall and decrease pleural pressure in the adjacent region, thereby increasing the transpulmonary pressure gradient and promoting alveolar filling in the lung units that are lagging. Collateral ventilation also promotes the synchronous emptying and filling of alveolar units. Even when the peripheral airways are completely obstructed, air may enter the alveoli through collateral channels, for example, the pores of Kohn. In emphysema, the resistance of the collateral channels is extremely low and may even be less than the airway resistance in some patients.[27]

Inhomogeneity in the distribution of ventilation (and the closing volume) can be determined with the *single-breath nitrogen washout* test.[28] After exhaling to residual volume the subject inhales 100 percent oxygen to total lung capacity; nitrogen concentration of the expired gas is continuously monitored during the ensuing exhalation of RV (Fig. 2-13). It should be recalled that during inspiration from RV, because of the compression of alveoli and potential airway closure at the lung base, the initial portion of the inspired gas, which consists of dead-space gas with a high nitrogen concentration, is distributed preferentially to the apexes.

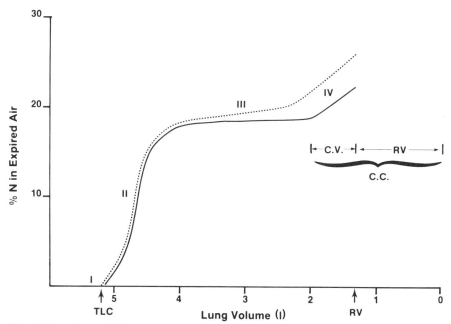

Fig. 2-13.   The single-breath nitrogen test of a normal subject (solid line) and a patient with small airway disease (dashed line). In the patient with airway disease the nitrogen concentration of expired air rises more steeply during the plateau phase (III) and the abrupt increase in nitrogen concentration, indicating airway closure (phase IV) occurs at a higher lung volume. CV, closing volume; RV, residual volume; CC, closing capacity (CV + RV); TLC, total lung capacity. (Reproduced with permission from Kinasewitz GT: The laboratory in pulmonary diseases. p. 119. In Mandell HN (ed): Laboratory Medicine in Clinical Practice, John Wright-PSG Inc., Boston, 1983)

Furthermore, the increase in alveolar volume during inspiration from RV to TLC is greater at the bases, so more oxygen is delivered here; consequently, the concentration of nitrogen is lower in the alveoli at the bottom of the lung.

During subsequent exhalation to residual volume, the first portion of the expired gas from the anatomic dead space contains only oxygen (phase I). Then, the concentration of nitrogen rapidly rises (phase II) as alveolar gas begins to appear. If gas enters and leaves all regions of the lung synchronously, this plateau phase (phase III) will be relatively flat, that is, nitrogen concentration will change by less than 2.5 percent/liter. However, if the distribution of ventilation is nonuniform, gas from different regions will have different nitrogen concentrations and the expired nitrogen concentration will rise during this phase. If airway closure occurs at low lung volumes, there will be an abrupt increase in expired nitrogen concentration (phase IV). The volume above RV at which this terminal increase in slope occurs is termed the *closing volume. Closing capacity* is the sum of the residual volume and closing volume. An increased closing volume is almost invariably found in those patients with chronic bronchitis and emphysema who have decreased expiratory flow rates.[29] Many cigarette smokers will have an increased closing volume, even when their spirometry is normal.[28] In addition to airway disease, however, loss of elastic recoil, which occurs with aging, will also increase the closing volume.[30] Thus, the demonstration of an abnormal closing volume is nonspecific and the potential usefulness of the closing volume test is undetermined at this time.

WORK OF BREATHING

In generating the pressure to move a volume of gas in and out of the lungs the ventilatory pump performs mechanical work. Although it is possible to measure the work performed in overcoming the elastic and flow-resistive elements of the lung by measuring intrapleural pressure and volume throughout the respiratory cycle, the amount of work expended on the entire respiratory system, including the chest wall and other muscles of respiration, is impossible to measure. Patients with lung disease adopt a respiratory pattern that minimizes their work of breathing.[31] Those with stiff, noncompliant lungs breathe at a rapid rate with a reduced tidal volume. This pattern maintains minute ventilation while reducing the work of expanding the lung. In contrast, patients with airflow obstruction often breathe slowly to reduce the work necessary to overcome increased airway resistance.

REFERENCES

1. Mead J: Measurement of the inertia of the lungs at increased ambient pressure. J Appl Physiol 9:208, 1956
2. Johanson WG, Pierce AK: Effects of elastase, collagenase and papain on structure and function of rat lungs in vitro. J Clin Invest 51:288, 1972

3. Sugihara T, Martin CJ, Hildebrandt J: Length-tension properties of alveolar wall in man. J Appl Physiol 30:874, 1971
4. Rahn H, Otis AB, Chadwick LE, Fenn WO: The pressure-volume diagram of the thorax and lung. Am J Physiol 146:161, 1946
5. Milic-Emili J, Mead J, Turner JM, Glauser EM: Improved technique for estimating pleural pressure from esophageal balloons. J Appl Physiol 19:207, 1964
6. Clements JA: Surface phenomena in relation to pulmonary function. Physiologist 5:11, 1962
7. Woolcock AJ, Vincent NJ, Macklem PT: Frequency dependence of compliance as a test for obstruction in the small airways. J Clin Invest 48:1097, 1969
8. Leaver DG, Tattersfield AE, Pride NB: Contributions of loss of elastic recoil and enhanced airways collapsibility to the airflow obstruction of chronic bronchitis and emphysema. J Clin Invest 52:2117, 1973
9. Turner JM, Mead J, Wohl ME: Elasticity of human lungs in relation to age. J Appl Physiol 25:664, 1968
10. Meneely GR, Kaltreider NL: The volume of the lung determined by helium dilution: Description of the method and comparison with other procedures. J Clin Invest 28:129, 1949
11. Darling RC, Cournard A, Richards DW Jr: Studies on the intrapulmonary mixture of gases. III. An open circuit method for measuring residual air. J Clin Invest 19:609, 1940
12. Dubois AB, Botelho SY, Bedell GH, et al: A rapid plethysmographic method for measuring thoracic gas volume: A comparison with a nitrogen washout method for measuring functional residual capacity in normal subjects. J Clin Invest 35:322, 1956
13. Gibson GJ, Pride NB: Lung distensibility: The static pressure-volume curve of the lungs and its use in clinical assessment. Br J Dis Chest 70:143, 1976
14. Leith DE, Mead J: Mechanisms determining residual volume of lungs in normal subjects. J Appl Physiol 23:221, 1967
15. Ferris BG, Mead J, Opie LH: Partitioning of respiratory flow resistance in man. J Appl Physiol 19:653, 1964
16. Macklem PT, Mead J: Resistance of central and peripheral airways by a retrograde catheter. J Appl Physiol 22:395, 1967
17. Dosman J, Bode F, Urbanetti J, et al: The use of a helium-oxygen mixture during maximum expiratory flow to demonstrate obstruction in small airways in smokers. J Clin Invest 55:1090, 1975
18. DuBois AB, Botelho SY, Comroe JH Jr: A new method for measuring airway resistance in man using a body plethysmograph: Values in normal subjects and in patients with respiratory disease. J Clin Invest 35:327, 1956
19. Fry DL Hyatt RE: Pulmonary mechanics: A unified analysis of the relationship between pressure, volume and gasflow in the lungs of normal and diseased human subjects. Am J Med 29:672, 1960
20. Mead J, Turner JM, Macklem PT, Little JB: Significance of the relationship between lung recoil and maximum expiratory airflow. J Appl Physiol 22:95, 1967
21. Pride NB, Permutt S, Riley R, Bromberger-Barnea B: Determinants of maximal expiratory flow from the lungs. J Appl Physiol 23:646, 1967
22. Kryger M, Bode F, Antic R, Anthonisen N: Diagnosis of obstruction of the upper and central airways. Am J Med 61:85, 1976
23. Daly WJ, Bondurant, S: Direct measurement of respiratory pleural pressure in man. J Appl Physiol 18:513, 1963
24. Milic-Emili J, Henderson JAM, Dolovich MB, et al: Regional distribution of inspired gas in the lung. J Appl Physiol 21:749, 1966
25. Otis AB, McKerrow CB, Bartlett RA, et al: Mechanical factors in distribution of ventilation. J Appl Physiol 8:427, 1956
26. Mead J, Takashima T, Leith D: Mechanical interdependence of distensible units in the lung. Fed Proc 26:551, 1967

27. Terry PB, Traystman RJ, Newball HH, et al: Collateral ventilation in man. N Engl J Med 298:10, 1978
28. Buist AS: The single breath nitrogen test. N Engl J Med 293:438, 1975
29. Rodarte JR, Hyatt RE, Rehder K, Marsh HM: New tests for the detection of obstructive pulmonary disease. Chest 72:762, 1977
30. Begin R, Renzetti AD, Bigler AH, Watanabe S: Flow and age dependence of airway closure and dynamic compliance. J Appl Physiol 38:199, 1975
31. Turino GM, Fishman AP: The congested lung. J Chronic Dis 9:510, 1959

3

Ventilation, Perfusion, and Gas Exchange

Gary T. Kinasewitz, M.D.

The primary function of the respiratory system is the exchange of oxygen and carbon dioxide across the alveolar-capillary membrane. The movement of oxygen from a region of high concentration, alveolar air, to a region of low concentration, the mixed venous blood returned to the lung, is passive and depends on the magnitude of the pressure gradient between alveolar air and blood. Similarly, the elimination of carbon dioxide from mixed venous blood into alveolar air is a passive process. To maintain O_2 and CO_2 concentration gradients, which facilitate gas transport across the alveolar capillary membrane, both the ventilatory and circulatory pumps of the respiratory system must be functioning properly. Each minute the ventilatory pump delivers fresh inspired air to maintain a high O_2 and low CO_2 concentration in the alveolar space. Simultaneously, the right ventricle pumps mixed venous blood with a low O_2 and high CO_2 content through the pulmonary capillaries. If either the ventilatory or circulatory pump fails to maintain an adequate output, or if the distribution of ventilation and perfusion is altered so there is inadequate exposure of alveolar gas to mixed venous blood, then gas exchange across the alveolar-capillary membrane will be impaired.

OXYGEN CONSUMPTION AND
CARBON DIOXIDE PRODUCTION

Oxygen is utilized by the tissues during aerobic metabolism; consequently, carbon dioxide is generated as a by-product of this metabolism. Under steady-state conditions, when the amount of oxygen contained within the blood and tissue stores is constant, the quantity of oxygen taken up from the alveolar gas by the blood in the pulmonary capillaries each minute is the oxygen consumption ($\dot{V}_{O_2}$); in a normal resting individual $\dot{V}_{O_2}$ is about 4 ml/(min)(kg) (STPD). Similarly, the quantity of CO_2 eliminated in the expired air each minute is the carbon dioxide production ($\dot{V}CO_2$), typically 3.2 ml/(min)(kg) (STPD). Because the generation of CO_2 is metabolically linked to the utilization of O_2, carbon dioxide production increases when the metabolic rate and oxygen consumption of the peripheral tissues increases, for example, during exercise. The respiratory quotient (RQ) is the amount of CO_2 produced per unit volume of oxygen metabolized; this will vary, depending on whether fat (RQ = 0.7) or carbohydrate (RQ = 1.0) is the primary organic substrate of aerobic metabolism. On an average American diet a mixture of fat and carbohydrate is utilized and the RQ is about 0.8.

The $\dot{V}CO_2$ can be determined by collecting a timed sample of expired gas in a Douglas bag and measuring the volume and fractional concentration (FE_{CO_2}) in the exhaled sample. Because the carbon dioxide concentration of the inspired air is essentially zero, the CO_2 present in the expired sample represents CO_2 production, which can be calculated as

$$K(FE_{CO_2}(\dot{V}E)) \tag{Eq. 3-1}$$

where $\dot{V}E$ is the minute ventilation or the volume of gas expired in 1 min (liters per minute, BTPS) and K is a constant that converts liters (BTPS) to milliliters (STPD).

The determination of oxygen consumption is somewhat more complicated because there is oxygen in inspired air and the total volume of gas expired ($\dot{V}E$) is slightly less than that inspired each minute ($\dot{V}I$). The difference between $\dot{V}I$ and $\dot{V}E$ occurs because when RQ = 0.8, only 8 ml CO_2 is added to alveolar gas for every 10 ml of O_2 removed from the alveolar gas by pulmonary capillary blood. Because nitrogen is not readily exchanged across the alveolar capillary membrane, the concentration of nitrogen in expired gas increases. If the expired minute volume is known, the inspired minute volume (liters per minute, BTPS) may be calculated as

$$\dot{V}I = \frac{\dot{V}E(FE_{N_2})}{(FI_{N_2})} \tag{Eq. 3-2}$$

where FI_{N_2} and FE_{N_2} are the concentrations of nitrogen in the inspired and expired gases, respectively. Once the inspired minute volume is known, oxygen consumption can be calculated as the difference between the amount of oxygen inspired and that expired each minute.

$$\dot{V}O_2 = K[(FI_{O_2}\dot{V}I) - (FE_{O_2}\dot{V}E)] \tag{Eq. 3-3}$$

The ratio $\dot{V}CO_2/\dot{V}O_2$ is the respiratory exchange ratio (R) that, under steady-state conditions, is the same as the respiratory quotient; normally, R equals 0.8.

ALVEOLAR VENTILATION

To understand the relationship between the concentration of a gas in air and its partial pressure in air and blood, it is helpful to consider the example of a gas

Fig. 3-1. On the left, gas molecules (closed circles) in contact with a liquid dissolve in it until the pressure of the gas in the liquid phase is equal to that in the gaseous phase. On the right, a mixture containing equal amounts of two gases (open and closed circles) exerts a total pressure equal to that of the single gas on the left; the partial pressure of each gas is 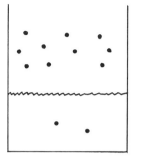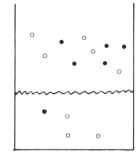 0.5 times the total pressure. The amount of each gas dissolved in the liquid depends on the solubility of the gases and need not be equal when the partial pressures of the two gases are equal.

mixture in an open container at sea level where the atmospheric pressure is 760 torr (Fig. 3-1). If the gas mixture contains 50 percent gas A and 50 percent gas B, then the partial pressure of gas A, the pressure exerted by the gas A molecules on the wall of the container, is the pressure that would result if only gas A occupied the container, or $760 \times 0.5 = 380$ torr. If there is a liquid in the bottom of the container, then molecules of A and B from the gas phase will enter the liquid until sufficient quantities of A and B have dissolved to produce a partial pressure (P_A and P_B) equal to that in the gas above the surface. The content of A and B in the liquid need not be equal; if gas A is more soluble in the liquid than gas B, then more molecules of gas A are in solution when $P_A = P_B$.

The sample of expired air we collect in a Douglas bag is a mixture of air from two areas, the gas-exchanging units of the lung (the alveoli and respiratory bronchioles), and that which remains in the trachea and conducting airways, the *anatomic dead space.* The volume of gas in these conducting airways is approximately equal to body weight in pounds, that is, about 150 ml in an average 150-lb adult. The portion of inspired air that reaches the gas-exchange area of the lung each minute is termed the alveolar ventilation (V_A); in a 150-lb person with a tidal volume of 500 ml, $\dot{V}_A$ is $500 - 150 = 350$ ml/breath, multiplied by the respiratory frequency. In a steady state, $\dot{V}_{CO_2}$ is the product of alveolar ventilation and the concentration of CO_2 in the expired alveolar gas. Note that the concentration of CO_2 in alveolar gas is greater than the CO_2 concentration of mixed expired gas because the mixed expired sample contains both alveolar and dead space gas, and the composition of the latter is essentially the same as inspired air. The partial pressure of CO_2 in alveolar gas ($P_{A_{CO_2}}$) is the product of its fractional concentration ($F_{A_{CO_2}}$) and barometric pressure (P_B), that is,

$$P_{A_{CO_2}} = F_{A_{CO_2}}(P_B) \qquad\qquad \text{(Eq. 3-4)}$$

Because CO_2 rapidly diffuses across the alveolar-capillary membrane and the dissociation curve for CO_2 is relatively linear in the physiological range, the partial pressure of CO_2 in alveolar air is approximately equal to that of arterial blood (Pa_{CO_2}). (The potential error in such an assumption must be small since the difference between arterial and mixed venous P_{CO_2} is only a few torr.) Thus it follows that

$$\dot{V}_{CO_2}(K) = \dot{V}_A(P_{a_{CO_2}}) \tag{Eq. 3-5}$$

where K is a constant (0.863) that converts liters (BTPS) to milliliters (STPD). It can be seen that doubling alveolar ventilation, for example, by voluntary hyperventilation, will reduce $P_{a_{CO_2}}$ by 50 percent if $\dot{V}_{CO_2}$ remains constant (Fig. 3-2). Similarly, if $\dot{V}_{CO_2}$ increases because of fever in a patient who is unable to increase $\dot{V}_A$, for example, the patient on controlled mechanical ventilation, $P_{a_{CO_2}}$ must rise.

Anatomic dead space may be determined from the curve of expired nitrogen concentration after a single breath of 100 percent O_2. The rapid increase in $F_{E_{N_2}}$ that occurs during phase II of the single-breath nitrogen washout is caused by the appearance of alveolar gas in the expirate (see Fig. 2-13). If this rapidly rising phase is bisected by a vertical line, the volume of gas to the left of the dividing line provides an estimate of the volume of the trachea and conducting airways.

Of far greater clinical importance than the measurement of this anatomic dead space is the determination of the *functional* or *physiological dead space* (VD), that is, the sum of the anatomic dead space plus the wasted ventilation to alveoli that are poorly perfused.[1] Patients with lung disease and diminished perfusion of alveolar capillaries in some areas of the lung, for example, the patient with bullous emphysema, have an increase in functional dead space, which means that to maintain the same level of alveolar ventilation they must increase the total volume of air moving in and out of the lung each minute ($\dot{V}_E$). This increases the work of breathing at any level of $\dot{V}_{O_2}$ and $\dot{V}_{CO_2}$, and if the increase in VD is large, the respiratory muscles will fatigue and respiratory failure will ensue. However, as long as the patient is able to increase his minute ventilation sufficiently to compensate for the rise in VD, then $\dot{V}_A$, and therefore, $P_{a_{CO_2}}$ may be normal.

Arterial P_{CO_2} is a measure of the adequacy of alveolar ventilation. Although we cannot measure inefficient or "wasted" ventilation directly, we can measure both minute ventilation and partial pressure of CO_2 ($P_{E_{CO_2}}$) in expired gas.[2] The

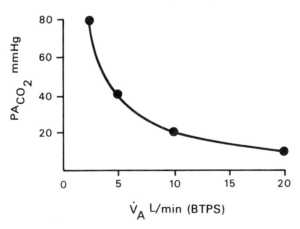

Fig. 3-2. Relationship between alveolar ventilation ($\dot{V}_A$) and $P_{A_{CO_2}}$ at a constant rate of CO_2 production (200 ml/min). An increase in CO_2 production would shift the curve to the right. [Reproduced with permission from George RB: Alveolar ventilation, ventilation-perfusion relationships, and gas transfer. p. 67. In George RB, Light RW, Matthay RA (eds): Chest Medicine. Churchill Livingstone, New York, 1983]

volume of CO_2 eliminated in the expired gas comes from alveolar gas, because the partial pressure of CO_2 in the inspired air that fills V_D during each breath is essentially zero. This can be expressed as

$$V_T(P_{E_{CO_2}}) = V_A(P_{A_{CO_2}}) + P_{I_{CO_2}}(V_D) \qquad \text{(Eq. 3-6)}$$

and since $P_{I_{CO_2}} \approx 0$ and $V_A = V_T - V_D$,

$$V_T(P_{E_{CO_2}}) = (V_T - V_D)P_{A_{CO_2}} \qquad \text{(Eq. 3-7)}$$

Substituting Pa_{CO_2} for $P_{A_{CO_2}}$ and rearranging yields the modified *Bohr equation,*

$$\frac{V_D}{V_T} = \frac{Pa_{CO_2} - P_{E_{CO_2}}}{Pa_{CO_2}} \qquad \text{(Eq. 3-8)}$$

The normal V_D/V_T ratio is 0.25 to 0.35 at rest; when the tidal volume increases during exercise, the relative increase in the volume of the trachea and large airways is less than the increase in alveolar gas so that the V_D/V_T ratio decreases and ventilation becomes more efficient.[3] In patients with lung disease, however, the proportion of wasted ventilation to poorly or nonfunctioning terminal respiratory units also increases as the tidal volume increases, so that the V_D/V_T ratio may remain high or even rise as ventilation is increased, for example, during hypoxia or exercise.[4]

GAS EXCHANGE

Arterial Blood Gases

The ultimate purpose of the respiratory system is to provide adequate oxygen for the body's needs and the simplest way to determine how well this is accomplished is to measure the P_{O_2} and P_{CO_2} of arterial blood. Normally, the Pa_{CO_2} of arterial blood is 40 torr (range 35 to 45 torr). Normal arterial P_{O_2} is greater than 90 torr in a young adult at sea level but, because of the increase in ventilation-perfusion mismatching that occurs with aging, the lower limit of normal for Pa_{O_2} declines with age and values of 80 torr are common in healthy 65-year-olds.[5] Far more information about the efficiency of arterial oxygenation can be obtained if one calculates the alveolar-arterial oxygen gradient $[P(A-a)_{O_2}]$. To determine the alveolar-arterial oxygen gradient we must first calculate the partial pressure of oxygen in alveolar gas ($P_{A_{O_2}}$) using the simplified ideal alveolar air equation, which is

$$P_{A_{O_2}} = F_{I_{O_2}}(P_B - 47) - (Pa_{CO_2}/R) \qquad \text{(Eq. 3-9)}$$

where $F_{I_{O_2}}$ is the fraction of oxygen in inspired air (0.209 for room air), P_B is the barometric pressure (760 torr at sea level), Pa_{CO_2} is the arterial P_{CO_2}, and R the respiratory exchange ratio, normally 0.8.[6]

Dry room air is composed of 79 percent nitrogen, 20.9 percent oxygen, and less than 0.1 percent carbon dioxide and inert gases. As we inspire and air moves through the upper airway, it is warmed and fully saturated with water vapor. At 37°C the partial pressure of water is 47 torr, so that the potential pressure each of the other gases can exert in the lungs is not 760 torr (atmospheric), but 760 minus 47, or 713 torr; thus, the Po_2 of inspired room air is $713 \times 0.209 \approx 150$ torr. In the ideal situation, after oxygen has been removed and CO_2 has been added, alveolar gas is equilibrated with arterial blood, and thus, has a mean PA_{O_2} of 100 torr and PA_{CO_2} of 40 torr. The volume of the tidal breath that enters the alveoli with Po_2 of 150 and Pco_2 of essentially zero torr is small compared to the volume of gas remaining in the chest at end-expiration (FRC); therefore, the fluctuation in alveolar gas tensions during each phase of the respiratory cycle is minimal. The simplified ideal alveolar air equation is the mathematical expression of the concept that the portion of the alveolar pressure (760 torr) which both O_2 and CO_2 can exert is limited to that not exerted by water (47 torr) and nitrogen (574 torr). If one hypoventilates so that Pa_{CO_2} rises, PA_{O_2} must fall, and, if the efficiency of gas exchange reflected by the alveolar-arterial O_2 gradient remains constant, Pa_{O_2} will also decrease (Fig. 3-3). Administering supplemental oxygen (increasing F_{IO_2}) increases the partial pressure that can be composed of oxygen and CO_2; if alveolar ventilation and Pa_{CO_2} remain constant, Pa_{O_2} must increase.

Even in normal individuals, gas exchange is rarely ideal. A small portion (<3 percent) of the arterial blood is returned to the left heart via the thebesian and bronchial veins and is never exposed to alveolar air (true anatomic shunt); a similar fraction is derived from alveolar-capillary units with low ventilation-perfusion ($\dot{V}/\dot{Q}$) ratios and is not fully oxygenated. Together, these comprise the *physiological shunt* that is present in everyone. As a consequence, arterial Po_2 is less than it would be if it were fully equilibrated with alveolar gas. The alveolar-arterial O_2 gradient, which is a sensitive index of the efficiency of gas exchange, is normally less than 10 torr in a 20-year-old. Normal $P(A-a)_{O_2}$ increases with age because of the increase in closing volume and lower $\dot{V}/\dot{Q}$ ratio at the lung bases

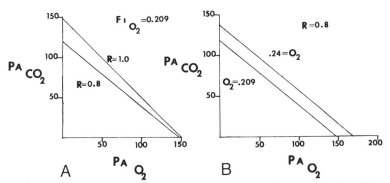

Fig. 3-3. (A) The relationship between PA_{CO_2} and PA_{O_2} when breathing room air at two different respiratory exchange ratios, 0.8 and 1.0, is illustrated. As PA_{CO_2} increases PA_{O_2} falls; the magnitude of the decrease in PA_{O_2} depends on the value of R. (B) The effect of increasing F_{IO_2} on the composition of alveolar gas is shown when R = 0.8. Increasing PA_{CO_2} still decreases PA_{O_2}, but, at any given level of PA_{CO_2}, the PA_{O_2} is greater when F_{IO_2} is increased.

in older people. Normal $P(A\text{-}a)_{O_2}$ may be as much as 20 torr in a 65-year-old individual.[5] In patients with abnormalities in gas exchange, whether from an increase in shunt flow, worsening of $\dot{V}/\dot{Q}$ matching, or diffusion impairment, this difference in oxygen tension between alveolar gas and arterial blood is increased.

Clinically, the alveolar-arterial O_2 gradient is extremely useful as an indicator of the severity of respiratory disease and also in following the response to therapy. If alveolar ventilation changes and Pa_{CO_2} and PA_{CO_2} fall, PA_{O_2} must rise and Pa_{O_2} will increase; determining $P(A\text{-}a)_{O_2}$ may enable us to diagnose an abnormality of gas exchange that is not reflected in Pa_{O_2}. For example, consider a 40-year-old patient with congestive heart failure who presents with these arterial blood gases: pH 7.50, Pa_{O_2} 88, Pa_{CO_2} 24. Despite the fact that the arterial Po_2 is normal, calculating $P(A\text{-}a)_{O_2}$ as

$$150 - \left(\frac{24}{0.8}\right) - 88 = 32 \text{ torr}$$

reveals an alveolar-arterial O_2 gradient that is about twice the normal limit, indicating a significant impairment in gas exchange.

Another patient may present in an obtunded state with these arterial blood gases: pH 7.21, Pa_{O_2} 60, and Pa_{CO_2} 64. Calculation of $P(A\text{-}a)_{O_2}$ in this individual,

$$150 - \left(\frac{64}{0.8}\right) - 60 = 10 \text{ torr}$$

reveals a normal value, indicating there is no impairment in gas exchange from intrinsic pulmonary parenchymal disease. The probable etiology of this patient's hypoventilation is depression of his respiratory drive secondary to his obtundation, as might be seen after an overdose of sedatives.

An increase in the arterial Pco_2 (>45 torr) indicates an inappropriately low level of alveolar ventilation for that patient's metabolic activity. This commonly occurs with severe obstructive lung disease, but may also occur with depression of the central nervous system or neuromuscular disorders that impair the respiratory muscles and reduce the level of alveolar ventilation.[7] An abnormally reduced arterial Pco_2 (<35 torr), indicating alveolar hyperventilation, occurs as the result of an increased respiratory drive and may be seen in a variety of disorders, such as anxiety, fever, acidosis, and infiltrative diseases of the lung, for example, pulmonary fibrosis.[7] The alveolar-arterial O_2 gradient should be calculated in all patients with a decreased Pa_{CO_2} because a significant abnormality in gas exchange may be obscured by a Pa_{O_2} that is in the normal range as a result of hyperventilation.

Etiology of Arterial Hypoxemia

Arterial hypoxemia can occur for five basic reasons (Table 3-1). At high altitudes atmospheric pressure is decreased, so that PA_{O_2} (by the ideal alveolar air equation) must fall. In Denver, where atmospheric pressure is only 690 torr, a

Table 3-1 Arterial Hypoxemia

Etiology	Example	Pa_{CO_2}	$P(A\text{-}a)_{O_2}$	Comment
Low FI_{O_2}	High altitude	$\downarrow$ or nl	nl	Etiology generally apparent
Hypoventilation	CNS depression	$\uparrow$	nl	$P(A\text{-}a)_{O_2}$ may be $\uparrow$ if coexistent lung disease present
$\dot{V}/\dot{Q}$ mismatching	Infiltrative and obstructive lung diseases	$\downarrow$, nl, or $\uparrow$	$\uparrow$	CO_2 retention uncommon unless *severe* obstructive dysfunction when hypoventilation may also be present
Diffusion defect	Interstitial fibrosis	$\downarrow$ or nl	$\uparrow$	Associated $\dot{V}/\dot{Q}$ mismatching is major cause of $\downarrow$ Pa_{O_2}
Right to left	Pulmonary arterio-venous mal-formation	$\downarrow$ or nl	$\uparrow$	$Pa_{O_2} < 600$ while breathing 100% O_2

nl = normal.

Pa_{O_2} of 70 torr is normal in a 20-year-old person. Alveolar hypoventilation will produce hypoxemia as previously discussed, but again, the alveolar-arterial O_2 gradient will be normal if the patient is free of intrinsic lung disease. In patients with an abnormal $P(A\text{-}a)_{O_2}$, hypoxemia may be produced by an increased right-to-left shunt, ventilation-perfusion mismatching, or diffusion impairment.

Ventilation/Perfusion Matching

Most of the arterial hypoxemia associated with an increased alveolar-arterial O_2 gradient encountered clinically is caused by ventilation-perfusion mismatching.[8,9] In a normal adult, alveolar ventilation is about 4 liters/min and pulmonary blood flow (cardiac output) is approximately 5 liters/min, resulting in an overall $\dot{V}/\dot{Q}$ ratio of 0.8. If each individual alveolar-capillary unit had a $\dot{V}/\dot{Q}$ ratio of 0.8, the matching of ventilation and perfusion would be ideal, and, in the absence of a physiological shunt, Pa_{O_2} would equal PA_{O_2}. However, because of the effects of gravity, relatively more blood than air goes to the lung bases, whereas conversely, ventilation of the apexes of the lung is greater than their perfusion.

In the preceding chapter the many factors that could alter the distribution of ventilation were discussed. In a normal individual the principal reason for differences in regional ventilation is the vertical gradient of pleural pressure produced by the effect of gravity on the lungs. Because of the effects of gravity on pulmonary circulation, the regional distribution of perfusion to the alveolar capillaries is also nonuniform. Hydrostatic pressures within the pulmonary vascular system behave like those within a continuous vertical column of fluid

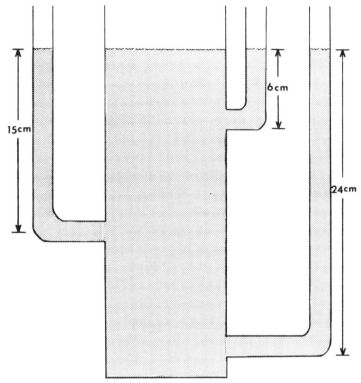

Fig. 3-4. The hydrostatic pressure gradient resulting from gravity. The mean pressure of the liquid indicated by the height of the column in the manometer on the left is 15 cm, but higher or lower pressures are obtained with the manometer at the bottom and top of the liquid, respectively. This occurs because the pressure of the liquid is increased by the weight of the fluid above it.

(Fig. 3-4). Although the mean pressure, measured in the middle of the column, may be 15 mmHg, the hydrostatic pressure at the bottom of the column will be increased by the weight of the fluid above it while the hydrostatic pressure at the top of the tube is less than the mean pressure. Although the mean pulmonary artery pressure (measured with a transducer referenced at the level of the right atrium) may be 15 mmHg, the pressure at the apexes will be less and the pressure at the bases will be greater than this mean value. Similarly, pulmonary venous pressure is greater at the base than the apex because of the influence of gravity. The hydrostatic pressure gradient from apex to base is greatest in the erect position when the distance from the top to the bottom of the lung is greatest.[10] When one assumes the supine position, the vertical distance between the top and bottom of the lung decreases, and consequently, the distribution of perfusion becomes more uniform.

As the hydrostatic pressure within the pulmonary vessels decreases when blood flows to the apexes, the intraluminal pressure distending the pulmonary

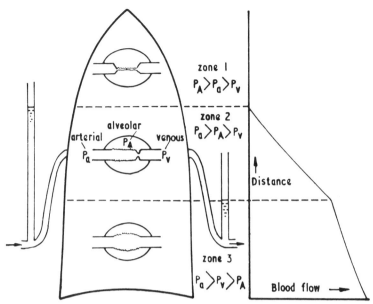

Fig. 3-5. Schematic representation of how arterial (Pa), alveolar (PA), and venous (Pv) pressure determine pulmonary blood flow in the different zones of the lung. See text for details. (Reproduced with permission from West JB, Dollery CT, Naimark A: Distribution of blood flow in isolated lung; relation to vascular and alveolar pressures. J Appl Physiol 19:713, 1964)

vessels also decreases; therefore, regional pulmonary vascular resistance increases at the top of the lung. Although pulmonary artery pressure is usually adequate to maintain some flow to the apexes, if hydrostatic pressure decreases, as with shock, or alveolar pressure increases, as with positive-pressure respiration, once alveolar pressure exceeds that in the pulmonary artery the intraalveolar vessels will be compressed and there will be no flow to this region of the lung.[11]

This region where alveolar pressure exceeds pulmonary artery pressure is commonly referred to as *zone 1* of the lung (Fig. 3-5). Beneath this zone is a region where alveolar pressure is less than pulmonary artery pressure but greater than left atrial pressure, called *zone 2*. The driving pressure for blood flow across this region of the lung is the difference between pulmonary arterial and alveolar pressure. Because hydrostatic pressure progressively increases down this zone, whereas alveolar pressure is the same throughout the lung, the driving pressure and therefore pulmonary blood flow also progressively increase from the top to the bottom of zone 2. Once pulmonary venous pressure exceeds alveolar pressure *(zone 3)*, the driving pressure for pulmonary blood flow through the lung is the difference between pulmonary arterial and left atrial pressure. Although this pressure difference between the pulmonary artery and left atrium remains fixed throughout zone 3, the absolute value of the hydrostatic pressure distending the capillaries increases down zone 3. The increased distention of the capillaries reduces the regional pulmonary vascular resistance; therefore, flow also increases progressively toward the bottom of this lung zone.

To understand the effect of variations in $\dot{V}/\dot{Q}$ on arterial blood gases, it is useful first to consider the extreme case of a $\dot{V}/\dot{Q}$ ratio of zero, for example, a totally unventilated but perfused alveolus. Blood coming from the capillary of this alveolus is mixed venous blood, that is, shunt, and because there is no ventilation to the alveolus, the gas within it will be equilibrated with mixed venous blood and have a $P_{A_{O_2}} = 40$ and $P_{A_{CO_2}} = 46$. If there is a small amount of ventilation relative to perfusion ($\dot{V}/\dot{Q} = 0.01$), $P_{A_{O_2}}$ will rise minimally while $P_{A_{CO_2}}$ falls only slightly with each tidal breath and there will be only a minimal change in the gas tensions of the capillary blood from this hypothetical alveolar unit.

The opposite extreme is the alveolus, which is ventilated but not perfused ($\dot{V}/\dot{Q} = \infty$), that is, alveolar dead space. The $P_{A_{O_2}}$ and $P_{A_{CO_2}}$ of this alveolus are 150 and 0, respectively, and any blood present in the pulmonary capillary of this unit will eventually equilibrate with the alveolar gas and have a $Pa_{O_2} = 150$ and $Pa_{CO_2} = 0$. If a small amount of perfusion is restored ($\dot{V}/\dot{Q} = 100$), then the amount of oxygen removed and the volume of carbon dioxide added to the alveolar air are small and alveolar gas tensions change minimally, so that the Pa_{O_2} and Pa_{CO_2} of the small amount of blood that passes through this unit will still be close to that of inspired air.

The effect of an abnormal distribution of $\dot{V}/\dot{Q}$ ratios on the P_{O_2} and P_{CO_2} of expired air and arterial blood is illustrated by a hypothetical lung with three alveolar-capillary units characterized by low ($1:10$), intermediate ($10:10$), and high ($10:1$) $\dot{V}/\dot{Q}$ ratios (Fig. 3-6). Expired gas collected in a Douglas bag will contain a total of 21 units of alveolar air; the 1 unit of gas from the low $\dot{V}/\dot{Q}$ alveolus will have a low $P_{A_{O_2}}$ and high $P_{A_{CO_2}}$, 10 units from the intermediate $\dot{V}/\dot{Q}$ alveolus will have normal gas tensions, whereas the 10 units from the high $\dot{V}/\dot{Q}$ alveolus will have an increased $P_{A_{O_2}}$ and low $P_{A_{CO_2}}$, reflecting the wasted ventilation. Arterial blood, on the other hand, will receive 10 of the 21 units of

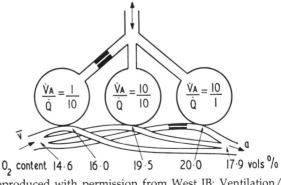

Fig. 3-6. Mismatching of ventilation and perfusion will produce arterial hypoxemia because the large volume of poorly oxygenated blood from the alveolus on the left ($\dot{V}/\dot{Q} = 1/10$) is not compensated by the small amount of well-oxygenated blood derived from the alveolus on the right ($\dot{V}/\dot{Q} = 10/1$). The P_{CO_2} of expired air falls because alveolar gas from the alveolus on the right contains very little CO_2. See text for details. (Reproduced with permission from West JB: Ventilation/Blood Flow and Gas Exchange. Blackwell, Oxford, 1970)

flow from the capillary with the low $\dot{V}/\dot{Q}$ ratio; blood from this alveolar-capillary unit will have a low oxygen content, producing arterial hypoxemia and increasing the alveolar-arterial O_2 gradient.

Diffusion

The movement of oxygen in alveolar gas across the alveolar-capillary membrane into the blood and the exchange of carbon dioxide in the reverse direction occur by diffusion. The rate at which a gas diffuses between a gas phase and a liquid phase, that is, between alveolar gas and capillary blood, is proportional to its solubility in the liquid.[12] Carbon dioxide is so much more soluble than O_2 that its transfer, even in severe lung disease, is relatively unaffected by an impairment in pulmonary gas diffusion. The *diffusing capacity* of the lung (DL) is defined as the volume of gas that enters the blood per minute per torr partial pressure difference of the gas between alveolar air and pulmonary capillary blood. Although it is the diffusion of oxygen into pulmonary capillary blood that is of clinical importance, carbon monoxide is used in the pulmonary function laboratory to determine the diffusing capacity of the lung (DL_{CO}) because it is easy to measure and its diffusing characteristics are similar to those of oxygen.

Two general techniques are commonly used to measure DL_{CO}. In the *single-breath* test, a single full breath of a gas containing a low concentration of CO and 10 percent helium is held for 10 sec, then exhaled completely. The inspired and expired concentrations of CO and helium are measured, alveolar volume determined from the helium tracer, and the rate of CO uptake calculated. In the *steady-state* method, a very low CO mixture is breathed until the rate of CO uptake from the lungs is constant. Although the single-breath test is simpler, breathholding is an artificial condition that is difficult for some patients who are short of breath. The steady-state method can also be used during exercise when breathholding is not feasible.

The effective barriers that the oxygen (or carbon monoxide) in alveolar gas must cross to combine with the hemoglobin in pulmonary capillary blood include the surface lining layer of the alveoli, alveolar epithelium, interstitium, pulmonary capillary endothelium, plasma, and red cell membrane. Normally, red blood cells spend 0.75 sec in the pulmonary capillary, which is an adequate period of time for oxygen to diffuse down its concentration gradient from the alveolus to the red blood cells and combine with hemoglobin (Fig. 3-7). Even when cardiac output is increased during heavy exercise so that the amount of time each red blood cell spends in the pulmonary capillary decreases to 0.25 sec, there is still sufficient time for complete equilibration in the healthy individual. In patients with a severe diffusional impairment, the normal red cell transit time through the pulmonary capillary (0.75 sec) is too rapid for O_2 to equilibrate between alveolar gas and capillary blood; thus, there will be a significant alveolar-pulmonary capillary O_2 gradient because of diffusion at rest. Patients with mild diffusion

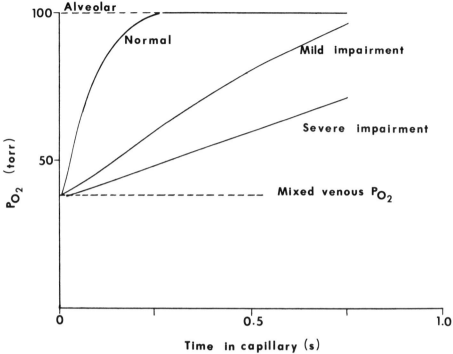

Fig. 3-7. Time course of oxygen transfer by diffusion into pulmonary capillary blood. In the normal individual oxygenation is complete within 0.25 sec, so the 0.75 sec the red blood cell spends in the pulmonary capillary represents a significant time reserve. Severe diffusion impairment will produce hypoxemia at rest, whereas a mild impairment may not be evident unless the transit time of the RBC through the capillary is decreased, e.g., when cardiac output increases during exercise.

defects may have sufficient time to oxygenate fully their pulmonary capillary blood at rest, but undergo profound desaturation during exercise when the transit time of the red blood cell through the pulmonary capillary is shortened.

The diffusing capacity of the lung is determined not only by the physical characteristics of the alveolar capillary membrane, that is, its surface area and thickness, but also by the rate at which the gas (oxygen or carbon monoxide) combines with hemoglobin. The rate at which O_2 and CO combine with the hemoglobin in pulmonary capillary blood is proportional to the speed at which the reaction occurs in 1 ml of blood (θ, milliliters of gas per minute per torr of pressure difference per milliliter of blood) and the total volume of blood in the pulmonary capillaries (Vc). Gas must diffuse from alveolar air to the inside of the red cell before it can combine with hemoglobin. Therefore, the D_L we measure in the pulmonary function laboratory is determined by the diffusion capacity of the alveolar capillary membrane (D_M) and the rate at which gas combines with hemoglobin, $\theta(Vc)$. Because the diffusing capacity is the flow of gas per unit pressure difference, the inverse, $1/D_L$, represents the resistance to gas transfer by diffusion that may be expressed as the sum of two resistances in series,

$$\frac{1}{D_L} = \frac{1}{D_M} + \frac{1}{\theta(V_C)} \qquad \text{(Eq. 3-10)}$$

In a normal individual, D_M and $\theta(V_C)$ contribute equally to D_L, so that disorders that decrease surface area or increase thickness of the alveolar capillary membrane, as well as those that reduce pulmonary capillary blood volume, will affect the diffusion capacity of the lung.

In essence, then, diffusing capacity is determined by the number of functioning alveoli in contact with red blood cells.[13] If the number of functioning alveolar-capillary units is reduced by pneumonectomy, $D_{L_{CO}}$ will be proportionately reduced. Yet, when the diffusing capacity per liter alveolar volume is calculated (D_L/V_A), it will be normal, indicating the remaining alveolar-capillary units are normal. Similarly, if the hemoglobin concentration of pulmonary capillary blood is reduced because of anemia, $D_{L_{CO}}$ will be reduced even though the alveolar-capillary membrane is normal. In diseases that destroy the alveolar septa, for example, emphysema, and those that obliterate the pulmonary capillary bed, such as pulmonary emboli, D_L/V_A is markedly reduced. While increased thickness of the alveolar-capillary membrane can theoretically increase the barrier to diffusion, most of the decreased $D_{L_{CO}}$ observed in pulmonary fibrosis is caused by loss of alveolar volume and fibrotic obliteration of the pulmonary capillary bed.

Disorders that expand the volume of blood in the pulmonary capillaries may actually increase $D_{L_{CO}}$. Early congestive heart failure is probably the most common cause of increased $D_{L_{CO}}$ encountered clinically.

Diffusion impairment is rarely the sole cause of hypoxemia. Although a decreased diffusing capacity is common in many of the diffuse infiltrative diseases of the lung, for example, pulmonary fibrosis, it is now recognized that the hypoxemia of the "alveolar-capillary block" syndromes is mainly a result of $\dot{V}/\dot{Q}$ mismatching rather than diffusion impairment.

Shunt Flow

There are two forms of shunt that reduce the oxygenation of arterial blood. The first is the normal anatomic shunt, caused by the shunting of blood from the thebesian and bronchial veins, which have no contact with alveoli. The second is the effective or relative shunt, caused by the flow of blood through areas that have a low $\dot{V}/\dot{Q}$ ratio. The combination of these two shunts is termed the physiological shunt or total venous admixture. The amount of oxygen delivered to the peripheral tissue is the product of the arterial oxygen content and the cardiac output. Total systemic blood flow may be thought of as being the sum of two components, the blood that flows through the lungs and is fully oxygenated with a P_{O_2} equal to that of alveolar gas, and that which is not exposed to alveolar gas and therefore has an oxygen content equal to that of mixed venous blood. In symbols,

$$Ca_{O_2}(\dot{Q}T) = Cc'_{O_2}(\dot{Q}c) + C\bar{v}_{O_2}(\dot{Q}s) \qquad \text{(Eq. 3-11)}$$

where $\dot{Q}c$ is ideal pulmonary blood flow, $\dot{Q}s$ is shunt flow, $\dot{Q}T$ is total cardiac output, and Cc'_{O_2}, Ca_{O_2}, and $C\bar{v}_{O_2}$ are the oxygen content of end-pulmonary capillary blood, arterial blood, and mixed venous blood, respectively. End-pulmonary capillary P_{O_2} is assumed equal to alveolar P_{O_2}, whereas mixed venous P_{O_2} can either be measured or an arterial-mixed venous content difference of 5 ml/dl is assumed (if the cardiac output is normal). Since

$$\dot{Q}c = \dot{Q}T - \dot{Q}s \qquad \text{(Eq. 3-12)}$$

the venous admixture at any given inspired oxygen concentration can be calculated from the shunt formula:

$$\frac{\dot{Q}s}{\dot{Q}T} = \frac{Cc'_{O_2} - Ca_{O_2}}{Cc'_{O_2} - C\bar{v}_{O_2}} \qquad \text{(Eq. 3-13)}$$

To understand the effect of an increased venous admixture on arterial blood gases, it is important to remember the different shapes of the O_2 and CO_2 dissociation curves in blood (Fig. 3-8). The relatively linear relationship between P_{CO_2} and CO_2 content in blood means that the content and P_{CO_2} of arterial blood is essentially the algebraic sum of the content and P_{CO_2} of pulmonary capillary and shunt blood; even if the venous admixture were to increase drastically, a modest increment in alveolar ventilation would maintain a normal Pa_{CO_2}. The sigmoid shape of the hemoglobin dissociation curve, however, means there is

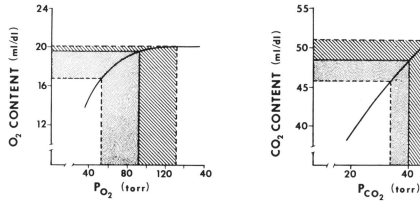

Fig. 3-8. Relationship between the partial pressure and content of O_2 (left) and CO_2 (right) in blood over the range of partial pressures encountered clinically. Regional hypoventilation produces a fall in O_2 content and an increase in CO_2 content; hyperventilation in another region of the lung can compensate for the change in CO_2 content, but the small increase in O_2 content produced by hyperventilation will not correct the decrease resulting from hypoventilation.

little increase in the oxygen content of pulmonary capillary blood with hyperventilation because hemoglobin is almost completely saturated at a Pa_{O_2} of 100 torr. Therefore, the Pa_{O_2} of arterial blood must fall as the shunt fraction increases.

The venous admixture measured while breathing room air includes the effect of $\dot{V}/\dot{Q}$ mismatching and diffusion impairment as well as that of true right-to-left shunts. When the hypoxemic patient inspires 100 percent oxygen for 20 min, thereby replacing nitrogen with oxygen and increasing PA_{O_2} in poorly ventilated lung units, hypoxemia from $\dot{V}/\dot{Q}$ mismatching or diffusion impairment will be relieved. Hypoxemia from a true right-to-left shunt, for example an arteriovenous malformation, will persist. Normally, the true shunt is about 3 percent of cardiac output.[6] A reasonable approximation of the true shunt fraction can be obtained from Pa_{O_2} measured after 20 min of oxygen breathing, using the formula

$$\% \text{ shunt} = (700 - Pa_{O_2})\frac{5}{100} \qquad \text{(Eq. 3-14)}$$

This estimation is relatively accurate for Pa_{O_2}'s greater than 100 torr while breathing 100 percent oxygen, assuming the patient's cardiac output is normal.

Approach to the Patient with Hypoxemia

Arterial hypoxemia can result from the five basic causes discussed (see Table 3-1). At high altitudes atmospheric pressure is decreased so that PA_{O_2} (by the ideal alveolar gas equation) must fall. Alveolar hypoventilation will produce hypoxemia but will not increase $P(A-a)_{O_2}$ in the patient free of lung disease. In patients with an abnormal alveolar-arterial O_2 gradient, hypoxemia may be the result of increased right-to-left shunt, $\dot{V}/\dot{Q}$ mismatching, or diffusion impairment. Having the patient inspire 100 percent oxygen for 20 min will correct the latter two causes of hypoxemia by replacing nitrogen with oxygen, thereby increasing PA_{O_2} in even poorly ventilated lung units; whereas, hypoxemia caused by a true right-to-left shunt will persist.

REFERENCES

1. Fowler WS: The respiratory dead space. Physiol Rev 35:860; Am J Physiol 154:405, 1948
2. Severinghaus JW, Stupfel M: Alveolar dead space as an index of distribution of blood flow in pulmonary capillaries. J Appl Physiol 10:335, 1957
3. Asmussen E, Nielsen M: Physiological dead space and alveolar gas pressures at rest and during muscular exercise. Acta Physiol Scand 38:1, 1956
4. Jones NL, McHardy GJR, Naimark A, Campbell EJM: Physiological dead space and alveolar-arterial gas pressure differences during exercise. Clin Sci 31:19, 1966
5. Mellemgaard K: Alveolar-arterial oxygen difference: Size and components in normal man. Acta Physiol Scand 67:10, 1966

6. Riley RL, Cournand A: "Ideal" alveolar air and the analysis of ventilation perfusion relationships in the lungs. J Appl Physiol 1:825, 1949
7. Kinasewitz GT: Regulation of ventilation. p. 103. In George RB, Light RW, Matthay RA (eds): Chest Medicine. Churchill Livingstone, New York, 1983
8. Wagner PD, Dantzker DR, Dueck R, et al: Ventilation-perfusion inequality in chronic obstructive pulmonary disease. J Clin Invest 59:203, 1977
9. Wagner PD: Ventilation-perfusion relationships. Ann Rev Physiol 42:235, 1980
10. Anthonisen NR, Milic-Emili J: Distribution of pulmonary perfusion in erect man. J Appl Physiol 21:760, 1966
11. West JB, Dollery CT, Naimark A: Distribution of blood flow in isolated lung; relation to vascular and alveolar pressures. J Appl Physiol 19:713, 1964
12. Forster RE: Exchange of gases between alveolar air and pulmonary capillary blood: Pulmonary diffusing capacity. Physiol Rev 37:391, 1957
13. Weinberger SE, Johnson TS, Weiss ST: Use and interpretation of the single-breath diffusing capacity. Chest 78:483, 1980

4

Gas Transport

Gary T. Kinasewitz, M.D.

Once the oxygen necessary for aerobic metabolism enters the blood in the pulmonary capillary, it is delivered by the arterial blood to the peripheral tissues where it is utilized. The amount of oxygen potentially available for aerobic metabolism is determined by both the O_2 content of arterial blood and the total peripheral blood flow each minute (cardiac output). If it were not for the remarkable ability of hemoglobin to bind oxygen and thereby increase the oxygen content of blood, the normal cardiac output of 5 liters/min would have to increase to more than 80 liters/min to maintain adequate oxygen delivery. Although some carbon dioxide also binds to hemoglobin and plasma proteins, most CO_2 in the blood is carried as bicarbonate. Only a small fraction of the CO_2 transported to the lungs each minute is carried in the plasma as dissolved CO_2.

OXYGEN TRANSPORT

The amount of oxygen dissolved in plasma at a Po_2 of 100 torr is 0.3 ml/dl, whereas the oxygen content of arterial blood at this Po_2 is 20 ml/dl, a 60-fold increase. The relationship between arterial Po_2 and the amount of oxygen dissolved in arterial plasma is linear; 0.0031 ml of oxygen is dissolved per torr of Po_2. In contrast, the relationship between arterial Po_2 and the total amount of oxygen in the blood is curvilinear (Fig. 4-1). The sigmoidal shape of the *oxyhemoglobin dissociation curve* is a result of the interaction between the four chains of the hemoglobin molecule, so that the uptake of oxygen by one of the heme groups facilitates further uptake by the other heme groups.[1] The maximal amount of oxygen that can be bound to 1 g of hemoglobin if all four heme groups are occupied by O_2 is 1.34 ml. The actual amount bound in relation to this maximal capacity is referred to as the percent saturation of hemoglobin (Sa_{O_2}), which can be determined as

$$Sa_{O_2} = \frac{\text{Amount } O_2 \text{ bound}}{[Hb](1.34)} \times 100 \qquad \text{(Eq. 4-1)}$$

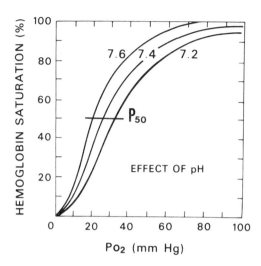

Fig. 4-1. The O_2 dissociation curve of blood. The effect of a change in pH on the position of the curve and the P_{50} of blood are shown. A doubling or halving of the normal 2,3-DPG concentration within the red blood cells would produce the same shift illustrated for pH = 7.2 and pH = 7.6, respectively.

where [Hb] is the concentration of hemoglobin in blood. It can be seen in Figure 4-1 that at normal arterial P_{O_2} arterial blood is approximately 98 percent saturated, whereas mixed venous blood with a P_{O_2} of 40 torr is about 75 percent saturated.

If we arbitrarily divide the oxyhemoglobin dissociation curve into an "association" curve, the upper flat portion of Figure 4-1, and a "dissociation" curve, the steep middle portion, it is easy to understand the physiological advantages of the sigmoidal shape of the curve. Even if the P_{O_2} of arterial blood falls because of lung disease, the association portion of the curve ensures that the saturation of arterial blood, and therefore its oxygen content, is well maintained. At a Pa_{O_2} of 60 torr hemoglobin is still 90 percent saturated. In contrast, the dissociation portion of the curve facilitates the unloading of oxygen in the peripheral capillaries where P_{O_2} approximates that of venous blood, that is, 40 torr.

The unloading of oxygen from hemoglobin is facilitated by the decrease in pH and addition of CO_2 which occur when the blood reaches the tissue capillaries, the *Bohr effect*.[2] An increase in the hydrogen ion concentration of the blood shifts the dissociation portion of the oxyhemoglobin curve to the right more than it changes the flat association portion of the curve, so that peripheral unloading of oxygen is enhanced even though the oxygen content of arterial blood is relatively constant. In addition to decreasing the pH of capillary blood, some of the CO_2 taken up in the peripheral capillary binds directly to hemoglobin and thus increases the release of O_2 from the hemoglobin molecule. When the blood returns to the lung, the excretion of CO_2 and increase in blood pH shifts the oxyhemoglobin dissociation curve back to the left and enhances O_2 uptake in the pulmonary capillary.

The binding of oxygen with hemoglobin is also affected by the concentration of 2,3-diphosphoglycerate (2,3-DPG) within the red blood cells.[3] Increased concentrations of this organic phosphate shift the oxyhemoglobin dissociation curve to the right, the same direction as does a decrease in pH. This rightward shift of the oxyhemoglobin dissociation curve occurs because the negatively charged 2,3-DPG molecule reduces the intracellular pH of the erythrocyte and binds to deoxyhemoglobin, thereby tending to maintain its reduced configuration. An increase in 2,3-DPG is an important compensatory mechanism to maintain adequate tissue oxygenation in the anemic patient whose arterial oxygen content is reduced because of a decrease in hemoglobin concentration.

The affinity of the hemoglobin molecule for oxygen can be determined by equilibrating blood with gas containing CO_2 and varying concentrations of oxygen and measuring hemoglobin saturation so an oxyhemoglobin dissociation curve can be constructed. More commonly, the pH, Po_2, and saturation of a sample of venous blood are measured and the Po_2 at which the blood would be 50 percent saturated (P_{50}) is calculated.[4] Normal P_{50} is about 26 torr. An increase in P_{50} indicates that the curve is shifted to the right, whereas a decrease indicates a leftward shift and an increased hemoglobin affinity.

CARBON DIOXIDE TRANSPORT

The solubility of carbon dioxide in plasma is greater than that of oxygen, but nonetheless more than 95 percent of CO_2 transported in the blood is carried as bicarbonate or bound to proteins, particularly hemoglobin. Most CO_2 in the blood is in the form of bicarbonate. The CO_2 that is dissolved in the plasma is converted into bicarbonate in the following sequence of reactions.

$$CO_2 + H_2O \overset{CA}{\rightleftharpoons} H_2CO_3 \rightleftharpoons HCO_3^- + H^+ \qquad \text{(Eq. 4-2)}$$

The initial reaction, the hydration of CO_2 into carbonic acid is extremely slow in plasma, but within the red cell it is accelerated by the presence of the enzyme carbonic anhydrase (CA). The second reaction, the ionic dissociation of carbonic acid, is rapid and the hydrogen ion that is generated binds to basic groups on the hemoglobin molecule while the bicarbonate diffuses down its concentration gradient out of the red blood cell and into the plasma. (In order to maintain electrical neutrality within the red blood cell, the outward movement of bicarbonate is accompanied by an inward flux of chloride ions, the *chloride shift*.) In addition to the CO_2 that is transported as bicarbonate in the blood, a small quantity of CO_2 is reversibly bound to the amino groups of hemoglobin to form carbamino compounds.

Deoxyhemoglobin is a weaker acid than oxyhemoglobin; therefore, more CO_2 can be carried in venous blood at any given Pco_2, the *Haldane effect*.[5] This occurs because the binding of the hydrogen ions liberated in the generation of bicarbonate and the binding of CO_2 to form carbamino groups is greater when hemoglobin is in its reduced or deoxygenated form. Thus, when oxygen is unloaded at the peripheral capillary the uptake of CO_2 is facilitated, while in the pulmonary capillary the reverse occurs.

The relationship between the amount of CO_2 in the blood and Pco_2 is the

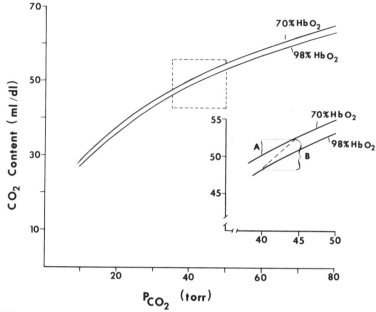

Fig. 4-2. The CO_2 dissociation curves of blood at two different levels of hemoglobin saturation. The magnified insert illustrates how the unloading of CO_2 in the lung that occurs because of the decrease in P_{CO_2} (bracket A) is enhanced by the concomitant oxygenation of the blood (bracket B), the Haldane effect.

dissociation curve for CO_2 (Fig. 4-2). Because the slope of the curve is quite steep, a CO_2 tension change of less than 10 torr will produce a difference in CO_2 content of 4 ml/dl, the normal arteriovenous difference. In contrast to the oxyhemoglobin dissociation curve, the CO_2 curve is almost linear over the range of P_{CO_2}'s encountered clinically; therefore, inadequate CO_2 elimination in some alveolar-capillary units because of unfavorable $\dot{V}/\dot{Q}$ ratios can be compensated for by increasing ventilation to units with normal $\dot{V}/\dot{Q}$ ratios.

The *CO_2 content* determined in the clinical laboratory measures CO_2 in blood in all its forms (as bicarbonate, dissolved, and in carbamino groups). Serum bicarbonate levels cannot be measured directly, but they can be calculated from the pH and P_{CO_2} of the blood.

SYSTEMIC GAS TRANSPORT

Systemic gas transport, that is, the delivery of oxygen to the peripheral tissue and the return of carbon dioxide to the lung, is dependent not only on the content of these gases in arterial and venous blood, but also on the cardiac output (C.O.). The delivery of oxygen to peripheral tissues can be calculated as

$$O_2 \text{ transport} = C.O.(Ca_{O_2}) \qquad \text{(Eq. 4-3)}$$

where Ca_{O_2} is the oxygen content of arterial blood. Ca_{O_2} is determined by both Pa_{O_2} and the hemoglobin concentration of the blood, that is,

$$Ca_{O_2} = 0.0031(Pa_{O_2}) + 1.34[Hb](Sa_{O_2}) \qquad \text{(Eq. 4-4)}$$

where Sa_{O_2} is the saturation, [Hb] is the hemoglobin concentration of arterial blood, and 0.0031 is the solubility constant or volume of oxygen dissolved per torr Pa_{O_2}. Because the amount of oxygen dissolved in plasma at a normal Pa_{O_2} is small compared with the quantity bound to hemoglobin, Equations 4-3 and 4-4 may be combined and simplified as

$$O_2 \text{ transport} = \text{C.O.} \times 1.34[Hb](Sa_{O_2}) \qquad \text{(Eq. 4-5)}$$

It is obvious from this relationship that O_2 transport is dependent on the integrated function of the cardiac (C.O.), respiratory (Sa_{O_2}), and erythropoietic systems ([Hb]) to maintain adequate delivery.

The oxygen consumption of a normal individual at rest is approximately 250 ml/min and his cardiac output is roughly 5 liters/min, so to meet the metabolic demand for oxygen, 50 ml of oxygen is extracted from each liter of blood every minute. Thus, the normal arteriovenous O_2 content difference is 5 ml/dl. Oxygen consumption then is the product of cardiac output and O_2 extraction, which may be written as

$$\dot{V}_{O_2} = \text{C.O.}[C(a-\bar{v})_{O_2}] \qquad \text{(Eq. 4-6)}$$

where $C(a-\bar{v})_{O_2}$ is the difference in oxygen content between arterial and mixed venous blood. This relationship, termed the *Fick principle,* is commonly employed to determine cardiac output. If oxygen consumption is calculated from a sample of expired gas and the oxygen content of arterial and mixed venous blood are determined, then cardiac output may be calculated as

$$\text{C.O.} = \frac{\dot{V}_{O_2}}{C(a-\bar{v})_{O_2}} \qquad \text{(Eq. 4-7)}$$

To obtain a sample of mixed venous blood it is necessary to pass a catheter via a peripheral vein into the pulmonary artery. Alternative methods of measuring cardiac output employ the indicator dilution technique. If an indicator substance is injected in a central vein proximal to the right ventricle and its concentration in the blood downstream from this large mixing chamber measured, cardiac output can be calculated. Indocyanine green dye is an indicator substance whose concentration in arterial blood can be determined with a densitometer. The development of balloon-tipped, flow-directed catheters with thermistors at the distal end has simplified the measurement of cardiac output. Cold saline or glucose solution is injected via the proximal port of the catheter into the vena cava; the change in blood temperature produced by this indicator is measured by a thermistor that is situated at the distal end of the catheter in the pulmonary artery. In addition to determining cardiac output, measurements of pulmonary artery pressure and pulmonary wedge pressure (a reflection of left atrial pressure) can be obtained with this catheter. Bedside monitoring of cardiac output is discussed further in Chapter 13.

Because the oxygen content of arterial blood with a Pa_{O_2} of 100 torr is 20 ml/dl and the normal ateriovenous O_2 difference is 5 ml/dl, only 25 percent of Ca_{O_2} is extracted by the peripheral tissues and there is a significant reserve of oxygen should the metabolic demands of these tissues increase. There is also a significant cardiac reserve in the normal individual and cardiac output may increase four- to fivefold to deliver sufficient oxygen to meet the body's needs. Acute increases in O_2 demand, for example, exercise or fever, are satisfied by an increase in both cardiac output and oxygen extraction.[6] The trained individual may utilize 4,000 ml oxygen per minute during maximal exercise, as 80 percent of the oxygen in arterial blood is extracted and his cardiac output reaches 25 liters/min.

Failure of the oxygen transport system can result from a deficiency in any of its three components. Even when Pa_{O_2}, hemoglobin concentration, and cardiac output are normal at rest, there may be an insufficient reserve to provide adequate O_2 delivery during periods of stress. The use of exercise testing to examine the integrated performance of the oxygen transport system and identify failure of the circulatory or respiratory components is discussed in Chapter 12.

REFERENCES

1. Bunn HE, Forget BG, Ranney HM: Human Hemoglobins. WB Saunders, Philadelphia, 1977
2. Hlastala MP, Woodson RD: Saturation dependency of the Bohr effect interactions among H^+, CO_2, and DPG. J Appl Physiol 38:1126, 1975
3. Klocke RA: Oxygen transport and 2,3-diphosphoglycerate (DPG). Chest 62, suppl. 2, 79, 1972
4. Lichtman MA, Murphy MS, Adamson JW: Detection of mutant hemoglobins with altered affinity to oxygen. Ann Int Med 84:517, 1976
5. Klocke RA: Mechanism and kinetics of the Haldane effect in human erythrocytes. J Appl Physiol 35:673, 1973
6. Thomas TM, Lefrak SS, Irwin RS, et al: The oxyhemoglobin dissociation curve in health and disease. Am J Med 57:331, 1974

Section II
TECHNIQUES OF ASSESSMENT

5

Pulmonary Function Testing Equipment

Steven A. Conrad, M.D.

The modern pulmonary function laboratory contains a multitude of instruments for assessing lung function. These include spirometers, flowmeters, gas analyzers, pressure transducers, plethysmographs, and often, computer systems. Although the cost of a large clinical or research laboratory can be considerable, a significant amount of information on pulmonary function can be obtained with the simple and relatively inexpensive spirometry equipment available in the community hospital. Recent advances in electronics and materials have reduced the size and cost of equipment while allowing increased automation of testing. Chemical methods of gas analysis have been largely supplanted by easier and more rapid physical methods, and the improved accuracy of modern instrumentation has increased reliability in test interpretation.

This chapter discusses the basic construction and operation of the instruments in use today. Little reference will be made to particular brands and individual characteristics, as such information is available from manufacturers. The emphasis instead will be on principles of operation.

VOLUME DISPLACEMENT SPIROMETRY

The principal function of a spirometer is the measurement of change in lung volume. Through measurement of lung volume change, the division of total lung volume into its component volume compartments is possible and assessment of dynamic lung function can be performed. Measurement of volume change is also necessary for the performance of other tests, such as gas distribution. Spirometers measure changes in lung volume by recording changes in volume of air exchanged through the airway opening. Because residual volume cannot be exhaled, spirometric measurements are limited to subdivisions of the vital capacity. Residual volume, or absolute lung volumes incorporating the residual volume, require additional methods.

Spirometers are of two basic types, *volume displacement* and *electronic integrating* spirometers. The latter incorporate pneumotachometers with special electronics and are discussed separately in the next section. Volume displacement spirometers are based on the concept of an expandable chamber into which the subject breathes. The chamber is designed to indicate changes accurately in its volume through changes in its dimensions.

Chamber design accounts for the differences among types of volume displacement spirometers. In general, however, the chamber must be sealed from the atmosphere, register its change in volume accurately, and provide little resistance to airflow. Spirometers for the measurement of a single exhalation have only a single connection with the chamber. If rebreathing studies are required, then separate intake and exhaust ports with a valve system for unidirectional flow help to minimize the dead space of the breathing circuit.

Several problems are associated with the use of volume displacement spirometers. When recording volume changes over a period of time during rebreathing, carbon dioxide can accumulate in the system and affect the respiratory pattern. To avoid this, CO_2 absorbers are used to remove exhaled CO_2. Because O_2 is consumed, the volume of the system will decrease over time during prolonged rebreathing studies. The spirometer is usually at room temperature and the change in exhaled air from body to ambient temperature is associated with a decrease in volume. This volume loss is predictable, however, and measurement of the temperature change allows one to correct for this volume loss. A spirometer chamber has inertia and the breathing circuit has a resistance, both of which can be significant; these can affect the accuracy of dynamic volume measurements. However, this is not a problem with static volume measurements.

Water-Seal Spirometers

A common approach to the construction of volume displacement spirometers is to use water as the seal between a movable cylindrical chamber and its base. The distance moved by the cylinder is proportional to the change in volume inside. To register the cylinder's displacement, and therefore the volume change, a pen connected by a mechanical linkage to the top of the bell records a graph on graduated paper. The graduated paper is rotated by a kymograph at a known speed, permitting volume to be recorded on one axis of the graph and time on the other.

Two principal designs are in use today. The counterweighted bell spirometer (most commonly the Collin's design)[1] has a metal bell inverted into its water seal over the base, as shown in Figure 5-1A. A pulley-counterweight mechanical system is used to balance the weight of the bell. The original designs had either a 9- or 13.5-liter reservoir capacity. Recent versions have capacities ranging from 7

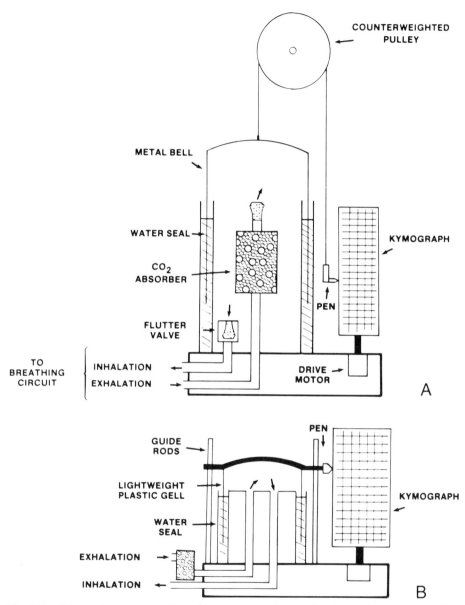

Fig. 5-1. Schematic representation of two common types of water-seal spirometers. (A) The metal bell spirometer uses an inverted, counterbalanced bell attached by a chain linkage to a kymograph recorder pen. A CO_2 absorber prevents accumulation of the gas, and flutter valves remove the dead space effect during rebreathing studies. (B) The Stead-Wells design has a lightweight plastic bell with a direct recording pen. No counterbalance is required. The design is similar in other respects to the metal bell spirometer.

to 14 liters, some of which have interchangeable bells for versatility in a single spirometer. A separate inhalation/exhalation breathing circuit with flutter valves and CO_2 canister permits rebreathing studies. One pen records volume change on moving graduated paper, while a second pen is geared to record the cumulative exhaled volume. The cumulative volume is used to calculate resting minute ventilation and maximal voluntary ventilation.

The Stead-Wells water-seal spirometer[2] has been developed more recently (Fig. 5-1B). It uses a lightweight plastic bell to circumvent the counterweight balancing system and a direct recording pen linkage in place of the pulley linkage. These design changes result in decreased inertia and improved response to rapid breathing.[3,4]

Water-seal spirometers are usually less expensive than other types, and require little maintenance or calibration. In spite of their mechanical simplicity, they generally have sufficient accuracy for use in clinical laboratories and are often considered the standard against which other spirometers are compared. They are difficult to move about because of the water bath, and therefore are unsuitable for bedside or portable use. Although measurements of lung volume with water-seal spirometers are accurate to approximately 25 ml, the inertia of the mechanical linkage has been shown to affect the measurement of flow and volume during rapid breathing; however, the Stead-Wells design has minimized this problem.

Dry Rolling-Seal Spirometers

Replacement of the water seal with a dry, flexible seal has resulted in lightweight, low inertia spirometers that require little maintenance. A piston is placed in a cylindrical chamber and sealed at its periphery by the dry seal, as shown in Figure 5-2. The seal used to close the system is a material positioned to roll back on itself. The material is airtight, chemically inert, and flexible. The assembly is usually suspended horizontally. The piston is made of a lightweight substance, such as aluminum. Displacement of the piston is recorded by an electronic potentiometer circuit that produces a voltage proportional to the volume in the spirometer. The voltage signal is electronically processed to calculate rate of volume change, or flow. This information is not available from the mechanical linkage used in the water-seal spirometers without modification of the linkage, but must be calculated from the volume tracings.

Dry rolling-seal spirometers are becoming increasingly popular. However, they are not portable, and their use is restricted to the clinical laboratory. They require little maintenance other than calibration of the electronic circuitry.

Bellows Spirometers

An expandable bellows is used as the basis of several volume displacement spirometers. Although they are less accurate than the water- and dry rolling-seal

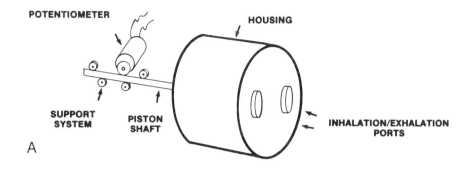

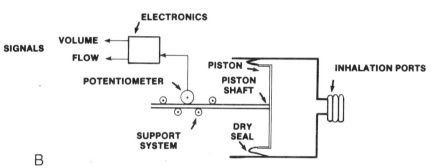

Fig. 5-2. Schematic of a dry rolling-seal spirometer. The lightweight piston is suspended horizontally on a low-friction suspension system. The spirometer chamber is sealed by a flexible rolling seal attached to the piston. The potentiometer provides an electrical signal proportional to volume, which can be further processed to provide flow.

types described previously, their design makes them suitable for portable or bedside spirometry. Common configurations are the wedge and box designs (Fig. 5-3). The expansion of the bellows chamber results in movement of one edge of the bellows through a distance proportional to the volume change of the spirometer chamber. An arm attached to the bellows records directly on paper. Alternatively, the paper moves against a pen. A motor drives the paper or pen along one axis at constant speed in order that timed volume recordings may be made.

PNEUMOTACHOMETRY

Pneumotachometers are instruments that generate an electrical signal in response to the instantaneous flow of respiratory gases. This signal may be used directly, or it may be electronically integrated or digitally integrated by computer to obtain a signal representing volume. In this manner, a pneumotachometer system may be used to replace volume displacement devices for spirometry. When combined with circuitry to obtain forced expiratory indexes electronically,

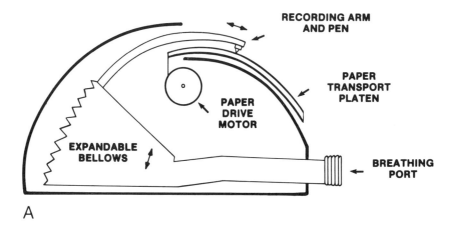

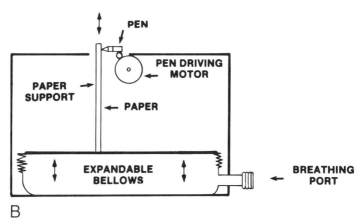

Fig. 5-3.   Sideview diagrams of two types of bellows spirometers. (A) The wedge bellows expands in an arc, driving a pen across the paper placed on a motor drive in the same arc. The motor drive moves the paper platen at a constant speed when activated. (B) The box bellows expands linearly. The paper is driven by the bellows, which is drawn against a pen driven perpendicularly by a motor at a constant speed.

they are called *electronic spirometers*. Their main use is in portable or bedside spirometry.

The advantages of pneumotachometers are that they are small, compact, and mechanically simple. The transducer itself is hand-held and the electronic monitoring circuitry is small. It has very little dead space and is an open system, so it may be used in prolonged inspiratory-expiratory studies without problems resulting from oxygen consumption and carbon dioxide accumulation. Disadvantages include dependence on a properly calibrated electronic circuitry (circuit performance can change with time) and a limited range of linear operation (with resulting limited range of dependable flow measurements). The transducers are often sensitive to environmental factors, such as humidity and temperature, and may be significantly affected by shaking or dropping.

Initial performance reports in the literature suggested that pneumotachometers were inaccurate and criticized their inability to generate a permanent record.[5] Improvements have led to development of electronic spirometers with acceptable accuracy and optional recorders to display the spirogram.[6] A graphic record is recommended in all spirometers to permit detection of performance problems and inconsistencies that electronic processing cannot detect.

In the clinical laboratory, pneumotachometers find their greatest use for flow measurements in body plethysmography. Volume displacement spirometers are generally preferred for clinical spirometry because most meet all the performance criteria of the American Thoracic Society.[7] Although many pneumotachometers do not meet these strict criteria, they are still suitable for portable and screening spirometry.

Differential Pressure Pneumotachometer

The relationship between flow, pressure, and resistance to flow in a conduit when flow is laminar is derived from Poiseuille's equation by simplification of the resistance term, so that

$$\dot{V} = \Delta P / R \qquad \text{(Eq. 5-1)}$$

where R represents the resistance term related to dimensions of the conduit and characteristics of the fluid. The differential pressure pneumotachometer is based on this principle. It consists of a rigid tube containing a small resistance to gas flow. The pressure difference across the flow resistance is measured by a differential pressure transducer. Since the resistance is constant, flow is proportional to the measured pressure difference. In practice, the pneumotachometer is constructed in the form of a tube in which a partial obstruction has been placed to create a resistance to airflow (Fig. 5-4). The resistance must be large enough to generate a measurable pressure difference, yet small enough so as not to add any significant resistance to that of the respiratory system. The *Fleisch pneumotachometer* uses a set of parallel capillary tubes to produce a laminar flow resistance.[8,9] Described in 1925, it is still in common use today. A fine wire mesh is used as the flow resistance in the *Silverman-Lilly* pneumotachometer.[10,11] Other designs have included a venturi tube,[12] concentric cylinders, and parallel plates. The pressure difference between two ports placed on either side of the resistance element is measured and converted to flow. The technique depends on laminar flow in the tube for accurate results. If turbulent flow occurs, the resistance of the tube is altered and flow is not directly related to pressure difference, but instead to the square root, so that

$$\dot{V} = \sqrt{\Delta P / R'} \qquad \text{(Eq. 5-2)}$$

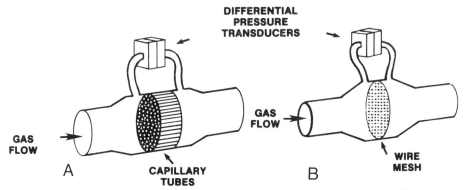

Fig. 5-4. Two types of the differential pressure pneumotachometer, in which a flow resistance produces a pressure difference proportional to the flow. The pressure difference is measured by a pressure transducer and converted to flow. (A) The Fleisch pneumotachometer design incorporates a set of parallel capillary tubes to provide flow resistance. (B) A fine wire mesh is used in the Silverman-Lilly pneumotachometer to provide flow resistance.

where R' represents a complex resistance term related to characteristics of the conduit and the fluid. In order to provide laminar flow, different size heads are designed for specific ranges of flow, with larger diameter heads used for greater flows.

Several problems are associated with the use of pneumotachometers.[13] One of the most common problems is the partial obstruction of the resistance element by exhaled water droplets or secretions. Although heating the resistance element evaporates condensation and helps to eliminate this problem, it also raises the gas temperature and may alter the flow characteristics of the unit. When airflow is turbulent the pressure differences are not linearly related to flow, so care must be taken not to exceed maximum rated flow. Adherence to calibrated specifications depends on gas composition and temperature, so calibrations should be performed using a gas mixture of similar temperature and composition as the one to be measured.

Thermal Dissipation Pneumotachometer

A gas or gas mixture has a constant specific heat, that is, it takes up or releases a given amount of heat for a given temperature change. The thermal dissipation or heated-element pneumotachometer utilizes this principle (Fig. 5-5). The device has an element heated by an electric current, with temperature controlled by varying the amount of current flowing to the element. The element is placed within a cylinder similar to that of other pneumotachometers. Temperature of the element and amount of current used to heat the element can be monitored. As gas flows around the element, heat is lost in proportion to the specific heat of the gas, and a greater current is required to maintain a constant element temperature. The change in current reflects the flow of gas in the

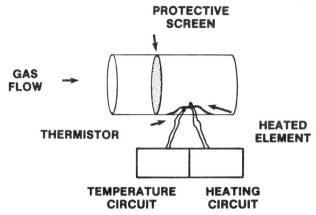

Fig. 5-5. The heat dissipation pneumotachometer, which uses a heated element. The greater the gas flow through the cylinder, the greater the amount of heat dissipated from the element, and the greater the current required to maintain a constant temperature. This current is proportional to gas flow. A protective screen is used to prevent foreign substances from altering the heat dissipation characteristics of the element.

pneumotachometer. Accuracy of this device can be affected by the water content and composition of exhaled air because water vapor and different gases have different specific heats. The response time is slower than most other types of pneumotachometers, as dissipation of heat in the element and changes in flow are not instantaneous. They are better suited for clinical applications requiring portability but not a great degree of accuracy. Because they are electronic, they can be made compact and are often used as portable or screening spirometers.

Ultrasonic Pneumotachometer

Ultrasound in the 100-mHz frequency range is used for measuring gas velocity and flow by one of two methods. In the first method, a small obstruction is placed in a cylinder that produces a controlled turbulence. An ultrasound beam directed across the turbulence is scattered by the turbulence. The degree of scattering is related to gas flow.

The second method is to measure laminar gas velocity by the augmented or retarded propagation of an ultrasound signal through the moving gas. By alternating transmission between a pair of opposed transducers, transit time differences between upstream and downstream flow are converted to a flow signal. The original designs had transducers placed at an angle to the flow, but a more recent version utilized a coaxial orientation of the transducers (Fig. 5-6).[14]

These devices generally have insufficient accuracy for clinical laboratory use and find their major use in screening and continuous monitoring devices.

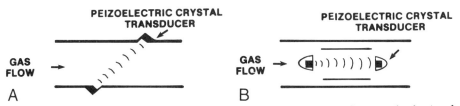

Fig. 5-6.   Ultrasonic pneumotachometer designs. These measure flow on the basis of wave velocity. Propagation speed of the ultrasound signal is enhanced or retarded by gas flow. A measurement consists of the signal transit times in each direction. The difference between transit times is proportional to flow. Models may use a tangential (A) or coaxial (B) arrangement of the transducers.

MECHANICAL FLOW MEASURING DEVICES

A rotating turbine to register flow forms the basis of a number of handheld flowmeters. The Wright respirometer is a very popular instrument for measuring exhaled volume, and variations in its design permit the measurement of flow, either through a mechanical linkage or by electronically converting turbine speed to flow. These instruments are suitable for bedside measurement of flow and volume, but because of the mechanical properties of the turbine they lack sufficient response and accuracy to permit their general use in the clinical laboratory. Their delicate mechanical structure requires that they be handled carefully, and condensed water vapor from expired air may interfere with rotation of the vanes.

PRESSURE MEASUREMENT

The measurement of pressure is indispensable to many pulmonary function tests. The differential pressure pneumotachometer described previously requires the measurement of pressure across a flow resistance. Total body plethysmography (to be described) requires measurement of airway pressure and pressure within the body plethysmograph. Lung compliance determinations require the measurement of esophageal pressure.

Measurements of pressure are made against a reference pressure. In most pressure measurements the reference is the atmospheric pressure. Some applications, such as the *differential pressure* pneumotachometer, require the measurement of the pressure difference between two sources, independent of atmospheric pressure. In the typical pressure transducer, the sensing element is placed between the pressure source and the atmosphere. In a differential pressure transducer, the sensing element is placed between the two pressure sources, as shown in Figure 5-7.

The standard for static pressure measurements is the mercury column

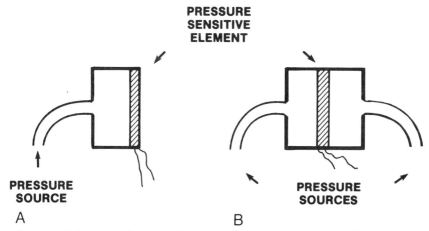

**PRESSURE
SENSITIVE
ELEMENT**

**PRESSURE
SOURCE**

A

**PRESSURE
SOURCES**

B

Fig. 5-7. Schematic of two configurations for the measurement of pressure. (A) A single-source pressure transducer has a single chamber and a pressure-sensitive element that uses atmospheric pressure as its reference. (B) A differential pressure transducer is dual-chambered, with the chambers separated by the pressure-sensing element and sealed from the atmosphere. Only a difference between the pressure sources, regardless of their absolute values, will be detected.

manometer. This manometer is constructed as a capillary tube filled with a uniform column of mercury (Fig. 5-8A). The pressure source is attached to the lower end of the tube and displaces the column upward against atmospheric pressure. The distance moved is read as pressure, and is given in the standard unit of pressure in use today (millimeters of mercury or torr). The device needs no calibration. It is limited to static pressure measurements because rapidly changing pressures are dampened by the system.

Pressure transducers that produce a permanent record of pressure are of two types, mechanical and electrical. Both use a rigid plastic or metal diaphragm that is displaced by the pressure source through a distance proportional to the applied pressure. The method for measuring the displacement of the diaphragm is through a mechanical linkage (mechanical transducer) or by conversion to an electrical signal (electronic transducer).

Mechanical Pressure Transducers

A mechanical linkage that can amplify small excursions of the diaphragm can indicate pressure through movement of a gauge or by recording on paper (Fig. 5-8B). They are subject to wear and other mechanical problems that can render them inaccurate. Therefore, except for static measurements, for which the mercury fluid manometer is in common use, mechanical pressure transducers have been largely replaced in the laboratory by electronic pressure transducers.

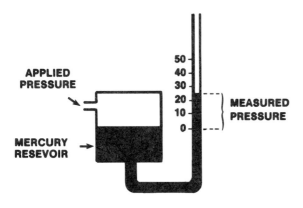

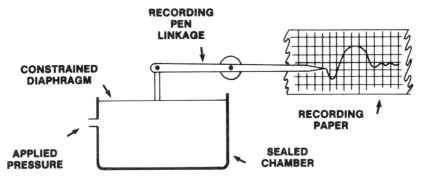

Fig. 5-8. Measurement of pressures through the use of a manometer or mechanical linkage. (A) A mercury column manometer measures pressure by the vertical displacement of a column of mercury. The reservoir is large in relation to the column diameter so that its level of mercury (the zero reference) does not significantly change. (B) A mechanical pressure transducer uses a pen linkage to record deflections of a constrained, rigid diaphragm. For small pressure changes, the pressure is proportional to the degree of deflection of the diaphragm.

Electronic Transducers

Electronic transducers use one of several principles to register displacement of the diaphragm. The *strain gauge* consists of a special resistive material bonded to a stiff diaphragm (Fig. 5-9A). Displacement of the diaphragm by the application of pressure results in stretching of the resistive material and a predictable change in its resistance. The change in resistance is electronically converted to units of pressure.

Other electronic transducers use *capacitance* or *inductance* to detect displacement of the diaphragm. In the former, the diaphragm forms one plate of a

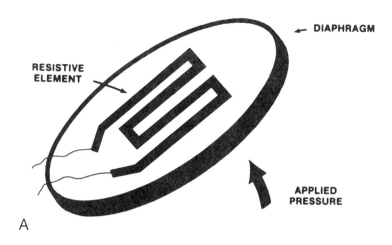

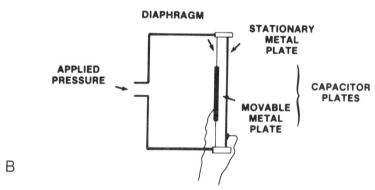

Fig. 5-9. Two principles of electronic pressure transducer operation. (A) The strain gauge incorporates a resistive film bonded to a semirigid diaphragm. Stretching of the resistive element through displacement of the diaphragm results in a predictable increase in resistance of the element. The change in resistance is converted to pressure. (B) A capacitance transducer uses a pair of metal plates, one stationary and the other fixed to a diaphragm. Displacement of the diaphragm by the application of pressure alters the distance between the two plates, and hence, the capacitance, which can be measured and converted to pressure.

capacitor; displacement of this plate relative to the other results in a measurable change in capacitance (Fig. 5-9B). The inductance type uses a wire coil through which a magnetic core connected to the diaphragm is placed. Movement of the diaphragm alters the relationship of the core and the coil, with a measurable change in the inductance properties of the coil.

Electronic transducers are small, lightweight, dependable, and have a rapid response; they are usually required for dynamic pressure measurements, as mechanical transducers do not have the necessary speed of response. They are sensitive instruments and require careful handling and regular calibration to assure accurate measurement of pressure.

TOTAL BODY PLETHYSMOGRAPHY

Plethysmography is a method for measuring variations in volume of an organ or limb, such as might occur from changes in blood volume. It is used in pulmonary function testing to measure *intrathoracic gas volume*. It is also capable of measuring changes in alveolar pressure for the measurement of *airway resistance*. To obtain these two measurements, the entire subject is placed into the plethysmograph for the testing. The plethysmograph is a rigid, airtight box; hence the term *total body plethysmograph*. The three types of plethysmographs available are: (1) pressure, (2) volume displacement, and (3) flow displacement plethysmographs. The difference between these types is the means by which the change in alveolar volume is estimated. The pressure type is probably the most popular.

The three types are similar in design (Fig. 5-10) and also operate similarly. The subject sits in a special box that is sealed from the atmosphere except through transducers for recording box pressure or volume change. The volume of the box is typically between 500 and 600 liters. A *flowhead* is located inside the plethysmograph for measuring flow and pressures at the airway opening (mouth). The flowhead has three components. A *pneumotachometer* with its own transducer is incorporated into the flowhead for the measurement of inspiratory-expiratory flow. Proximal to the pneumotachometer is an electrically activated *shutter* that, when activated by the technician, occludes the lumen of the flowhead and prevents airflow. Just proximal to the shutter is another *pressure transducer* for the measurement of pressure at the airway opening. When the shutter is closed with the glottis open, alveolar pressure becomes equal to the pressure measured at the airway opening.

The differences between the three types of plethysmographs in the estimation of alveolar volume and pressure are discussed in the following sections.

Pressure Plethysmography

The pressure-type body plethysmograph employs a constant volume box in which changes in box pressure are used to estimate changes in alveolar volume for the determination of thoracic gas volume. The relationship between a volume change within the box (such as results from a change in lung volume in a subject inside the box) and box pressure is dependent on the pressure-volume characteristics of the box. The box is "calibrated" for the subject by placing the subject inside and determining these characteristics. A known volume of gas is cyclically

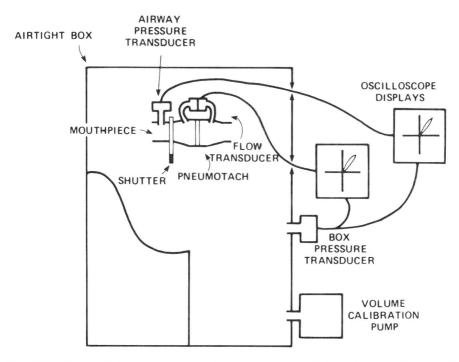

Fig. 5-10. Body plethysmograph for the measurement of thoracic gas volume and airway resistance. The type shown is a pressure plethysmograph, which uses pressure changes in the box to estimate lung volume changes. Pressure transducers are used to monitor the box and mouth pressures. A flow transducer allows simultaneous recording of flow at the mouth. From these measurements, thoracic gas volume and airway resistance may be calculated using the techniques outlined in Chapters 6 and 7. The volume and flow displacement plethysmograph design is similar; differences are explained in text. [Used with permission from Conrad SA and George RB: Clinical pulmonary function testing. p. 161. In George RB, Light RW, Matthay RA (eds): Chest Medicine. Churchill Livingstone, New York, 1983]

resulting pressure change is recorded. The box compliance C_{box} (volume change divided by the resulting pressure change) remains relatively constant for small changes in lung volume. The volume change in the subject's lungs (ΔV_L) may then be determined from the change in box pressure (ΔP_{box}) by the relation:

$$\Delta V_L = C_{box}(\Delta P_{box}) \qquad \text{(Eq. 5-3)}$$

The change in alveolar pressure used in the measurement of airway resistance may be determined from box pressure in a similar manner, by using a constant of proportionality. Alveolar pressure is measured at the airway opening with the shutter closed and is related to the change in box pressure. After this calibration, box pressure may be used to estimate alveolar pressure during active breathing if flow is slow and constant.

In actual measurement the transducer outputs of airway opening pressure, flow, and box pressure are displayed on a recording X-Y oscilloscope. Under control of the technician, the mouth pressure is displayed on the y axis with box pressure on the x axis. The oscilloscope may also be used to display flow on the y axis with box pressure on the x axis. These displays facilitate measurement of thoracic gas volume and airway resistance. These measurement techniques are presented in Chapters 6 and 7, respectively.

Volume Displacement Plethysmography

With this technique, volume change in the lungs can be measured directly by incorporating a spirometer into the box wall rather than measuring it indirectly from box pressure. There is no need to calibrate box pressure readings in order to estimate volume changes. In estimating alveolar pressure, calibration similar to that for a pressure box is used, but the box volume change is used in place of box pressure change for this purpose. The major limitation here is the inability to record volume changes accurately with rapid respiratory rates or expiratory flows.

Flow Plethysmography

Replacement of the spirometer in the volume displacement plethysmograph with a pneumotachometer permits measurement of volume change through integration of the flow signal. This allows direct measurement of volume displacement with good performance at higher respiratory frequencies. In other respects, the operation is similar to the volume displacement plethysmograph.

ANALYSIS OF EXPIRED GASES

Two approaches to the determination of gas concentration or partial pressure in a gas mixture or body fluid are chemical analysis and the use of physical attributes. *Chemical analysis* of a gas mixture involves use of reagents to absorb the gas under study, after which the change in volume of the gas mixture is measured and related to the concentration. These methods have been almost universally replaced by *physical methods,* in which characteristics like infrared absorption or particle mass are quantitatively related to concentration. Physical methods are easily performed in the laboratory. The most common methods in use today are summarized in Table 5-1 and will be described in the sections that follow.

Table 5-1 Common Methods of Gas Analysis

Gas	Tests	Analysis Method	Interfering Gases	Response Time
N_2	Nitrogen washout (single and multibreath)	Emission spectroscopy by ionization	CO_2, H_2O	Rapid
He	Helium dilution	Thermal conductivity	CO_2, H_2O	Slow
CO_2	Expired gas analysis	Infrared absorption	CO, H_2O	Rapid
	Blood gas	CO_2-induced change in pH	None	Slow
CO	CO diffusion	Infrared absorption	CO_2, H_2O	Rapid
O_2	Expired gas analysis	Electrolytic fuel cell	None	Rapid
	Blood gas	Polarography	Halothane	Slow
All	On-line respiratory gas monitoring	Mass spectrometry	Variable	Rapid

Emission Spectroscopy by Ionization

Ionization of certain gases by high voltage in a near-vacuum results in the emission of light of characteristic wavelengths. Nitrogen emits light in the ultraviolet spectrum when ionized, with principal wavelengths between 300 and 480 nm. Under conditions of constant low pressure and ionization current, the intensity of emitted light is related to the concentration of nitrogen in the chamber.

The analyzer is composed of a chamber containing two electrodes driven by a constant current source and an applied voltage of about 1 kV (Fig. 5-11). The chamber is maintained under low pressure by a vacuum pump. A needle valve allows a small but controlled amount of sample gas to bleed into the analysis chamber. The light emitted during ionization is filtered to remove undesirable wavelengths, including those from H_2O and CO_2, and permit those wavelengths primarily from N_2 to pass to the detector. The filtered light is sensed by a phototube, amplified, and converted to an electrical signal representing gas concentration. The response time is rapid, on the order of 50 msec, permitting monitoring of instantaneous concentration on a breath-by-breath basis. The meter must be calibrated at zero percent and 80 to 100 percent nitrogen at frequent intervals to ensure accurate results.

Sources of error include particle collection in the needle valve, leaks in the vacuum system, or significant concentrations of interfering gases. The system requires regular calibration and checks to determine correctable sources of error and to correct for electronic drift.

The principal use of this analyzer is for multibreath and single-breath nitrogen washout studies where instantaneous concentration of nitrogen concentration is plotted as a function of volume.

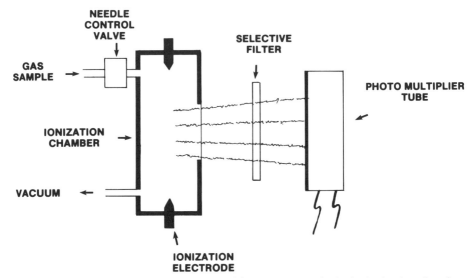

Fig. 5-11. Emission spectroscopy unit used for nitrogen analysis. An ionization chamber is maintained at near-vacuum by a pump. A needle valve bleeds a small, controlled amount of the sample gas into the chamber. The gas is ionized by a high voltage, constant current source. The emitted light is first filtered to select out wavelengths most specific for nitrogen. The photomultiplier tube converts the filtered light to a current that represents fractional concentration of nitrogen. The greater the nitrogen concentration, the greater the amount of ionization and the larger the current produced by the phototube.

Thermal Conductivity

Gases as well as other substances conduct heat according to molecular weight, and this physical characteristic can be used to detect small changes in concentration of certain gases. This method assumes that the change in concentration of the gas is small and that interfering gases do not change in concentration. The instrument used compares thermal conductivity by means of temperature change of a sample gas exposed to a heat source in relation to a reference gas. The latter has a composition similar to the test gas.

The most sensitive means of detecting differences in temperature is by the use of two thermistors placed in a *Wheatstone bridge,* a sensitive circuit for measuring small differences in resistance. Changes in temperature result in changes in the resistances of the thermistors, producing a voltage representing the difference in temperature. The sample and reference gases are heated and passed over separate thermistors in the bridge. Differences in gas concentration result in different rates of heat exchange with the thermistors, reflecting the concentration of the sample gas in relation to the reference gas.

This method is suited for measurement of helium concentration because there is a large difference between the thermal conductivity of this gas and other common respiratory gases. Its response is slow, making it useful for helium dilution measurements at equilibrium but not for dynamic measurements.

Infrared Absorption Spectroscopy

The absorption of energy in the infrared spectrum is a property of chemical species often used in identification of compounds in analytical chemistry procedures. This property is used in pulmonary function testing to measure low concentrations of carbon monoxide and carbon dioxide in respiratory gases. The principle of operation is based on the difference in infrared energy absorption between the sample gas and a reference gas.

The instrumentation used is depicted in Figure 5-12. The three basic components are a dual-path pulsed infrared source, two gas chambers, and a detector cell. The infrared sources produce energy within the 4.0 to 5.0 μm wavelength range. Each beam is directed through its respective gas chamber. The sample gas chamber holds the gas mixture containing a gas species of interest, for example, CO_2, whose concentration is to be determined. The reference gas chamber contains a gas mixture similar to the sample gas, except that the gas species of interest is absent or exists in known concentration. The infrared beams are identical in energy when they enter the gas chambers. Infrared energy is ab-

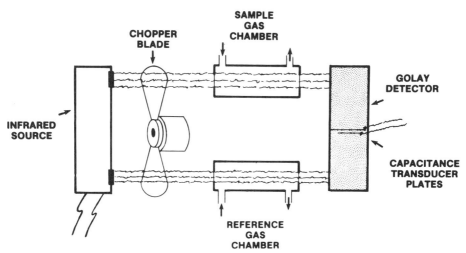

Fig. 5-12. Infrared absorption spectroscopy unit used for monitoring of CO_2 and CO concentration in respiratory gases. The chopper blade provides synchronized pulses of infrared radiation to the gas chambers. Differences in gas concentration between the sample and reference chambers results in a difference in energy in the two beams as a result of absorption. This results in a difference in the energy of the infrared light that strikes the detector, with the generation of a signal proportional to the difference in gas concentration.

sorbed by the gas species of interest in each chamber, resulting in a decrease in the energy of each beam. The loss of energy is related to the concentration of the gas species in the chamber, and the difference between the energies of the emerging beams is related to the difference in concentrations between the reference and sample gases. This energy difference is quantitated by the detector to provide a measure of the gas species concentration in the sample gas.

The detector is designed to measure the difference between the two infrared beams emerging from the gas chambers. It consists of two sealed compartments separated by a diaphragm. Each detector compartment is filled with a substance that expands when struck by infrared energy, as it absorbs the energy and converts it to heat. If one compartment receives more energy in its incident beam than the other, then the diaphragm will deflect away. The degree of deflection is proportional to the difference between the energies of the two beams, and hence, to the difference in gas concentrations. The deflection is measured by a capacitative transducer similar to that used in pressure transducers, and converted to gas concentration for display. The infrared beams are pulsed at a rate of 60 times/sec to permit the detector compartments to return to their static states in between pulses, thus preventing overexpansion of the detector compartments.

An alternative approach is to use an infrared detector with compartments containing the gas of interest, such as CO_2. This makes the detector specific for that gas, eliminating the need for a reference gas chamber, which is replaced by an optical balance to permit calibration at zero concentration.

The infrared method is limited to the measurement of low gas concentrations in which the concentration of only one gas species varies significantly. The method is sensitive to changes in H_2O, CO_2, and CO, so a variation in the concentration of more than one gas may interfere with the process and produce spurious results. In the pulmonary function laboratory, carbon monoxide used in diffusion studies is usually measured by this method. In exercise testing and other forms of expired gas analysis, CO_2 concentration is measured by this method, usually to determine CO_2 production. The method has a rapid response time (100 msec) and may be used for on-line gas analysis.

Electrolytic Fuel Cell

The need for rapid-response oxygen analysis has led to the popularity of the fuel cell, which uses a solid electrolyte for an electrochemical reaction. The cell consists of a cylinder of calcia-stabilized zirconium oxide. The interior and exterior surfaces are coated with porous platinum electrodes, to which platinum lead wires are attached. The gas circuit admits the sample gas into the interior of the cylinder. The reference gas is circulated at its exterior surface and the ends of the cylinder are sealed to prevent contact of the two gases. Then it is heated to allow the solid solution electrode to behave as an ideal electrolyte, permitting diffusion of oxygen into the solid. The reference gas is usually atmospheric air because its oxygen concentration is known.

The cell is responsive to oxygen partial pressure, according to the following equation pair occurring at the surfaces:

$$O_2 + 4e^- \rightarrow 2O^{-2}$$
$$2O^{-2} \rightarrow O_2 + 4e^-$$

(Eq. 5-4)

The cell produces a voltage proportional to the log of the ratio of the partial pressures of the sample and reference gases. A logarithmic amplifier is used to provide a reading of the oxygen partial pressure in the sample gas.

The response time is rapid (50 msec), permitting on-line oxygen monitoring. Its greatest use is in exercise testing.

Mass Spectroscopy

The mass of a gas is a physical property that can be used for identification and measurement of its concentration. Mass spectroscopy is a method in which a gas sample is ionized, then separated into an ion spectrum on the basis of weight. Detectors then quantitate the species with the mass of interest. Several gases may be analyzed simultaneously, facilitating the monitoring of respiratory gases.[15]

There are several types of mass spectrometers, and three are in common use. One of the earliest developed is the *magnetic sector* mass spectrometer. The basic construction of a magnetic sector mass spectrometer is shown in Figure 5-13. The sample gas is drawn through a controlled port into an ionization chamber maintained at near-vacuum. The gas is ionized by electrons generated by a controlled current, accelerated by an electric potential, and then focused into a beam by electromagnetic lenses. The ions are subjected to a constant acceleration. A second magnetic field then causes the ions to deflect away from the original path, with the radius of curvature of deflection dependent on the mass of the ion. The ions are thus spacially separated on the basis of their mass. Ion detectors placed at precise locations within the spectrum sense the current generated by the ions and produce a signal proportional to the concentration of the ions. The detectors themselves are not specific for a given species, but rather, the method depends on their location in the spectrum to differentiate ions of different gases. If two gases ionize into species of identical mass, they cannot be distinguished.

The *time-of-flight* mass spectrometer identifies a gas by using the time required for the ion to travel a preset distance under a precise acceleration. A deflection magnet is not used; instead, a sensitive timing circuitry is employed. The *quadripole* mass spectrometer sends an accelerated beam of ions though the midst of four equally spaced cylinders lying on parallel axes. By appropriate electromagnetic activation of the cylinders, only ions of a certain mass are permitted to emerge, which can then be quantitated with a detector. Details of the fundamental principles of mass spectroscopy are available in the literature.[16]

Sources of error include obstruction to the metering of gases into the chamber and the presence of interfering substances of identical mass. The mass

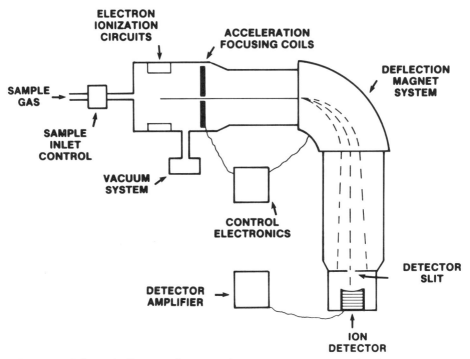

Fig. 5-13.   Schematic diagram of a magnetic-sector mass spectrometer. A vacuum pump maintains a high vacuum to avoid interference with ionization and ion acceleration. Ions are generated from the sample gas by bombardment with electrons from the electron source. The ions are accelerated to a predetermined velocity and collimated. The deflection magnet alters the trajectory of the ions into a spatial spectrum based on mass. Only those ions of a particular mass will strike the detector. The current produced by the ion detector is related to the concentration of the gas producing the ion.

spectrometer has a rapid response (100 msec) and is ideal for simultaneously monitoring instantaneous concentrations of several respiratory gases on-line, but its cost and maintenance requirements are usually prohibitive for most laboratories.

ANALYSIS OF BLOOD GASES AND pH

pH

The pH of blood (or other solution) is measured in the laboratory by using an electrode that produces a voltage proportional to pH.[17] The electrode contains a special glass membrane that is polarized (producing a voltage difference across the membrane) when the pH of the solution inside the electrode differs from the sample solution or blood on the other side. The magnitude of the voltage difference is proportional to the pH difference. A reference electrode using Ag-AgCl or calomel (Hg_2Cl_2) with an interposed voltmeter completes the circuit. The sensitive voltmeter registers the voltage across the membrane and converts it to pH units.

The electrode is subject to drift and must be frequently calibrated. Most analyzers use calibration standards of 6.841 and 7.383 pH units, which encompass most of the physiological range of blood pH.

Po$_2$ by Polarography

Polarography is an electrochemical method used for measurement of oxygen partial pressure in fluids, with its principal application found in blood gas analysis. Oxygen undergoes a reduction reaction when subjected to a polarization voltage of about 0.7 volts. Electrons are consumed in small quantity by the electrode as oxygen is reduced. This consumption results in a current that is proportional to the O_2 concentration. Reduction takes place at a platinum cathode according to the following equations[17]:

$$O_2 + 2H_2O + 4e^- \rightarrow 2H_2O_2 + 4e^- \rightarrow 4OH^-$$
$$4OH^- + 4KCl \rightarrow 4KOH + 4Cl^- \qquad \text{(Eq. 5-5)}$$

A silver-silver chloride (Ag-AgCl) anode and a bridge of KCl electrolyte solution form the rest of the electrode. The anode equation is

$$4Ag + 4Cl^- \rightarrow 4AgCl + 4e^- \qquad \text{(Eq. 5-6)}$$

resulting in the four electrons for the reduction process.

The electrode contains a membrane permeable to oxygen to prevent exposure to contaminating substances.

The currents generated are small (picoamperes to nanoamperes), requiring the use of sensitive amplification instruments. These small currents are sensitive to measurement error so the equipment must be regularly calibrated, using at least two concentrations of oxygen. Although the response is linear over most concentrations, large changes in concentration may result in nonlinear output. For this reason, the electrode is calibrated at physiological oxygen tensions. If Po$_2$ is high, for example, over 300 torr, the electrode will require recalibration at the higher Po$_2$.

This principle is used for oxygen measurements in blood gas electrodes and oxygen monitors. The response time of most polarographic electrodes is on the order of seconds to minutes, so it is not rapid enough for on-line monitoring.

Pco$_2$ by CO$_2$-Induced Change in pH

The partial pressure of carbon dioxide in blood is measured by the Severinghaus' principle, in which CO_2 diffuses into a buffer solution and produces a measurable change in pH.[17,18] The reaction takes place behind a semipermeable membrane in a solution of $NaHCO_3$:

$$CO_2 + H_2O \rightarrow H_2CO_3 \rightarrow H^+ + HCO_3^- \qquad \text{(Eq. 5-7)}$$

The pH change is detected by a glass pH electrode with a calomel or Ag-AgCl reference electrode (described previously). The pH change is proportional to the change in log P_{CO_2} concentration. An amplifier gives a signal representing P_{CO_2}. As in polarography, the response time is slow and the method is usually limited to sample blood gas analysis.

COMPUTER SYSTEMS

A recent addition to the pulmonary function laboratory has been the integration of dedicated computer systems with pulmonary function testing equipment. These systems perform a number of tasks that automate testing procedures. There are a number of advantages in using computer-based testing equipment. Technical errors are reduced by controlling the sequence of the test and by avoiding the hand analysis required of manual systems. This results in a reduction in variability of results among laboratory personnel and increased consistency in test results. By removing the need for graphical analysis and manual calculations, a reduction in testing time is usually achieved. Transcription errors in reporting results are eliminated. Data storage and retrieval is simplified by the use of magnetic storage media, from which new reports can be easily generated, and access to the data of a large number of patients is readily achieved.

Components of a Laboratory Computer System

A typical computer system for pulmonary function testing equipment consists of several distinct functional components. The hardware consists of the computer system equipment, whereas the software is the collection of programs for operating the computer and testing equipment.

The *hardware* has several components. The equipment interface contains converters that enable the computer to sense and control the equipment. The *analog-to-digital converter* (ADC) samples voltages produced by the equipment. Such voltages represent the operation or state of the equipment, such as spirometer volume, expiratory flow, or nitrogen concentration. The voltages are converted to numerical values in computer format so they can be processed by the computer. The *digital-to-analog converter* (DAC) enables the computer to control the operation of the equipment, such as activating a solenoid or enabling a test function. The *console terminal* permits interaction with the software for data entry and program control. The *central processing unit* (CPU) contains the memory and processing circuitry to execute the program and store the data.

Magnetic memory permits large amounts of data to be recorded and stored for future use. It also stores the programs when the computer system is shut down.

The two common forms of inexpensive media for storage are the diskette and cassette tape. The diskette, or "floppy disk," is a flexible magnetic disk the size of a small phonograph record capable of storing up to 1 million characters of information. A cassette tape can hold a similar amount at lower cost but at some disadvantage. A disk drive can rapidly store and retrieve information from anywhere on the disk, but a cassette tape is slow because the entire tape has to be read before data can be stored or retrieved from one end of the tape.

Software is of two types. *System software* consists of the general-purpose programs used to operate the basic functions of the computer. It contains master programs that enable the creation of application programs to perform specific tasks and maintenance functions on programs and data. *Application software* consists of special-purpose programs, like those used for acquiring, processing, and reporting pulmonary function data.

Functions of a Computer System

Several functions are performed by computer-based systems (Table 5-2). Automatic *data acquisition* is the conversion of information generated by the laboratory testing equipment to computer-readable form where it is recorded as data in the computer. An example would be the recording of the entire spirogram or flow-volume loop at 10-msec intervals, from which the spirogram can be constructed later or other measurements obtained.

Data reduction is the process of extracting information of clinical interest from raw data, such as the extraction of forced expired volumes from the total number of points comprising the stored spirogram. After this is done, the raw data can be discarded, greatly reducing storage requirements from, for example, 500 spirogram data points to less than a dozen indexes of forced expiration.

The next principal function is *data analysis,* in which calculations are performed on acquired data, such as calculation of predicted equations, and interpretation of the results through the computer's decision-making capabilities.

Once all the final data have been collected or calculated, they are organized and printed by the *report generation* capabilities of the computer. Such a report is usually suitable for inclusion into the medical record. For purposes of serial comparison or use in research the system is capable of *data storage.* This usually

Table 5-2 Computer System Functions

1. Data acquisition
2. Data reduction
3. Data analysis
4. Report generation
5. Data storage and retrieval
6. Equipment control

takes place using inexpensive magnetic tapes or disks. These magnetic media are capable of storing the data of several hundred patients on each tape or disk.

The last function is *equipment control.* The computer system can be programmed to control the operation of equipment using a special interface incorporating DACs, including such functions as shutter operation in the plethysmograph or inspired gas control in the single-breath nitrogen test. This is an expensive feature of computer systems and is not commonly employed.

In summary, a computer system can offer greater throughput with a lower incidence of errors. Its cost is justified only by its use for a large number of patients; therefore, it is usually limited to large clinical or research laboratories. The falling prices of hardware, however, might make feasible more widespread use of computer systems in the pulmonary function laboratory. It can be expected that future pulmonary function equipment will have computer systems built in as integral components, with much of their operation made transparent to the technician.

REFERENCES

1. Clinical Spirometry. Warren E. Collins, Braintree, Mass, 1967
2. Wells HS, Stead WW, Rossing TD, Ognanovich J: Accuracy of an improved spirometer for recording fast breathing. J Appl Physiol 14:451, 1959
3. Stead WW, Wells HS, Gault NS, Ognanovich J: Inaccuracy of the conventional water-filled spirometer for recording rapid breathing. J Appl Physiol 14:448, 1959
4. Kory RC, Hamilton LH: Evaluation of spirometers used in pulmonary function studies. Am Rev Resp Dis 87:228, 1963
5. Fitzgerald MX, Smith AA, Gaensler EA: Evaluation of "electronic" spirometers. N Engl J Med 289:1283, 1973
6. Shanks DE, Morris JF: Clinical comparison of two electronic spirometers with a water-sealed spirometer. Chest 69:461, 1976
7. Gardner RM: ATS statement — Snowbird workshop on standardization of spirometry. Am Rev Resp Dis 119:831, 1979
8. Fleisch A: Der pneumotachograph — ein apparat zur beischwindigkeit-registrierung der atemluft. Arch Ges Physiol 209:713, 1925
9. Turney SZ, Blumenfeld W: Heated Fleisch pneumotachometer: A calibration procedure. J Appl Physiol 34:117, 1973
10. Silverman L, Whittenberger JL: Clinical pneumotachograph. p. 104. In Comroe JH (ed): Methods in Clinical Research. Vol. 2. Yearbook Publishers, Chicago, Ill, 1950
11. Lilly JC: Flow meter for recording respiratory flow of human subjects. p. 113. In Comroe JH (ed): Methods in Clinical Research. Vol. 2. Yearbook Publishers, Chicago, Ill, 1950
12. Wigertz O: A low-resistance flow meter for wide-range ventilatory measurement. Resp Physiol 7:263, 1969
13. Grenvik A, Hedstrand U, Sjogren H: Problems in pneumotachography. Acta Anaesth Scand 10:147, 1966
14. Blumenfeld W, Turney SZ, Denman RS: A coaxial ultrasonic pneumotachometer. Med Biol Eng 13:855, 1975
15. Fowler KT: The respiratory mass spectrometer. Phys Med Biol 14:185, 1969
16. Watson JT: Introduction to Mass Spectrometry: Biomedical, Environmental, and Forensic Applications. Raven Press, New York, 1976

17. Hicks R, Schenken JR, Steinrauf MA: Laboratory Instrumentation. Harper & Row, Hagerstown, Md, 1974
18. Severinghaus JW: Blood gas concentrations. p. 1475. In Fenn RO, Rahn H (eds): Handbook of Physiology. Vol. 2, Respiration. American Physiological Society, Washington, D.C., 1965

6

Lung Volumes

Steven A. Conrad, M.D.

Hutchinson first described the measurement of vital capacity in his original description of spirometry in 1844.[1] These measurements of lung volume formed the foundation of modern pulmonary function tests. The lung volumes measured by the methods to be described represent anatomic or physiological limits and are *static*, or independent of time. These limits are often altered in many diseases, although the alterations are not specific. Serial volume determinations are often useful in documenting the progression or response to therapy of particular diseases. Volume measurements are also used in calculation of other test results, such as diffusing capacity and the ratio of forced expiratory volume to vital capacity. This chapter discusses four approaches to volume measurement: spirometry, gas dilution, plethysmography, and radiographic methods. The basis for each of the methods will be presented, then the clinical application of each approach to measurement of specific volumes will be discussed, with details given on the individual tests. The factors that affect the volumes in health and disease comprise the last section.

Total lung capacity (TLC), for the purposes of volume measurement, may be divided into two major compartments. Vital capacity is the maximal amount of gas that can be exhaled with effort following full inspiration. Vital capacity (VC) and its subdivisions therefore comprise that portion of total lung volume that can be measured directly by recording changes in lung volume during breathing through the use of *spirometry*. Residual volume (RV) is that portion of TLC that remains in the thorax after maximum exhalation, and its measurement requires the use of *gas dilution* or *plethysmographic* methods. In practice, although it is feasible to measure RV, functional residual capacity (FRC) rather than RV is usually measured because it is the resting volume at the end of a normal expiration. In this state transthoracic pressure is zero; because no effort is required to maintain this volume, it is a more reproducible value. RV can then be calculated from FRC by subtracting the expiratory reserve volume (ERV) measured by spirometry. *Radiographic methods* for estimating TLC have a limited but special place in the assessment of pulmonary function.

SPIROMETRIC METHODS

Spirometry is the measurement of the volume of gas passing through the airway opening. Two methods are in common use. With the simplest, oldest, and most established method, the patient breathes through a mouthpiece into a closed spirometry system, allowing the volume change to be accurately recorded on graph paper. Measurements are not significantly affected by oxygen consumption or carbon dioxide production because they are made over brief intervals of time. Correction is required for temperature change because exhaled volume decreases with the drop in temperature from the lungs to the spirometer.

A second method of measuring static lung volumes employs a pneumotachometer system. A bidirectional pneumotachometer is used to detect respiratory gas flow, and the flow signal is electronically integrated to obtain volume. Electronic spirometers (see Chapter 5) employ this principle. Because the system is open to the atmosphere, accumulation of carbon dioxide does not occur and prolonged studies do not require CO_2 removal.

Single-Stage Vital Capacity

The spirometer is prepared for use and checked for leaks. If a volume displacement spirometer is used, it should be checked for restriction of movement. The water level should be checked if it is a water-seal type. The procedure is explained to the subject, who is seated comfortably in front of the spirometer with all restrictive clothing loosened and the nose occluded with a noseclip. He is encouraged to practice the maneuver if he has not performed the test previously. With the bell in midposition the kymograph is started at a slow speed (32 mm/sec for the Collins water-seal spirometer). The subject breathes normal tidal breaths to establish a constant end-tidal volume; then he is instructed to inhale maximally to total lung capacity, then to exhale slowly and completely to residual volume, followed by a return to tidal breathing. A typical tracing of this *single-stage vital capacity* maneuver is given in Figure 6-1. Vital capacity is measured as the volume change between the maximal end-inspiratory and end-expiratory limits. The upper and lower limits of the resting breathing excursions are averaged over a stable portion of the tracing. The volume between these limits is the *tidal volume* (TV). The volume between the tidal end-inspiratory level and maximal end-inspiratory limit is the *inspiratory reserve volume* (IRV). The volume between the resting tidal end-expiratory level and maximal end-expiratory limit is the *expiratory reserve volume* (ERV). The sum of IRV and TV is the *inspiratory capacity* (IC).

The volumes may be read directly from the graph paper. It is standard practice to correct the volumes obtained by spirometry, which are recorded as ambient temperature and pressure, saturated (ATPS), to body temperature and

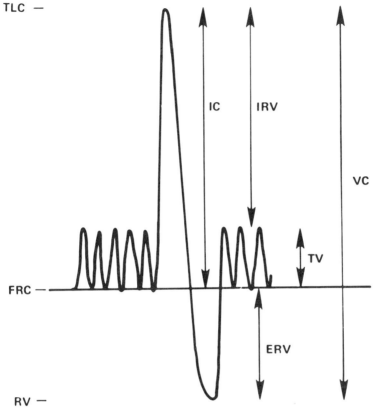

Fig. 6-1. Spirometer tracing from a single-stage vital capacity maneuver, showing the lung volumes and compartments measured from the tracing. The tracing is obtained by having the subject breathe quietly for a brief period of time, followed by a maximal inspiration, and then a slow, complete expiration. The subject then returns to tidal breathing. Total lung capacity (TLC), functional residual capacity (FRC), and residual volume (RV) are shown for orientation. Measurements include tidal volume (TV), inspiratory reserve volume (IRV), expiratory reserve volume (ERV), inspiratory capacity (IC), and vital capacity (VC). [Reprinted with permission from Conrad SA and George RB: Clinical pulmonary function testing. p. 161. In George RB, Light RW, Matthay RA (eds): Chest Medicine. Churchill Livingstone, New York, 1983]

pressure, saturated (BTPS). This correction estimates the volumes as they exist in the subject. The calculation is

$$V_{BTPS} = V_{ATPS} \left(\frac{310}{T}\right) \left(\frac{P_B - P_{H_2O}}{P_B - 47}\right) \qquad \text{(Eq. 6-1)}$$

where T is the temperature of the spirometer in degrees Kelvin (273 + T °C), and

Table 6-1 Water Vapor Pressures and Factors to
Convert ATPS to BTPS

Temperature (°C)	P_{H_2O}[a]	f[b]
37	47.0	1.000
36	44.6	1.007
35	42.2	1.013
34	39.9	1.020
33	37.7	1.026
32	35.7	1.033
31	33.7	1.039
30	31.8	1.045
29	30.0	1.051
28	28.3	1.057
27	26.7	1.063
26	25.2	1.068
25	23.8	1.074
24	22.4	1.080
23	21.1	1.085
22	19.8	1.091
21	18.7	1.096
20	17.5	1.102

[a] Data from Weast RC (ed): Handbook of Chemistry
and Physics. 56th Ed. CRC Press Cleveland, Ohio, 1975
[b] Calculated from Equation 6-1 for $P_B = 760$ mmHg.

P_{H_2O} is the water vapor pressure at the spirometer temperature, determined from Table 6-1.

The conversion to BTPS is facilitated by the use of a table of factors that combine the temperature and water vapor pressure factors into a single factor.

$$V_{BTPS} = V_{ATPS}(f) \qquad \text{(Eq. 6-2)}$$

where f at the ambient temperature is also obtained from Table 6-1.

Two-Stage Vital Capacity

An alternative to the single-stage technique is the *two-stage vital capacity* maneuver in which inspiratory and expiratory maneuvers are performed separately. The equipment and the subject are prepared as for the single-stage test. After initial tidal breathing, a full inspiration to TLC is made, followed by a return to tidal breathing. After several tidal breaths, a full expiration to residual volume is made (Fig. 6-2). IRV, ERV, TV, and IC are determined as for the single-stage test, but vital capacity is calculated as the sum of ERV and IC since the vital capacity maneuver is recorded in two separate phases. Separate measurement of the inspiratory and expiratory phases has been shown occasionally to yield higher values for vital capacity than the single-stage method, most commonly in the elderly and in those with chronic obstructive disease where loss of elasticity or trapping of air during expiration from TLC is thought to be responsible.[2,3]

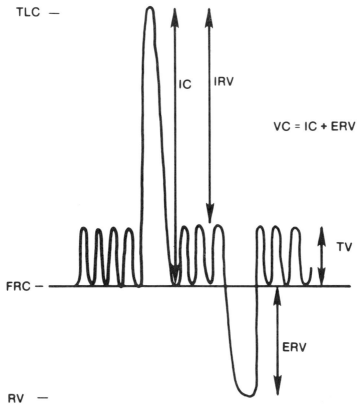

Fig. 6-2. Spirometer tracing from a two-stage vital capacity maneuver, showing the lung volumes and compartments measured from the tracing. The tracing is obtained by having the subject breathe quietly for a brief period of time, followed by a maximal inspiration, and then a return to tidal breathing for three to four breaths. Next, the subject makes a slow, maximal expiration. The patient then returns to tidal breathing. Total lung capacity (TLC), functional residual capacity (FRC), and residual volume (RV) are shown for orientation. Measurements include tidal volume (TV), inspiratory reserve volume (IRV), expiratory reserve volume (ERV), and inspiratory capacity (IC). Vital capacity (VC) is computed as the sum of ERV and IC rather than being measured from the tracing. This separation of vital capacity into two phases reduces air trapping in the subject with obstructive lung disease.

Sources of Error in Spirometry

Spirometric volume measurements, especially those obtained with volume displacement spirometers, are subject to little inherent error. The common causes of error can usually be readily identified. In the presence of obstruction to airflow rapid exhalation may result in air trapping, which causes a decrease in measured

VC, particularly as a result of a reduced expiratory reserve volume. Another source of error can arise if the subject performs tidal breathing irregularly, making it difficult to define the FRC level and the boundary between TV and IRV. This error can be minimized by careful instruction and by allowing the subject to become familiar with the equipment during an extended period of quiet breathing. The test should not be rushed, as this leads to poor subject performance and increased error. Correction of volumes to BTPS with careful measurement of ambient and body temperatures reduces volume error caused by contraction that results from the temperature change. Other potential sources of underestimation of volumes are leakage of air from the spirometer system and volume loss because of increased system compliance. The latter plays a more significant role in forced ventilatory maneuvers.

GAS DILUTION METHODS FOR FUNCTIONAL RESIDUAL CAPACITY

In common practice, FRC is measured and ERV is subtracted from it to derive RV. Two simple yet reasonably accurate approaches to the measurement of functional residual capacity are the *gas dilution* methods and *body plethysmography*. The latter method is based on the changes in thoracic gas volume that occur with pressure changes; FRC calculated from gas dilution methods may differ from plethysmographically measured FRC. There is a physiological basis to this difference, and in many labs both methods are routinely used to measure FRC.

Basic Principles

In general, gas dilution volume measurements involve the addition of a tracer gas to a closed or open system, part of which includes the lungs. By studying the dilution of the tracer gas within the system, one may determine the absolute volume of the lungs. The two approaches are the *equilibration* and the *washout* or *elimination* techniques, used when the lungs form part of a closed, rebreathing, or an open, nonrebreathing system, respectively. The basic principles of the two approaches are presented in the following sections.

Equilibration Method   When a subject rebreathes from a spirometer system containing a known volume and concentration of tracer gas, the gas will distribute from the spirometer into both the lungs and spirometer. By measuring the change in tracer gas concentration after equilibrium, the new volume of distribution composed of the lungs and spirometer combined can be calculated. Because the final volume of the system consists of the volume of spirometer plus the lungs, lung volume (V_L) is determined according to the following equation:

$$V_L = \left(V_S \frac{F_i}{F_f} \right) - V_S \qquad \text{(Eq. 6-3)}$$

where Vs is the volume of the spirometer and connecting conduits, and F_i and F_f are the initial and final fractional concentrations of tracer gas.

The equilibration method requires a tracer gas that can be distributed quickly throughout the lungs. Such a gas must be biologically inert with little significant absorption or diffusion, and its concentration easily measured. Helium is most commonly used, although argon, xenon, or hydrogen may be substituted.

Resident Gas Washout Method A concept similar to the equilibration method is the washout method, in which a tracer gas resident in the lungs is eliminated or "washed out" by breathing a gas mixture free of the tracer gas. One of two techniques may be employed. In the *reservoir technique*, the expired gas is collected into a large reservoir, such as a Tissot spirometer, over a period of time long enough to render intrapulmonary concentration nearly zero. The mixed expired gas is analyzed for the concentration of the tracer gas. The principle is similar to the equilibration method and employs the following equation:

$$V_L = \frac{F_E}{F_i - F_f} \times V_S \qquad \text{(Eq. 6-4)}$$

where F_E is the fractional concentration of the tracer in the mixed expired gas, and F_i and F_f are the initial and final end-tidal (alveolar) fractional concentrations of the tracer gas. Nitrogen is usually used as the tracer gas because it is already present in the alveolar gas and only slowly diffuses from blood and tissue into the alveolar gas. This technique requires a large-capacity gas collecting system and has been largely replaced by the *open analyzer technique,* in which exhaled gas is not collected, but rather, nitrogen volume and concentration are continually monitored and from which the volume and average nitrogen concentration of mixed expired gas may be computed.

Although residual volume is the only lung compartment that cannot be directly measured with a spirometer, it is common practice to measure functional residual capacity in place of residual volume, then compute residual volume by subtracting the expiratory reserve volume.

$$RV = FRC - ERV \qquad \text{(Eq. 6-5)}$$

ERV is obtained independently by spirometry. FRC is more reproducible than RV because it is measured at end-expiration during tidal breathing, a lung volume that results when the subject is completely relaxed.

Helium Equilibration Method

The closed-circuit helium equilibration or dilution method for determining FRC, which was first described for clinical use in 1941,[4] is still in common use today. Helium is used as the tracer gas because it is inert, readily obtained, and its concentration is easily measured. The equipment required is a spirometer system with separate inspiratory and expiratory ports modified to enable rebreathing and a sensor for measuring helium concentration in the system. A blower in the conduit keeps the gases well mixed. Carbon dioxide accumulation is prevented with a canister of CO_2 absorbent. Oxygen from an external source can be added to the system under control of the technician. Two approaches are the *constant volume* and *decreasing volume* techniques.

Constant Volume Technique   Herrald and McMichael first described a method for measuring FRC using oxygen dilution in a constant volume system.[5] Meneely and Kaltreider[6] modified the constant volume technique to use helium as the dilution tracer. Helium has thermal characteristics quite different from nitrogen or oxygen, permitting continuous analysis by the thermal conductivity method. Hydrogen, which was employed prior to this, has physical properties similar to helium but is dangerous when mixed with oxygen.

Prior to analysis, the dead space of a given spirometer system is determined by gas dilution if it is not known or specified by the manufacturer. After this step, the subject is connected to the system containing air while the flow rate of added oxygen is adjusted to maintain a constant end-tidal volume. The flow rate ranges from 250 to 300 ml/min. The subject is disconnected from the system and the oxygen cut off temporarily. Helium is added to the spirometer to bring the system's gas concentration to 12 to 15 percent, and the blower mixer is activated. After the helium concentration has equilibrated in the spirometer system, the measured helium concentration is recorded as the initial helium concentration. The subject is then switched into the circuit at the end of expiration (FRC) and rebreathes the mixture with a normal tidal pattern. The oxygen line is turned on coincident with the switching, delivering about 250 ml/min of oxygen. After 7 min (or when the helium concentration has stabilized), the subject is switched from the circuit at the end-tidal point, and the final helium concentration is recorded. FRC is calculated as

$$FRC = Vs \left(\frac{F_iHe - F_fHe}{F_fHe} \right) \qquad \text{(Eq. 6-6)}$$

where F_iHe and F_fHe are the initial and final fractional concentrations of helium, and Vs is the volume of the spirometer system and dead space. The volume loss from helium is only a few milliliters and may be considered negligible. The FRC obtained should be corrected to BTPS according to Equation 6-1.

Modern instrumentation has automated and simplified most of this procedure. Pushbuttons initiate automatic spirometer filling, helium injection, constant oxygen injection, and calculation of results, but the principle of operation is identical.

Decreasing Volume Technique   The decreasing volume technique avoids the necessity of bleeding oxygen into the system throughout the procedure. The method permits the volume of the spirometer system to decrease with time, and makes an important assumption that the well-mixed spirometer system is in equilibrium with the lungs during oxygen consumption. Although the method is simpler to perform than the constant volume technique, it is not as commonly employed because the assumption is not entirely valid and requires correction for accurate results.

The method described by Meneely and coworkers[7] with a Collins-type spirometer system is to add 1 liter of helium to an empty spirometer system, then

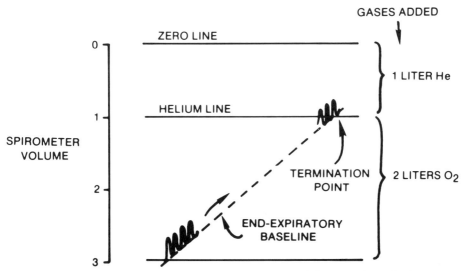

Fig. 6-3. Spirometer tracing during the measurement of functional residual capacity (FRC) by the decreasing volume technique of the helium equilibrium method. The spirometer is emptied and the zero line is transcribed. Then 1 liter of helium is added, and the helium line is transcribed. Next, about 2 liters of oxygen are added, mixed, and the initial helium concentration measured. The subject is then switched into the system and begins rebreathing. When the end-expiratory line crosses the helium line, the test is stopped, and the final helium concentration is measured. Calculations for FRC are given in text.

inscribe this volume as the "helium line" on the kymograph (Fig. 6-3). Next, 2 liters of oxygen are added to the system (sufficient to last 7 to 10 min during rebreathing). The patient is switched into the system at end-expiration and the volume excursions are recorded during rebreathing. The end-expiratory baseline will decrease at about 250 ml/min because of oxygen consumption. When the baseline of the tracing crosses the helium line, the spirometer system volume is equal to the initial volume after only helium was added. The helium concentration is recorded at the helium line crossing (Fig. 6-3). The equation for FRC is

$$FRC = \frac{V_{He}}{F_f He} - (V_{He} + V_D) \qquad \text{(Eq. 6-7)}$$

where V_{He} is the volume of helium added to the system, $F_f He$ is the final helium concentration, and V_D is the system dead space (a constant determined beforehand, as for the constant volume technique).

Nitrogen Equilibration Method

Nitrogen may be used in place of helium for closed-circuit equilibration measurement of FRC. The constant volume or decreasing volume techniques may be applied; they are identical with the helium method with two major differences:

1. Nitrogen is present in the lungs as the tracer gas, and the spirometer is filled with oxygen instead of air. A foreign gas need not be introduced. Gas equilibrates from the lungs into the spirometer instead of the spirometer to the lungs. The initial tracer gas concentration is measured as the end-tidal N_2 concentration while breathing room air.
2. Nitrogen, unlike helium, diffuses across the alveolar-capillary membrane at a rate great enough to affect calculations. The rate of diffusion of nitrogen into the lungs is about 40 ml/min (0.04 liter/min). For a 7-min test this is approximately 0.28 liter.

The calculation thus has the following form:

$$FRC = \frac{Vs(F_fN_2) - V_tN_2}{F_iN_2 - F_fN_2} \qquad \text{(Eq. 6-8)}$$

where Vs is the spirometer system volume at the end of the test, F_iN_2 and F_fN_2 are the initial and final fractional nitrogen concentrations, and V_tN_2 is the volume of nitrogen that diffused from the tissues into the lungs.

$$V_tN_2 = 0.04(\text{test time, min}) \qquad \text{(Eq. 6-9)}$$

Since the advent of rapid response nitrogen analyzers, the nitrogen equilibration method has largely been replaced by nitrogen washout methods.

Multibreath Nitrogen Washout Method

In this method, nitrogen normally present in the alveoli is washed out by repeated inhalations of a nitrogen-free gas, usually oxygen. As in the N_2 equilibrium method, no foreign tracer gas is required.[8] The nitrogen normally present in the lungs is used as the tracer gas. Two techniques have been used. The reservoir technique was the first developed, but has been largely replaced by the open analyzer technique.

Reservoir Technique Oxygen is inhaled while exhaled gas is collected in a Tissot spirometer (160 liter) or a large Douglas bag. The process begins with switching into the system at FRC and continues for 7 to 10 min, after which time it is assumed that the alveolar nitrogen concentration has been reduced to a negligible level (less than 1 percent). For analysis, FRC represents the initial volume at the start of the test and the change in alveolar nitrogen concentration is determined by the difference between the initial and final alveolar tracer concentrations. The final volume is the volume of gas collected in the spirometer or bag and its nitrogen concentration constitutes the final tracer concentration. The following formula is used for the test:

$$FRC = \frac{V_E(F_{E_{N_2}}) - V_tN_2}{F_iN_2 - F_fN_2} \qquad \text{(Eq. 6-10)}$$

where V_E is the total exhaled volume and system dead space, $F_{E_{N_2}}$ is the fractional nitrogen concentration in the mixed expired gas, V_tN_2 is the volume of nitrogen lost by diffusion from tissue into the lungs, and F_iN_2 and F_fN_2 are the initial and final end-tidal (alveolar) fractional nitrogen concentrations. Connection to oxygen for washout must occur precisely at end-tidal level to reflect FRC accurately. Correction must be made for the small amount of nitrogen (V_tN_2) that leaves the body tissues and diffuses into the lungs when alveolar nitrogen concentration decreases (Eq. 6-9).

Open Analyzer Technique The development of rapid-response nitrogen sensors has enabled a modification of the reservoir technique that eliminates the need for a bulky reservoir to collect the expired gas. Instantaneous expiratory flow and nitrogen concentration are continuously measured and the test continues until the end-tidal nitrogen concentration is less than 1 percent. The instantaneous product of expiratory flow and fractional nitrogen concentration is integrated, giving the total cumulative volume of exhaled nitrogen. FRC is calculated by

$$FRC = \frac{V_{E_{N_2}} - V_tN_2}{F_iN_2 - F_fN_2} \qquad \text{(Eq. 6-11)}$$

where $V_{E \cdot N_2}$ is the cumulative volume of exhaled nitrogen, V_tN_2 is the correction for nitrogen diffusion from the blood (Eq. 6-9), and F_iN_2 and F_fN_2 are the initial and final end-tidal (alveolar) fractional nitrogen concentrations, respectively.

Measurement of Residual Volume by Single-Breath Nitrogen Elimination

In practice, residual volume is usually calculated from FRC and ERV, as FRC is a more reproducible measurement. RV may be measured by multibreath gas dilution methods in a manner similar to FRC by having the patient begin the test at his residual volume. These methods are difficult, prone to error, and are not used in the clinical laboratory. An alternative to obtaining RV by calculation from FRC is to measure it by the single-breath nitrogen method. The method is useful because the single-breath nitrogen test is commonly used to measure closing volume and for gas distribution studies.

The single-breath nitrogen method for RV is based on the principle of the open-circuit multibreath nitrogen washout method. The subject exhales completely down to residual volume; therefore, the nitrogen in his lungs is present only in the residual volume. The subject then inhales nitrogen-free gas (oxygen) to total lung capacity and momentarily holds his breath, during which time the nitrogen in the residual volume redistributes itself into a new volume, TLC. Then, the subject exhales while nitrogen concentration and volume of the expirate are measured (see Fig. 7-15). The equation for RV is

$$RV = V_E \left(\frac{F_{E_{N_2}}}{F_iN_2 - F_{E_{N_2}}} \right) \qquad \text{(Eq. 6-12)}$$

Final nitrogen concentration, $F_{E_{N_2}}$, is the mean expired nitrogen concentration. Because concentration varies widely over the exhalation, it must be calculated by measuring the area under the N_2 curve and dividing by the expired volume, V_E. Initial N_2 concentration, F_iN_2, is assumed to be approximately the same as the atmosphere (0.81) or is measured as the end-expiratory concentration of nitrogen while breathing room air. The exhaled volume must equal the inhaled volume. No correction for nitrogen excretion is required. The method has a very important assumption, that equilibrium distribution of nitrogen occurs during a single inspiration. This may be valid for normal lungs, but does not hold for lungs with obstruction where air trapping and inhomogeneous gas distribution occur.

Measurement of Total Lung Capacity by Single-Breath Nitrogen Elimination

In practice, total lung capacity is most often calculated as the sum of measured functional residual capacity (FRC) and inspiratory capacity (IC) in place of direct measurement, as FRC is a more reproducible measurement. FRC is measured by gas dilution or plethysmographic methods and IC by spirometry.

It is also possible to measure TLC by a gas dilution method. For subjects without significant obstructive disease a simple modification of the single-breath method for RV results in

$$TLC = V_E \left(\frac{F_iN_2}{F_iN_2 - F_fN_2} \right) \qquad \text{(Eq. 6-13)}$$

The test is performed in an identical fashion to the single-breath RV method.

Selection of a Gas Dilution Method

A laboratory may limit its gas dilution studies to one gas, usually helium or nitrogen.

When helium is used, FRC is usually measured by the constant volume equilibrium technique. The advantages of helium are that it is readily available and the instrumentation needed is generally not as expensive as that for faster nitrogen analyzers. Its disadvantages are that dynamic washout studies are not possible and helium must be supplied in tanks.

Nitrogen methods are usually preferable if costs permit, as nitrogen washout methods and single-breath tests, which can be performed with the same instrumentation, are complementary and provide more information. In addition, because the atmosphere is the source of nitrogen, only oxygen need be supplied.

Sources of Error in Gas Dilution Methods

Five main sources of error in gas dilution studies have been identified[4]:

1. Incomplete mixing of gases in the lungs and spirometer will result in over- or underestimation of equilibrium gas concentration, depending on the method used. This can be partially compensated for by extending the time for equilibrium in patients with obstruction, or by continuously observing the tracer gas concentration during the test.
2. Technical errors in measuring gas concentrations can reduce accuracy, but careful calibration and maintenance reduce this source of error.
3. Diffusion of gases between the lung and blood can produce an error. The error can be partially controlled by adding correction factors to the calculations.
4. Switching the subject into the system must occur at the resting end-expiratory level or the value measured will not be the FRC. Careful attention to technique will minimize this error.
5. The "nitrogen lag" effect occurs when the decreasing volume variation of the closed-circuit equilibrium method is used, resulting in unequal concentration of tracer gas in the alveoli and spirometer system.

PLETHYSMOGRAPHIC METHOD FOR FUNCTIONAL RESIDUAL CAPACITY

Principles of Plethysmography

The body plethysmograph is a large, airtight box that allows the simultaneous determination of pressure-volume relationships in the thorax of a person placed inside the apparatus. These pressure-volume relationships are used to estimate intrathoracic lung volume. The principle is applied in one of three ways: pressure, volume, or flow plethysmography.

Pressure plethysmography, the most commonly employed method, is based on Boyle's law, which is derived from the behavior of ideal gases as described by the ideal gas law. The basic plethysmograph equation for thoracic gas volume, derived in Appendix C, is

$$V_{TG} = P_B \left(\frac{\Delta V_L}{\Delta Pao} \right) \qquad \text{(Eq. 6-14)}$$

In order to estimate the gas volume of the thorax (VTG) we must know the atmospheric pressure (PB) plus the pressure-volume relationship of the gas contained within the thorax. We can measure the pressure change in the thorax by the pressure gauge at the airway opening or mouth (ΔPao), since alveolar pressure is equal to mouth pressure when gas flow is blocked by a closed shutter. Measuring the volume change of the thorax (ΔVL) is not straightforward because the container is closed and no air is allowed to be exchanged. Volume change can be estimated with a pressure-type body plethysmograph from the pressure change within the box. The pressure-volume relationship of the box is established by calibrating the box, in which a known volume (ΔV_{box}) is cyclically injected at the expected respiratory frequency with the subject in place and the box pressure change (ΔP_{box}) noted. The acoustic compliance of the box (C_{box}) is defined by

$$C_{box} = \frac{\Delta V_{box}}{\Delta P_{box}} \qquad \text{(Eq. 6-15)}$$

An unknown volume change of the thorax within the box ($\Delta V'_{box}$) can then be determined from the pressure change.

$$\Delta V'_{box} = C_{box}(\Delta P_{box}) \qquad \text{(Eq. 6-16)}$$

The final equation, as used in the pressure plethysmograph, is in the following form:

$$V_{TG} = P_B \left(\frac{\Delta P_{box}}{\Delta Pao} \right) \times C_{box} \qquad \text{(Eq. 6-17)}$$

The ratio of box-to-mouth pressures is easily measured if the box and lung pressure signals are displayed on the X-Y oscilloscope. The slope of the resulting line corresponds to the ratio of pressures and VTG is easily calculated. Equation 6-17 is based on a number of assumptions about gas behavior, but nonetheless provides a good estimate of volume. The clinical application of Equation 6-17 to lung volume measurement is discussed in the next section.

Volume and flow displacement plethysmographs are a more recent development that allows measurement of volume change directly through use of sensitive instrumentation, obviating the need for calibration of the box to determine its acoustic compliance. The instrumentation is generally more complex than that for pressure plethysmography and does not provide any significant increase in accuracy for clinical purposes.

Functional Residual Capacity by VTG

Body plethysmographic determination of gas volume is frequently applied to determine functional residual capacity.[9] The method is simple and rapid but differs in principle from gas dilution methods. Proper interpretation necessitates an understanding of these differences. The body plethysmographic method measures all gas contained within the thoracic cavity (thoracic gas volume, V_{TG}), in contrast to the gas dilution methods, which do not measure "trapped gas" (gas not in communication with the airways). As a result, V_{TG} estimation of FRC may differ from FRC measurement by gas dilution methods in certain disease states. This is discussed in more detail in the next section.

Body plethysmography requires cooperation from the subject; therefore, the operation of the equipment and the details of the procedure should be explained to the subject. The subject is placed in the box and the door sealed. Temperature equilibrium takes place with the box vent open for the next 3 to 5 min or until the end-expiratory baseline stabilizes. The oscilloscope is switched to the flow-box pressure mode ($\dot{V}/P_{box}$) with the shutter open, and the subject is asked to start normal tidal breathing. He is encouraged to relax so that end-expiration corresponds to FRC. Attainment of a stable breathing pattern is detected by development of a stable oscilloscope trace in the form of a loop that retraces itself (Fig. 6-4A). At the end of an expiration the shutter is closed, the oscilloscope switched to the mouth pressure-box pressure mode (Pao/P_{box}), and the subject is asked to breathe several times against the shutter. The resulting trace of mouth pressure versus box pressure is nearly linear (Fig. 6-4B). The tangent of the angle with the baseline θ (tan θ) is recorded with the aid of a commercial protractor, which corresponds to the uncalibrated slope of the curve. The thoracic gas volume is calculated as follows:

$$V_{TG} = \frac{(P_B - P_{H_2O})}{\tan \theta} \left(\frac{V_{box}CAL}{Pao\ CAL} \right) \qquad \text{(Eq. 6-18)}$$

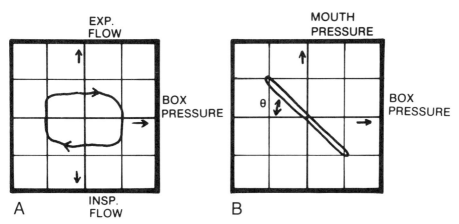

Fig. 6-4. Oscilloscope tracings obtained during the measurement of V_{TG} by body plethysmography. (A) Initial tracing with the shutter open during quiet tidal breathing in the flow-box pressure mode. Once the loop has stabilized, the shutter is closed at end-expiration and the system switched to the mouth pressure-box pressure mode, and the subject begins panting. (B) The loop with the shutter closed approaches a line, the slope of which is proportional to the V_{TG}. Calculations are given in text.

The pressures are expressed in centimeters of H_2O with ($P_B - P_{H_2O}$) equal to 970 cm H_2O at sea level. The value tan θ corresponds to the slope $\Delta Pao/\Delta P_B$ and is read from the protractor on the screen. The two calibration values represent the mouth pressure and box volume values corresponding to a single division on the x and y axes of the oscilloscope grid, respectively. These are assumed to be constant and are usually calibrated by the manufacturer, but if the subject is larger than average a correction for his extra displacement must be made. The correction is either specified by the manufacturer or must be determined experimentally, as described previously, with a volume pump.

Comparison of Plethysmography with Gas Dilution (The Trapped Gas Concept)

Gas spaces in the normal lung are *communicating* spaces because they are well ventilated via the airways. Gas dilution methods and thoracic gas volume (plethysmographic) methods give comparable results for FRC in normal subjects. In the diseased lung there may be "trapped gas" that is either totally isolated from the airways or is very slow to equilibrate. The isolated gas spaces are termed *noncommunicating* because the gas within them does not readily exchange with the air carried by the airways.

Noncommunicating spaces may be extrapulmonary or intrapulmonary. *Extrapulmonary* gas is of two types. A pneumothorax is one type of extrapulmonary gas. Because it is within the pleural cavity it is compressible; it is included in measurements of V_{TG}, but not the FRC measured by gas dilution methods because the gas is not in communication with the airways and therefore does not equilibrate. A second type of extrapulmonary gas is gas contained within abdominal organs, which may be detected in the measurement of V_{TG}, even though the contribution is usually negligible.[10]

Intrapulmonary noncommunicating gas spaces are also of two types. The first includes cysts, bullae, and cavitary lesions, as well as the gas within a pulmonary segment or lobe behind a bronchial obstruction. Such spaces represent truly "trapped gas." Trapped gas resulting from noncommunicating spaces accounts for a significant difference between the FRC determined by plethysmography and by gas dilution methods. The second type of intrapulmonary trapped gas is that contained within *slowly communicating* spaces. Ventilation of these areas of diseased lung is retarded (but not prohibited) by parenchymal destruction or airway disease. The 7-min equilibrium time limit routinely used for gas dilution methods may not permit adequate gas equilibrium with the slow spaces; hence, these spaces behave as trapped gas. Extending the time limit of the gas dilution test (prolonged washout or equilibration) permits improved gas dilution within the slow spaces. The difference between gas dilution FRC and FRC by plethysmography in emphysematous subjects can be minimized by extending equilibration time.

The *volume of trapped gas,* or difference in FRC determined by gas dilution and plethysmography, is often reported by laboratories. It is most often a result of slow-communicating intrapulmonary spaces[11] and helps to assess the degree of disturbed intrapulmonary gas mixing.

Sources of Error in Plethysmography

Technical and procedural errors are easily introduced if care is not taken. Small pressure changes must be monitored, necessitating sensitive equipment. Careful calibration is required on a frequent basis. Leaks in the box will alter its pressure-volume relationship and possibly affect measurement. A common procedural error is caused by the patient's inability to relax, resulting in an unconscious increase in FRC. This can be minimized by careful instruction and practice with the subject.

An unavoidable source of error results from the physical properties of the lungs. Plethysmography is based on Boyle's law, which assumes *isothermal* volume changes in which temperature equilibrium is reached. Panting maneuvers occur rapidly; therefore; temperature equilibrium may not occur in the lungs. In normal subjects with normal alveolar structure with high surface area, the error is minimal. In diseased lungs with dilated air spaces, expansion and compression may be *adiabatic*, with incomplete temperature equilibrium and underestimation of volumes. This error can be reduced to some extent by avoiding high panting frequencies during the test procedure.

RADIOGRAPHIC METHODS

Several investigators have shown that analysis of chest radiographs permits reasonably accurate estimation of static lung volumes. All these methods require measurement of certain lung field dimensions and subsequent calculation of volume. The many assumptions about the shape of the lungs, volume of capillary blood and pulmonary tissue, and volume of mediastinal tissues required to perform the calculations limit the accuracy of these methods. They do not replace conventional volume measurements, but are useful in situations in which the subject is unable to perform the routine tests; they are also valuable for current or retrospective determinations when pulmonary function tests have not been or cannot be performed but chest radiographs are available. All methods require standardized techniques for obtaining the radiographs. Each method has a specified technique regarding patient position, posture, and tube-to-film distance. Several methods for determining TLC will be briefly introduced, and one will be detailed for use.

Early Approaches

The first attempt at volume determination from radiographs was reported by Hurtado and Fray.[12] A planimeter was used to measure the frontal area of the lungs from a 6-ft posteroanterior chest radiograph. The area was multiplied by the thickness of the thorax, giving a value called the *radiological chest volume* (RCV). A correction factor of one-third (obtained from regression analysis) is applied to estimate TLC.

Another radiographic approach introduced by Kovach and coworkers[13] treated the lungs as if they had the shape of a paraboloid of revolution, a solid derived by revolving a parabola around its principal axis. This shape, with the mediastinal structures excluded, has the appearance of a pair of lungs. However, it offers no increase in precision over other methods.

The most widely used technique is the ellipsoid method of Barnhard and coworkers.[14,15] It represents the lungs as a stack of five elliptical cylindroids from apex to base, with dimensions obtained from 6-ft posteroanterior and lateral radiographs. The volume of the cylindroids are individually calculated and summed to give the final volume. Use of computer techniques makes this method rapid as well as accurate. Application of this method will be discussed in the next section.

Another planimetric method using posteroanterior and lateral films has been reported by Harris and coworkers.[16] It does not have the accuracy of the ellipsoid method, but has the advantages of simplicity and speed of calculation.

Total Lung Capacity by the Barnhard Method

The ellipsoid method of Barnhard and associates[14] is described in more detail in this section. Standard 6-ft posteroanterior and left lateral chest films at full inspiration are required. The lung fields are outlined and divided into five segments by six horizontal lines in the following manner (Fig. 6-5):

1. The apex of the lungs
2. A line 2.75 cm below line 1
3. A line 2.75 cm below line 2
4. A line at the higher dome of the diaphragm
5. A line midway between lines 3 and 4
6. A line at the posterior sulcus on the lateral view, extending the same distance below line 4 on the PA view

The volume of each segment is computed as the volume of an elliptical structure.

$$Vseg = \frac{\pi}{4} \times diam_{PA} \times diam_{TR} \times ht \times 0.73 \qquad \text{(Eq. 6-19)}$$

where $diam_{PA}$ and $diam_{TR}$ represent the posteroanterior and transverse diameters, respectively, of the middle of the lung fields, and ht the height of the segment. All measurements are made in centimeters. The constant 0.73 corrects for divergence of the x-ray beam. The five segment volumes are summed to give the total thoracic volume (TTV).

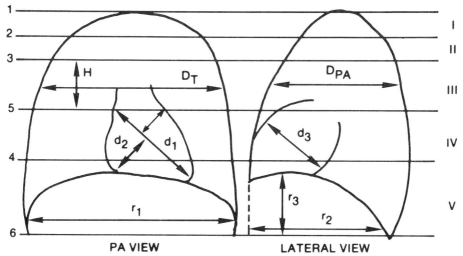

Fig. 6-5. Outline of the lungs and heart from standard posteroanterior and lateral chest radiographs used in the calculation of total lung capacity (TLC) by a radiographic method. Horizontal lines 1 through 6 were drawn according to the directions given in text, dividing the lung fields into five segments (I through V). The segment volumes are calculated and summed to give the total thoracic volume (TTV). TTV is corrected by subtracting the calculated volume of the heart, the volume of the lung parenchyma, and the estimated pulmonary blood volume to give TLC. Calculations are detailed in text.

The volume of the heart is computed as the volume of an ellipsoid using the dimensions shown in the Figure 6-5. The long axis (d_1) is drawn from the junction of the superior vena cava and the right atrium to the apex of the heart. The transverse diameter (d_2) is the sum of the two longest radial distances from the long axis, and the anteroposterior diameter (d_3) is the largest distance in the lateral projection perpendicular to the long axis of the heart. The heart volume is calculated as

$$V_H = \frac{\pi}{6} \times d_1 \times d_2 \times d_3 \times 0.73 \qquad \text{(Eq. 6-20)}$$

The volume of each hemidiaphragm is computed separately, using the dimensions outlined in Figure 6-5, according to the following formula:

$$V_{DI} = \frac{\pi}{6} \times \frac{r_1}{2} \times r_2 \times r_3 \times 0.73 \qquad \text{(Eq. 6-21)}$$

The lung parenchymal volume is estimated as 130 ml. The pulmonary blood volume is estimated as 15 percent of the total blood volume (TBV). In the initial report the volume was obtained from a table, but a quick estimate for TBV is

$$\begin{aligned} TBV_{male} &= \text{wt (kg)} \times 77 \text{ ml} \\ TBV_{female} &= \text{wt (kg)} \times 67 \text{ ml} \end{aligned} \qquad \text{(Eq. 6-22)}$$

The pulmonary blood volume (PBV) is estimated as

$$PBV = TBV(0.15) \qquad \text{(Eq. 6-23)}$$

The final calculation for TLC is

$$TLC \simeq TTV - V_H - 2V_{DI} - 130 - PBV \qquad \text{(Eq. 6-24)}$$

SIGNIFICANCE OF LUNG VOLUMES

Lung volumes can be altered by disease, but may also be affected by several factors in healthy individuals. Abnormal volumes alone are not diagnostic of a specific etiology, but can lend support to clinical diagnoses and aid in the assessment of the severity of disease and response to treatment.

Factors Affecting Volumes in Health

The repeated measurement of a biological variable, such as lung volume, is associated with an inherent variability. Vital capacity is a volume that, for a given subject, is highly repeatable with a small standard deviation if the test is properly performed. Repeat measurements of vital capacity have been shown to approximate a normal distribution.[4] Mean vital capacity has been shown to increase when performed repeatedly and frequently over long periods of time.[17] This may represent a training effect.

The effect of age on VC has been documented. VC is greatest when an individual is about 25 to 30 years old,[18] with a gradual decrease thereafter of about 200 ml per decade. RV and the RV/TLC ratio tend to increase as VC falls. TLC itself decreases less than 100 ml per decade.[19]

Posture affects lung volumes; for this reason all subjects should be tested in the erect position. The abdominal organs exert a negative pressure on the diaphragm in the erect position, and a positive pressure in the supine position. FRC undergoes the largest decrease with the supine position; TLC falls as well. Studies of VC show conflicting results, but most agree that VC decreases in the supine position.[20,21] These changes are caused by changes in the position of the diaphragm and in chest wall dimensions. The volume of blood in the thorax has also been shown to increase.[22]

Subconscious alteration during testing may affect FRC measurements. When trying to perform a test according to directions, the subject is made aware of his breathing pattern and may initiate or perform the FRC test at a lung volume slightly different from his true FRC. Having the subject relax tends to minimize this effect.

Lung Volume Patterns in Disease

Obstructive and restrictive disease processes tend to alter lung volumes in characteristic ways, regardless of the specific etiology causing the dysfunction.

Obstructive Disease Acute reversible obstruction, such as occurs in asthma, is associated with difficulty in exhalation that tends to reduce vital capacity at the expense of an increase in FRC and RV. This is a form of dynamic air trapping. TLC is slightly increased, as shown on radiographs, by depression of the diaphragms. Tests of vital capacity may underestimate true VC because a VC maneuver may be interrupted by air hunger. These changes are reversible with return of baseline lung function.

Chronic obstruction results in similar but permanent changes. TLC increases by enlargement of the chest wall dimensions as well as flattening of the diaphragm. RV is increased out of proportion to an increase in TLC because of chronic air trapping. The RV/TLC ratio thus increases with RV. These changes are largely irreversible because of the chronicity of the disease. TLC expansion reaches an anatomic limit with time, but continuation of the disease process results in progressive loss of VC in the face of increasing RV. Measured VC can be reduced to 0.5 liter or less in severe disease.

Restrictive Disease Restrictive dysfunction is characterized by volume loss from space-occupying lesions, such as masses or bullae, by loss of volume from lung tissue resection, by restriction of chest wall movement from musculoskeletal disease, or by restriction of lung expansion by loss of compliance from parenchymal disease. Because all volumes are affected in restrictive disorders, a reduction in vital capacity is associated with a reduction in RV and TLC. Airway function is maintained, so tests of forced expiratory mechanics are normal provided they are corrected for the decrease in VC.

REFERENCES

1. Hutchinson J: Pneumatic apparatus for valuing the respiratory powers. Lancet 1:390, 1844
2. Christie RV: The lung volume and its subdivisions. I. Methods of measurement. J Clin Invest 11:1099, 1932
3. Cournand A, Richards W, Darling RC: Graphic tracings of respiration in study of pulmonary disease. Am Rev Tuberc 4:487, 1939
4. Meneely GR, Kaltreider NL: Use of helium for determination of pulmonary capacity. Proc Soc Exper Biol Med 46:266, 1941
5. Herrald FJC, McMichael J: Determination of lung volume: A simple constant volume modification of Christie's method. Proc Roy Soc Lond 126:491, 1939
6. Meneely GR, Kaltreider NL: The volume of the lung determined by helium dilution. J Clin Invest 28:129, 1949
7. Meneely GR, Ball COT, Kory RC, et al: A simplified closed circuit helium dilution method for the determination of the residual volume of the lungs. Am J Med 28:824, 1960

8. Darling RC, Cournand A, Richards DW Jr: Studies on the intrapulmonary mixture of gases. III. An open circuit method for measuring residual air. J Clin Invest 19:609, 1940
9. Dubois AB, Botelho SY, Bedell GN, et al: A rapid plethysmographic method for measuring thoracic gas volume: A comparison with a nitrogen washout method for measuring functional residual capacity in normal subjects. J Clin Invest 35:322, 1956
10. Brown R, Hoppin FG, Ingram RH Jr, et al: Influence of abdominal gas on the Boyle's law determination of thoracic gas volume. J Appl Physiol: Resp Environ Exer Physiol 44:469, 1978
11. Rechel G: Differences between intrathoracic gas measured by the body plethysmograph and functional residual capacity determined by gas dilution methods. Prog Resp Dis 4:188, 1969
12. Hurtado A, Fray WW: Studies of total pulmonary capacity and its subdivisions. II. Correlation with physical and radiologic measurements. J Clin Invest 12:807, 1933
13. Kovach JC, Avedian V, Morales G, Poulos P: Lung compartment determination. J Thorac Surg 31:452, 1956
14. Barnhard HJ, Pierce JA, Joyce JW, Bates JH: Roentgenographic determination of total lung capacity. Am J Med 28:51, 1960
15. Ferris BG: Epidemiology standardization project. Standardized radiologic measurement of TLC. Am Rev Resp Dis 118:99, 1978
16. Harris TR, Pratt PC, Kilburn KH: Total lung capacity measured by roentgenograms. Am J Med 50:756, 1971
17. Mills JN: Variability of the vital capacity in the normal human subject. J Physiol (Lond) 110:76, 1949
18. Bergland E, Birath G, Bjure J, et al: Spirometric studies in normal subjects. I. Forced expirograms in subjects between 7 and 70 years of age. Acta Med Scand 173:185, 1963
19. Needham CD, Rogan MC, McDonald J: Normal standards for lung volumes, intrapulmonary gas-mixing and maximum breathing capacity. Thorax 9:313, 1954
20. Svanberg L: Influence of posture on the lung volumes, ventilation and circulation of normals. Scand J Clin Lab Invest, suppl., 25:1, 1957
21. Moreno F, Lyons HA: Effect of posture on lung volumes. J Appl Physiol 16:27, 1961
22. Sjostrand T: Determination of changes in the intrathoracic blood volume in man. Acta Physiol Scand 22:114, 1951

7

Mechanics of the Respiratory System

Steven A. Conrad, M.D.

Measurement of static and dynamic properties of the respiratory system is useful in identifying various types of dysfunction. Static properties are assessed while the lungs and chest wall are at rest, that is, in the absence of airflow or muscle contraction, and are used to determine the *elastic properties* of the lung parenchyma. Dynamic properties are assessed during active breathing or respiratory muscle contraction. By recording exhaled gas volume and flow during a forced expiration, several indexes of *airflow dynamics* can be measured; they are used principally for the detection and characterization of obstructive airway diseases. More sensitive assessment of *resistive properties* of the tracheobronchial tree and respiratory system can be made using special techniques. *Maximal respiratory pressures* provide information on respiratory muscle function. In addition to these static and dynamic measurements, characterization of *small airway function* is described in this chapter.

ELASTIC PROPERTIES

The inherent elasticity of the lungs may be altered by disease, and lung elasticity is measured by determination of *static pulmonary compliance,* a measure of the distensibility of the lungs. It is defined as the ratio of the change in lung volume to a change in transpulmonary pressure applied in the absence of airflow, or

$$Cst(L) = \frac{\Delta V_L}{\Delta P_L} \qquad \text{(Eq. 7-1)}$$

A high compliance (greater distensibility) means that application of a given pressure results in a relatively large volume change. A low compliance means that a smaller volume results from the given pressure, or that a higher transpul-

129

monary pressure is required to inflate the lungs to the same volume. Both high and low compliances may represent abnormality.

The compliance of the respiratory system is not constant over the entire range of vital capacity (see Chapter 2). Plotting volume-pressure relationships over the range of vital capacity results in a curve rather than a straight line (see Fig. 2-1). For consistency in measurement, compliance is taken at a particular volume, conventionally, functional residual capacity, a reproducible volume at which point the curve is most nearly linear.

The two components of total *static respiratory system* compliance are the *static pulmonary* [Cst(L)] and *static chest wall* [Cst(w)] compliances. The relationship between them is

$$\frac{1}{Cst(\text{RS})} = \frac{1}{Cst(\text{L})} + \frac{1}{Cst(\text{w})} \qquad \text{(Eq. 7-2)}$$

because the reciprocal of compliance, termed *elastance*, is additive.

Because elastic properties are assessed in the absence of a forced expiration, airway and extrapulmonary factors are not involved. Static pulmonary compliance reflects inherent properties of the pulmonary parenchyma. Pulmonary compliance is usually of more clinical interest than chest wall compliance because the majority of diseases affect the lungs rather than the chest wall. The measurement of chest wall compliance, however, may implicate the chest wall as the etiology of a restrictive ventilatory dysfunction when the parenchyma is normal.

Static Pulmonary Compliance

Pulmonary compliance is obtained from a static volume-transpulmonary pressure curve constructed from simultaneous measurements of lung volume and transpulmonary pressure. The testing apparatus consists of a spirometer system with a shutter mechanism at the mouth, and a differential pressure transducer for the measurement of transpulmonary pressure as the difference between mouth and esophageal pressures (Fig. 7-1). Changes in *esophageal pressure* (Pes) approximate changes in the pleural pressure.[1,2]

Direct measurement of pleural pressure is an invasive procedure with potentially serious complications. Esophageal pressure measurements are made using a small-diameter catheter with a thin-walled balloon on the distal end that measures 10 cm in length and several millimeters in diameter. The balloon is partially inflated and pressures are measured through a port at the proximal end of the catheter. The balloon capacity is about 10 ml; distention of the balloon does not occur until about 5 ml of air is injected. The volume injected for measurement ranges from 0.5 to 2.0 ml, depending on balloon size, so pressure generated by tension within the balloon wall may be avoided.[3]

Alveolar pressure is estimated by measurement of pressure at the mouthpiece proximal to the shutter, since during static conditions the pressure at the airway

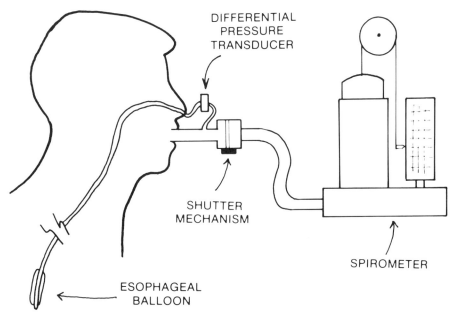

Fig. 7-1. Diagram of apparatus for the measurement of static compliance. The differential pressure transducer measures transpulmonary pressure as the difference between esophageal pressure and proximal airway pressure. The shutter is used to stop expiration at volume increments of about 500 ml to collect a series of volume-pressure points. The spirometer records the exhaled volume increments.

opening (Pao) equals alveolar pressure. *Transpulmonary pressure* (PL) is therefore obtained by measuring the difference between esophageal and mouth pressures when the glottis is closed and the respiratory system has come to rest:

$$P_L = P_A - Ppl \approx Pao - Pes \qquad \text{(Eq. 7-3)}$$

A volume-pressure curve may be constructed during inspiration or expiration. The static volume-pressure curve measured during an expiration from total lung capacity (TLC) is different from one measured during inspiration from residual volume (RV). This difference results from *hysteresis*. It is believed to be the result of differences in alveolar surface tension. Because the volume history of the lungs affects the volume-pressure relationship,[4] it is conventional to construct a curve during expiration. If hysteresis is to be studied, then both curves must be constructed. Measurements are made in the upright position.

Posture can affect the relationship between esophageal and pleural pressures. Esophageal pressure changes have been shown to approximate pleural pressure changes well in the upright, lateral, or prone positions, with little difference between them. The supine position should be avoided because it results in overestimation of pleural pressure, presumably from esophageal compression by the heart.[5] The esophageal catheter is lubricated and passed through a topically anesthetized naris for a distance of 36 to 40 cm to a position in the distal third of the esophagus. Placement of the catheter is somewhat unpleasant initially, but once in place it causes little discomfort and is usually well tolerated. A differential pressure transducer is placed between the catheter and a port on the mouthpiece.

After initial placement, the balloon is distended to capacity to remove any distortion incurred during placement, then opened to the atmosphere and deflated by having the subject perform a Valsalva maneuver. A syringe is attached, and while the subject relaxes, the required volume of air for measurement is injected into the balloon. Proper balloon placement is assured by noting negative pressure changes with inspiration. Positive pressure swings indicate balloon placement in the stomach. An alternative method of insertion is to place the balloon in the stomach, then withdraw it 10 cm past the point that pressure swings indicate it has moved into the esophagus.

The procedure begins by having the subject inhale fully to TLC with the mouthpiece in place, followed by closure of the shutter. Pressure is measured at TLC, then the shutter is opened and expiration initiated. The shutter is closed at volume decrements of approximately 0.5 liter, during which time the subject relaxes and transpulmonary pressure is recorded. This continues to residual volume. One of the measurement points should be at functional residual capacity (FRC). Several curves should be constructed to assure uniformity of results. Esophageal contractions can raise esophageal pressure and invalidate the results. Curves with contractions evidenced by higher pressures should be disregarded.

Static pulmonary compliance [Cst(L)] corresponds to the slope of the curve at a given point. The measurement is made near FRC, a reproducible point within the range where the compliance curve is most linear. Compliance is calculated by dividing the volume change (ΔV_L) between FRC and the volume approximately 0.5 liter greater by the difference in transpulmonary pressure [$\Delta P(ao\text{-}es)$] at these two volumes. The compliance value is reported in liters per centimeter of H_2O.

The volume of the lung at which compliance is measured affects the value of the compliance. The compliance per liter of absolute volume or *specific pulmonary compliance* [Cst(L)/V_L] is relatively constant in the normal lung, and permits comparison of lungs of different sizes.[6] By convention V_L is taken to be FRC. Cst(L)/FRC is obtained by dividing the compliance measured at FRC by the FRC. A less commonly employed alternative to normalizing compliance to FRC is to normalize compliance to the predicted vital capacity, giving the value Cst(L)/ VC_{pred}. It has been shown that static pulmonary compliance varies linearly with vital capacity.[7]

Normal values for static pulmonary compliance have a mean value of approximately 0.30 liter/cm H_2O with a range of about 0.15 to 0.45 liter/cm H_2O.[8,9] The development of interstitial fibrosis or interstitial pulmonary edema will decrease static compliance, as will a loss of surfactant. Closure of airways or airway obstruction by a foreign body or secretions will reduce alveolar volume available for expansion and therefore also decrease compliance. Loss of elastic fibers in the interstitium of the lungs, such as occurs in emphysema, will result in increased compliance.

Total Respiratory System Compliance

The technique for measuring total *static respiratory system compliance* [Cst(RS)] is similar to that for pulmonary compliance, except that the pressure difference measured is between the airway opening and the body surface P(ao-bs), so that there is no need for intraesophageal pressure measurement. The technique does not allow the separation of pulmonary and chest wall components. Its primary usefulness in the clinical laboratory lies in the ability to determine static *chest wall compliance* [Cst(w)] by subtracting the pulmonary component:

$$\frac{1}{Cst(w)} = \frac{1}{Cst(RS)} - \frac{1}{Cst(L)} \qquad \text{(Eq. 7-4)}$$

This measurement may be useful if chest wall abnormalities like kyphoscoliosis are thought to contribute to a restrictive ventilatory dysfunction. Another major use is to follow changes in lung compliance in patients on mechanical ventilation (Chapter 13). Acute changes in total compliance reflect changes in lung compliance, as chest wall compliance changes little over brief intervals.

DYNAMICS OF AIRFLOW

Spirometry, with measurement of expired volume or flow at the mouth during forced breathing, provides a rapid and simple means of characterizing airway function. Three methods are in use. The *forced expiratory spirogram* is a graphic recording of volume exhaled as a function of time. A simple spirometer with a kymograph is the only equipment required. The *flow-volume loop* is a graph of inspiratory and expiratory flow as a function of exhaled volume. More instrumentation is required, but it offers a few advantages over the simple spirogram. *Maximal voluntary ventilation* has a role in the evaluation of respiratory muscle endurance in patients with lung disease. It may also be useful for demonstrating air trapping in the presence of airway obstruction.

Forced Expiratory Spirogram

The spirometer is prepared by checking the breathing circuit for proper attachment and absence of leaks. If the spirometer is a water-seal or dry-rolling type, the bell or piston is manually moved from the empty to full positions to assure smooth operation. If a water-seal spirometer is used, the water level should be checked and directional flutter valves removed to minimize resistance to breathing.

The procedure is explained to the subject, who is comfortably seated with the mouthpiece at the level of his mouth. Although no clinically significant difference results from the standing position,[10] it is customary to use the sitting position; in any case, the same position should be used at each visit. Restrictive clothing should be loosened. The spirometer bell is placed in midposition and the kymograph or X-Y recorder started at a slow speed.

The subject begins natural tidal breathing. When a stable pattern is noted, the subject is asked to take a full inspiration to TLC, then exhale forcefully into the spirometer. Just prior to exhalation the rotational speed of the kymograph (or pen speed of the X-Y recorder) is manually (or automatically) increased for better resolution. Because accurate results depend on proper performance of the test, the procedure requires continuous verbal encouragement throughout expiration. It is helpful to practice with the subject on the first session if he is unfamiliar with the test, unless the subject has severe obstructive lung disease or muscle wasting. Excessive testing in these groups can lead to fatigue and inability to complete the tests.

Once a spirogram is recorded, its beginning and ending limits are identified and indexes of forced expiration are measured from the graph. Several spirograms are obtained in this fashion and one or two are selected as representative on the basis of predetermined criteria. Graphical and selection techniques are discussed in the sections that follow.

Defining the Limits of the Spirogram   The initial portion of a forced expiration consists of a rapid rise to maximal flow, represented on the spirogram by the section with the greatest slope. This is followed by a gradual reduction in flow, during which the spirogram shows a gradual leveling off to a plateau. Because the start of the test during the generation of peak flow may not be abrupt, determination of the starting point of the tracing is not straightforward. The most common technique for determining the starting point, recommended by the Epidemiology Standardization Project, is *back-extrapolation*, in which the initial maximal flow is extrapolated to the end-inspiratory baseline (Fig. 7-2).[11,12] The intersection of these two lines is considered the start of the tracing.

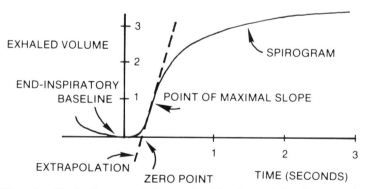

Fig. 7-2.   The back-extrapolation method for determining the start of a forced expiratory spirogram. A line tangent to the curve at the point of maximum slope is extrapolated to the end-inspiratory baseline. The point where it crosses the baseline is the start of timing for the test. The end-inspiratory baseline is the baseline for the volume measurements.

The back-extrapolation method cannot be used with portable electronic spirometers that lack the capability of storing the entire spirogram. An alternative method suitable for these devices, which agrees relatively closely with back extrapolation, is to start the timing of the test on the end-inspiratory baseline at a point corresponding to 200 ml exhaled volume on the tracing.[11]

The end of the tracing is more difficult to define. In the normal person the maximally exhaled volume is easily determined because exhalation is completed within 3 to 4 sec and the terminal limb of the spirogram is flat. In subjects with obstructive lung dysfunction, however, the time required for complete exhalation is significantly prolonged; patients often fatigue or develop air hunger and stop the test before exhalation is complete. The end of the test is considered the point of maximal volume, but one must realize that results may vary depending on the length of time the patient can exhale before taking the next breath. For automated testing, the FVC may be defined as the point at which flow has decreased to 0.05 liter/sec, sustained for 0.5 sec, and only after exhalation has continued at least 6 sec.[12] These criteria may not be met in severe obstruction; then FVC must be reported as the maximum value obtained, regardless of the time required for exhalation.

Spirogram Selection   The forced expiratory spirogram should be performed repeatedly in any given testing session to assure selection of a tracing with maximal effort. The precise number of tracings needed and a method for selecting a representative tracing have not been firmly established. Most laboratories obtain between three and five tracings, depending on their consistency. Variability in measurements of more than 10 percent among the tracings suggests patient fatigue or poor cooperation. Even with consistent tracings, however, there will be some variability, and selection of the single tracing from which to make measurements can be difficult.

The topic of spirogram selection has received considerable attention. A recommended approach is to obtain three tracings of reasonable effort, then record the maximal FEV_1 and FVC whether or not they are from the same tracing.[13,14] One of these tracings must be chosen to obtain timed flows, which come from a single tracing.

Another approach that has been shown not to be significantly different from the one just discussed is to select the single tracing with the largest sum of FEV_1 and FVC for analysis.[15,16] This method is most suitable for measurement of all timed expiratory volumes and for computer-based systems with automatic spirogram selection.

After a spirographic curve is selected for analysis and its limits defined, a number of measurements are made from the curve, including a series of timed volumes (forced expiratory volumes) and a series of time- or volume-averaged flows (forced expiratory flows). Many of these measurements are redundant, however, and not all are required for assessing airflow obstruction.

Forced Expiratory Volumes   The maximal volume that a patient can exhale, independent of the time required to achieve it, is recorded and is known as the forced vital capacity (FVC). It corresponds to the slow vital capacity in healthy lungs, and is usually reached within 3 or 4 sec of starting forced exhalation. Airway obstruction prolongs the time required to reach residual volume; in cases of severe obstruction the subject may cease exhalation because of dyspnea or fatigue before true residual volume is reached.

Volumes are also obtained from the spirogram at 0.5, 1, and 3 sec (Fig. 7-3). These are indicated as FEV_t, where the subscript t represents the time at which the measurement is made, that is, FEV_1 is the forced expired volume in 1 sec.

Forced expiratory volumes convey information on airflow obstruction because of their time dependence. $FEV_{0.5}$ is measured when the absolute lung volume is large, FEV_1 when lung volume is usually more than half exhaled, and FEV_3 when lung volume is usually near residual lung volume. The timed volumes are also low in restrictive disease, but are decreased in proportion to the decrease in FVC. For this reason, forced expired volumes should be interpreted in light of FVC.

Forced Expiratory Volume Ratios   Airway conductance increases with lung volume; therefore, individuals with large lung volumes will have large timed volumes. The dependence of forced expired volumes on body size and vital capacity can be minimized by normalizing forced expiratory volumes to forced vital capacity and expressing the ratio as a percentage.[17] This reduces the variability between normal individuals and permits comparison between indi-

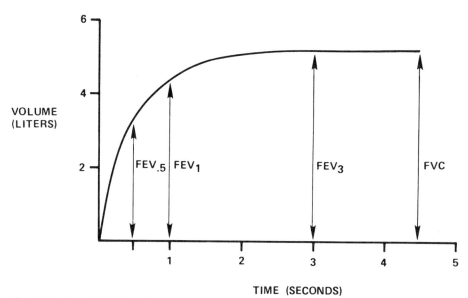

Fig. 7-3.   A typical forced expiratory spirogram showing the timed volumes obtained from the tracing. $FEV_{0.5}$, FEV_1, and FEV_3 represent the forced expired volumes at 0.5, 1.0, and 3.0 sec, respectively. Forced vital capacity (FVC) is the maximum volume that can be forcefully exhaled. [Reproduced from Conrad SA, George RB: Clinical pulmonary function testing. p. 161. In George RB, Light RW, Matthay RA (eds): Chest Medicine. Churchill Livingstone, New York, 1983]

viduals of different body size. It also reduces variation from changes in vital capacity in any given individual. Timed FEV-to-FVC ratios provide information similar to the ratios of airway conductance to lung volume, and changes tend to reflect proportional changes in airway conductance.[18] For these reasons, timed FEV-to-FVC ratios are the preferred method of diagnosing obstructive airway disease.

These ratios are abbreviated $FEV_t/FVC\%$, where t is conventionally 0.5, 1, or 3 sec. They are not entirely constant in normal groups, but decrease linearly to a small degree with age. $FEV_{0.5}/FVC\%$ assesses airflow at relatively large lung volumes with major contributions from the larger airways, and its value is usually greater than 50 percent. $FEV_1/FVC\%$ assesses airflow over most of FVC, with a significant contribution from small airways. It is greater than 75 percent in most normal individuals. $FEV_3/FVC\%$ is normally above 95 percent, and may reflect function of the small airways.

Use of forced vital capacity (FVC) to form the ratio, although conventional, may underestimate the degree of obstruction. Because FVC can vary with bronchomotor tone in an individual, using slow vital capacity to form the ratio ($FEV_t/VC\%$) tends to reduce variability and allows more consistent results in assessing dynamic airflow. This method, which requires a separate spirometric determination of slow vital capacity, has not gained universal acceptance.

Forced Expiratory Flows Expiratory flow averaged over preselected segments of the spirogram are used in assessment of dynamic airway function, and provide information comparable to that obtained from forced expired volumes. Three measurements are commonly obtained from the spirogram by measuring volume and time changes over these segments, and calculating an average flow:

$$FEF = \frac{\text{change in volume}}{\text{change in time}} \qquad \text{(Eq. 7-5)}$$

Forced expiratory flows are abbreviated $FEF_{x\text{-}y}$, where the subscript represents the volume range over which the measurement is made (Fig. 7-4). For $FEF_{0.2\text{-}1.2}$, flow is calculated over the segment from 200 to 1,200 ml of exhaled air. Two other commonly measured expiratory flows are obtained from 25 to 75 percent of exhaled vital capacity ($FEF_{25\text{-}75\%}$) and from 75 to 85 percent of exhaled vital capacity ($FEF_{75\text{-}85\%}$).

$FEF_{0.2\text{-}1.2}$ measures average flow over 1 liter of the initial part of the spirogram. The measurement begins at 200 ml to permit attainment of peak flow. The absolute lung volume is large at the time of measurement, and most of the resistance to flow assessed by this test is caused by obstruction in larger airways. The test has a large variability, caused in part by its effort dependence, and is not useful for detecting disease in the medium or small airways, or for assessing response to treatment.

$FEF_{25\text{-}75\%}$ is a frequently performed measurement and was formerly termed the midhalf flow rate or maximal midexpiratory flow (MMEF). It assesses airway function over the middle half of vital capacity and is a sensitive indicator of airway obstruction in the clinical setting.[19,20]

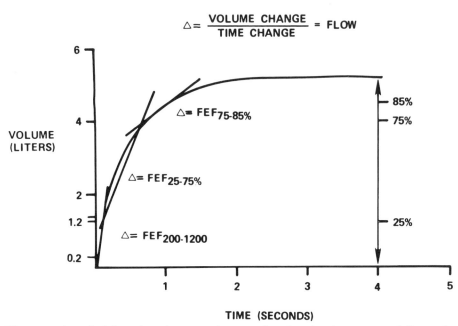

$$\triangle = \frac{\text{VOLUME CHANGE}}{\text{TIME CHANGE}} = \text{FLOW}$$

Fig. 7-4. A typical forced expiratory spirogram showing the time-averaged flows obtained from the tracing. The flow between 200 and 1,200 ml exhaled air ($FEV_{0.2-1.2}$) is taken at a high lung volume near TLC. The average flow between 25 and 75 percent of exhaled vital capacity ($FEV_{25-75\%}$) measures flow in the midportion of the exhaled vital capacity. The average flow between 75 and 85 percent of exhaled vital capacity ($FEV_{75-85\%}$) measures flow at low lung volume, when small airway resistance is dominant. [Reproduced from Conrad SA, George RB: Clinical pulmonary function testing. p. 161. In George RB, Light RW, Matthay RA: Chest Medicine. Churchill Livingstone, New York, 1983]

$FEF_{75-85\%}$, or maximal end-expiratory flow, assesses airway function at low lung volumes and may be a sensitive indicator of early small airway dysfunction before these changes are severe enough to be reflected as a decreased $FEF_{25-75\%}$.[21]

Forced expiratory flows are highly dependent on vital capacity. Prolongation of the exhalation in a subject with obstructive airway disease will result in a reduction in $FEV_{25-75\%}$, even though airway characteristics have not changed. Administration of a bronchodilator can result in a paradoxical decrease in $FEV_{25-75\%}$[22] if VC is significantly improved, or if exhalation can be maintained for a longer period of time. By adjusting $FEV_{25-75\%}$ to the subject's TLC instead of VC, this problem of postbronchodilator assessment is avoided.[23,24] A simple means of doing this is to choose two points on the postbronchodilator tracing corresponding to the same two volumes above the end-inspiratory point on the prebronchodilator tracing, and measure the slope of the line.

Flow-Volume Studies

The relationship between flow and volume during forced breathing and the determinants of expiratory flow were presented in detail in Chapter 2. This relationship can be analyzed in the pulmonary function laboratory by obtaining *flow-volume tracings.*[25,26] Instrumentation that simultaneously measures flow and volume is used with an X-Y recorder to plot flow on the ordinate and volume on the abscissa. A dry rolling-seal spirometer is well adapted to this because it offers little resistance to breathing, and flow and volume can be electronically obtained. A pneumotachometer system can also be used, as volume can be obtained by integration of flow. Modification of water-seal spirometers by addition of a potentiometer to provide volume and flow is frequently performed, but these spirometers may have enough inertia and resistance to reduce the fidelity of the flow-volume loop. Expiratory flow is conventionally recorded as being above the baseline and inspiratory flow below it. The subject makes a forced expiratory maneuver, as in conventional spirometry, followed by a maximal inspiratory maneuver back to total lung capacity. The recorder plots the simultaneous flow and volume. The result is a loop in which expiratory flow rises rapidly then declines to zero flow at residual volume, creating the expiratory section of the curve, followed by the inspiratory section. The latter begins at residual volume and traces below the baseline back to total lung capacity (Fig. 7-5).

The expiratory and inspiratory curves have different shapes because of differences in the mechanisms of flow limitation during inspiration and expiration. The initial portion of the expiratory flow-volume curve is a rapid, effort-dependent rise to peak flow. Limitation of peak flow is primarily caused by effort and upper airway resistance because the peripheral airways are at maximal dilatation at full inspiration and thus offer miminal resistance. Once peak flow is attained, flow decreases with volume. If sufficient effort is used, this latter portion of the curve represents an envelope of maximal flow that is dependent on airway and elastic characteristics and cannot be increased with greater effort. This is exemplified by having the subject make a series of expiratory flow-volume curves, starting from decreasing lung volumes (see Fig. 2-7A). Peak flow can only rise up to the envelope, then follows it as if the subject had started at TLC. Lung volume changes do not affect flow-volume relationships as long as airway function is not affected. This implies that restrictive lung diseases have normal flow-volume relationships, whereas obstructive airway diseases would alter the relationship.

Maximal Expiratory Flows The expiratory flow-volume curve is routinely quantitated by measuring maximal flows after 25 percent, 50 percent, and 75 percent of vital capacity has been exhaled. These measurements are labeled $FEF_{xx\%}$, where xx represents the percentage of vital capacity exhaled when the measurement is made (Fig. 7-6). In addition, the peak or maximal flow is measured (FEFmax). These values give an indication of flow at high, middle, and low lung volumes, and can be compared with predicted values for objective

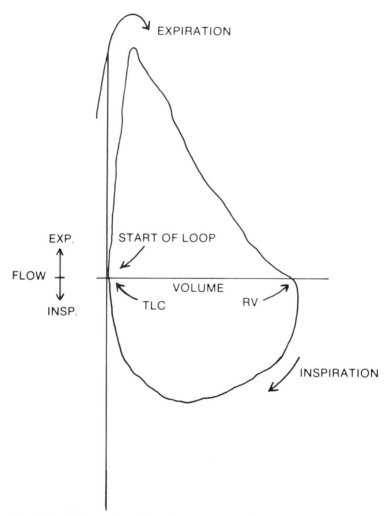

Fig. 7-5. A flow-volume loop demonstrating the expiratory (upper) and inspiratory (lower) limbs. The maneuver starts with the subject exhaling from TLC down to RV, then inhaling back to TLC. The tracing starts at zero flow on the left and courses clockwise, with expiration ending at zero flow on the right. The inspiratory limb courses back to the starting point.

assessment of airway function, in particular, the volume-dependence of airway function.

The flow-volume curve provides a significant amount of information in graphic form. Flow and volume assessment can be performed simultaneously. Although no time information is inherent in the graph, the equipment can be designed to place tic marks at 0.5, 1, and 3 sec so that $FEV_{0.5}$, FEV_1, and FEV_3 can be obtained without the need for a separate spirogram.

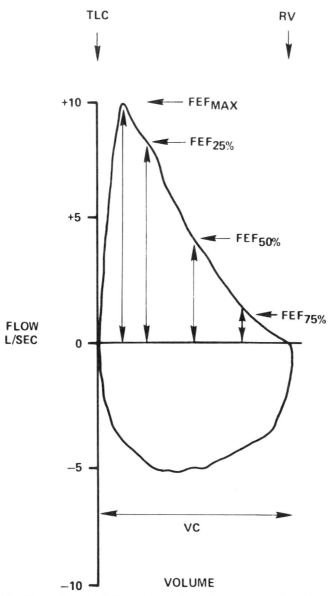

Fig. 7-6. A typical flow-volume loop from a normal subject. Instantaneous flows are measured after 25 percent ($FEF_{25\%}$), 50 percent ($FEF_{50\%}$), and 75 percent ($FEF_{75\%}$) of VC has been exhaled. The peak flow (FEFmax) is easily measured as the flow at the peak of the graph. [Reproduced from Conrad SA, George RB: Clinical pulmonary function testing. p. 161. In George RB, Light RW, Matthay, RA (eds): Chest Medicine. Churchill Livingstone, New York, 1983]

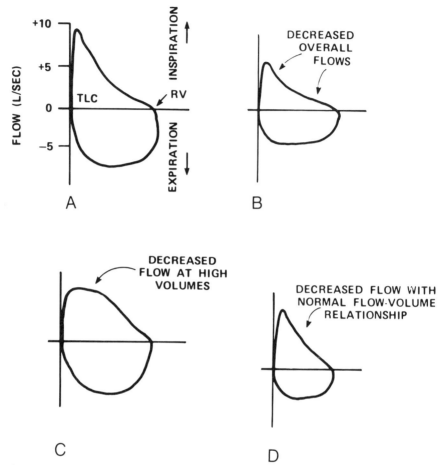

Fig. 7-7. Examples of abnormal flow-volume loops. (A) Mild obstructive airway disease characterized by decreased flow at low lung volume when elastic support is reduced. (B) Significant obstructive airway disease characterized by decreased overall flows, with a further decrease at low lung volumes. (C) Variable intrathoracic large airway obstruction in which peak flow is decreased at higher lung volume with preservation of normal flow-volume relationships at lower lung volumes. (D) Restrictive pulmonary disease with decreased vital capacity and flows, but preservation of normal flow-volume relationship. [Reproduced from Conrad SA, George RB: Clinical pulmonary function testing. p. 161. In George RB, Light RW, Matthay RA (eds): Chest Medicine. Churchill Livingstone, New York, 1983]

Patterns of the Flow-Volume Loop   Several patterns can be identified for restrictive and for upper and lower airway dysfunctions (Fig. 7-7). In *restrictive* diseases caused by decreased lung volumes, the flow-volume relationship remains normal in the face of a decreased vital capacity. In *obstruction* of peripheral airways the flow-volume relationship is altered. With this type of dysfunction, the overall flow envelope is decreased. In severe disease with significant airway closure, the tail of the curve may show severe and sudden decreases in flow.

In obstruction of the upper airways (i.e., the larynx, trachea, and mainstem bronchi) a characteristic decrease occurs in the peak flow on inspiration, expiration, or both (see Fig. 10-8).[27] If the obstruction is *fixed*, that is, it does not change caliber during breathing, then the peak flow of both the inspiratory and expiratory curves are decreased with a flattening of the initial portion of the loop. A *variable* obstruction manifests differently, depending on whether it is intrathoracic or extrathoracic. If it is extrathoracic (above the suprasternal notch), expiratory flow is unimpeded but inspiratory flow tends to worsen the obstruction. The inspiratory flow-volume curve in this case shows the characteristic flattening. Likewise, an intrathoracic (below the suprasternal notch) variable obstruction is manifested as peak expiratory flow limitation with less inspiratory effect, since positive pressure within the thorax during forced expiration tends to collapse the airways.

Because the shape of the flow-volume curve carries significant information, and often in a subtle manner, it is important to visually examine the curves and avoid strict reliance on numbers extracted from it.

Maximum Voluntary Ventilation

Maximum voluntary ventilation (MVV) is defined as the largest minute ventilation that a subject can achieve with effort. This test is performed with a spirometer or integrating pneumotachometer system that cumulatively measures exhaled volume. A high flow (10 liters/sec) pneumotachometer is required. The subject is instructed to breathe as hard and fast as possible. The test is maintained for 12 sec and MVV, reported in liters per minute, is calculated by multiplying the 12-sec volume by 5. Additional information on respiratory muscle fatigue is obtained by comparing MVV extrapolated from the 5-sec volume to that extrapolated from the 10-sec volume. Normal individuals can sustain MVV during the testing interval, whereas someone with muscular weakness might tire easily with his extrapolated MVV falling markedly with time.

Maximum voluntary ventilation depends on a multitude of factors. First, and of great importance, is patient effort, which may account for the large variability in the normal range. Airway function plays a prime role. Chest wall and diaphragmatic muscle function and compliance, as well as pulmonary tissue resistance, are contributing factors. MVV is a simple means of assessing ventilatory reserve, and as such, MVV has been recommended as a useful screening test for patients who require upper abdominal or thoracic surgery. MVV has a place in preoperative pulmonary function assessment (see Chapter 10) because it measures patient cooperation, muscle endurance, and other extrapulmonary factors as well as lung function.

RESISTIVE PROPERTIES

Resistance to gas flow during breathing has several sources. *Airway resistance* (Raw) is resistance to airflow in the upper airways and the tracheobronchial tree. Further resistance, equal to about 20 percent of Raw, is offered by tissue deformation and is termed *tissue resistance* (Rti). The sum of the airway and tissue resistances is *pulmonary resistance* (RL). Total resistance to breathing includes chest wall resistance in addition to pulmonary resistance and is termed *total respiratory system resistance* (Rrs). Typical values for the components of Rrs are given in Figure 7-8.

Airway resistance is altered in obstructive pulmonary diseases. Separation of the flow-resistive properties of the airways themselves from other factors that limit expiratory flow requires special measurement.

Resistance to gas flow through a conduit is defined as the pressure difference between the ends of the conduit divided by the resulting flow, or

$$R = \frac{\Delta P}{\dot{V}}$$

(Eq. 7-6)

Measurement of resistance is therefore performed by simultaneously measuring pressure difference and flow.

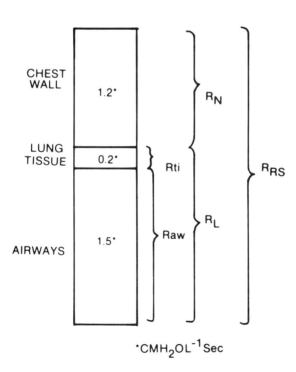

CHEST WALL   1.2* R_N

LUNG TISSUE   0.2*   Rti R_{RS}

AIRWAYS   1.5*   Raw R_L

*$CMH_2OL^{-1}Sec$

Fig. 7-8. The relative contributions of component resistances to total respiratory system resistance (Rrs). Rrs is composed of the total pulmonary (RL) and chest wall (Rw) resistances. RL is composed of the airway resistance (Raw) and tissue resistance (Rti).

Table 7-1 Methods for Assessing Resistance in the Respiratory System

Name	Abbreviation	Source	Method
Airway resistance	Raw	Upper and lower airways	Body plethysmography
Pulmonary resistance	R_L	Airway and tissue resistances	Esophageal pressure-flow method
Total resistance	Rrs	Airway, tissue, and chest wall resistances	Forced oscillation

Several methods have been developed for assessing respiratory resistance in human subjects (Table 7-1):

1. Airway resistance is measured through the use of body plethysmography, enabling simultaneous measurement of thoracic gas volume, and therefore permitting standardization for lung volume.
2. Pulmonary resistance is measured with an esophageal balloon placed to record transpulmonary pressure. Because of the invasiveness of the procedure, and the limited information obtained in addition to airway resistance, the test has limited application.
3. Total respiratory resistance is measured by the forced oscillation technique. It requires less effort on the part of the patient, does not require expensive equipment, and is not as dependent on cooperation, but does not allow volume measurement or the separation of airway resistance from tissue and chest wall resistances.

The most common method in use today is the measurement of Raw with plethysmography because airway resistance is the component of most clinical interest. The forced oscillation method has value in subjects who cannot cooperate or undergo plethysmography. Although it does not measure airway resistance it may be used to follow changes in airway resistance, as it is this component that accounts for nearly all acute variations in total respiratory system resistance.

Airway Resistance by Plethysmography

The measurement of flow and alveolar pressure required for calculation of airway resistance can be performed in a body plethysmograph, or body box. The use of the pneumotachometer, shutter mechanism, and panting manuever are carefully explained to the subject prior to the test because cooperation is essential for accurate results.

The subject is seated in the body box and the door is sealed. The box vent is opened for 3 to 5 min during temperature equilibrium, then closed. The X-Y storage oscilloscope is placed in the flow-box pressure mode ($\dot{V}/P_{box}$) and the subject is asked to begin small rapid breathing movements (panting) at the end of

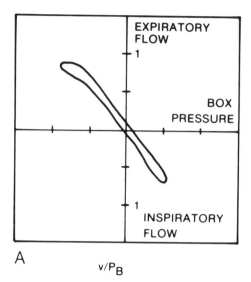

A   v/P_B

Fig. 7-9. Examples of the two loops obtained in the measurement of Raw. (A) Plot of flow-versus-box pressure. (B) Plot of mouth pressure versus box pressure. Airway resistance is proportional to the ratio of the slope of loop B to the slope of loop A. A more detailed introduction is given in text.

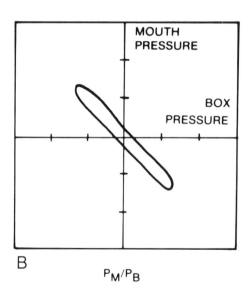

B   P_M/P_B

a normal expiration (FRC). The curve is observed for development of a stable pattern and to monitor maximal expiratory flow, which should not be permitted to exceed 1 to 2 liters/sec to prevent dynamic airway compression. A stable pattern is nearly linear, especially at lower flows, and should nearly retrace itself (Fig. 7-9A).

If the loop is not closed to a line, the panting frequency is increased until the loop is nearly linear. Once a stable pattern develops, two or three loops are recorded on the storage oscilloscope. The flow-box pressure slope is later mea-

Fig. 7-10. The measurement of the slope of the flow-box pressure curve during Raw determination during plethysmography is critical to the accurate assessment of Raw. In most subjects the loop will approximate a line, the slope of which is easily determined (A). In cases of severe obstructive airway disease, there is separation of the expiratory and inspiratory limbs with development of a nonlinear relationship at higher flows (B). In this case, the slope is taken along the expiratory limb at a flow of 0.5 liter/sec.

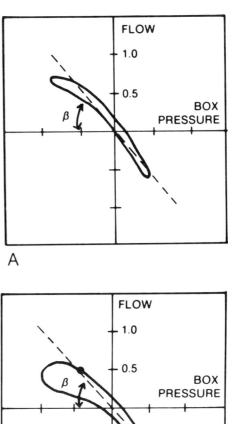

A

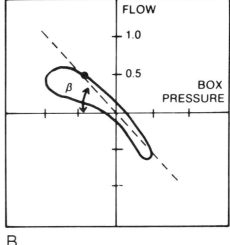

B

sured from the tracing by the method described in the next section. While the subject is still panting, the oscilloscope is switched to the mouth pressure-box pressure (Pao/P_{box}) mode and the shutter is closed at end-expiration to occlude the airway. Two or three loops of the Pao/P_{box} curve are recorded (Fig. 7-9B). Because airflow is prevented by the shutter, the mouth pressure is equivalent to alveolar pressure, and Pao/P_{box} is a measure of PA/P_{box}.

Measurement of Slopes The slopes of the $\dot{V}/P_{box}$ and Pao/P_{box} curves stored on the oscilloscope must be accurately measured. In place of direct measurement of the slope as $\Delta y/\Delta x$, a built-in protractor is used to easily measure the angle between the curve and the baseline (Fig. 7-10A). The tangent of an angle θ (tan θ) with the baseline is equal to the slope of the curve:

$$\tan \theta = \frac{\Delta y}{\Delta x} \qquad \text{(Eq. 7-7)}$$

The measurement of the angle is quicker than the measurement of the individual changes in the two variables.

Measurement of the angle of the flow-box pressure curve may not be straightforward, since in subjects with obstructive lung disease this curve may not appear linear at higher pressures (Fig. 7-10B). Because the point chosen in this instance can greatly influence the value of Raw, it is conventional to use the initial portion of the expiratory limb of the curve near the origin, between flows of -0.5 to 0.5 liter/sec. The nonlinear behavior of the curve at higher flows is thought to reflect dynamic compression of the airways.[28]

Calculation of Raw Dividing the mouth pressure-box pressure slope by the flow-box pressure slope (measured under identical conditions in the body box) forms the basis for calculation of airway resistance:

$$\frac{\Delta Pao/\Delta P_{box}}{\dot{V}/\Delta P_{box}} = \frac{\Delta P_m}{\dot{V}} = \frac{\Delta P_A}{\dot{V}} = Raw \qquad \text{(Eq. 7-8)}$$

Two corrections are required, the calibration of the oscilloscope tracing and the correction for pneumotachometer resistance. The calibration factor is determined beforehand, usually at the factory, for given oscilloscope settings. It is equal to the mouth pressure (centimeters of H_2O) per oscilloscope division divided by the flow in liters per second per division:

$$k = \frac{\Delta Pao/division}{\dot{V}/division} \qquad \text{(Eq. 7-9)}$$

The pneumotachometer resistance (Rpneu) is also determined beforehand. In the calculation of Raw, the angles of $Pao/P_{box}(\alpha)$ and $\dot{V}/P_{box}(\beta)$ curves are used, resulting in the final equation for Raw:

$$Raw = k\left(\frac{\tan \alpha}{\tan \beta}\right) - Rpneu \qquad \text{(Eq. 7-10)}$$

The results are expressed in centimeters of H_2O per liter per second.

Normal Values In healthy adults, airway resistance ranges from 0.5 to 2.0 cm H_2O/liter/sec, with a mean of 1.5. Much of the variation is from the dependence of airway resistance on lung volume. This intrinsic variability can be reduced by converting airway resistance to specific airway conductance. Another source of variation is the difficulty of obtaining the true slope in oscilloscope tracings that are not linear.

Airway Conductance

The inverse of airway resistance is *airway conductance,* or flow per unit pressure change. It has a linear relationship to absolute lung volume.[29,30] If conductance measurements are made at several lung volumes in a given patient, they would fall near a line over most of the range of lung volume. Resistance, on the other hand, has a nonlinear relationship to lung volume (see Fig. 2-6).

This linear relationship of conductance with lung volume permits the standardization of conductance measurements, enabling comparisons between subjects of different size. This reduces the intersubject variability of the test and the range of normal values is reduced. This adjustment of conductance for the volume at which it is measured (Gaw/V_L) is termed *specific airway conductance,* also abbreviated SGaw.

The normal value of specific conductance ranges from approximately 0.20 to 0.30 liter/sec per cm H_2O per liter V_{TG} with a mean value of approximately 0.25.

Total Pulmonary Resistance by Esophageal Pressure

Placement of an esophageal balloon, as for measurement of pulmonary compliance, enables measurement of pulmonary resistance. The equipment consists of a pneumotachometer with associated transducers for measurement of flow and a differential pressure transducer for measuring the difference between esophageal and airway opening pressure (transpulmonary pressure). Measurement is facilitated by displaying flow and pressure on an X-Y oscilloscope.

The balloon is placed and adjusted in a manner identical to that for measurement of static compliance. The subject breathes quietly for a few breaths until the pattern stabilizes, then pants at approximately 2 cycles/sec, with maximal flow limited to 0.5 liter/sec. The oscilloscope tracing is similar to the flow-box pressure tracing obtained in plethysmography (Fig. 7-9A). The slope of the curve obtained from the tracing is equal to R_L. If a discrepancy exists between the inspiratory and expiratory limbs, then the slope of the expiratory limb between 0 and 0.5 liter/sec is used.

Total Respiratory Resistance by Forced Oscillation

The combined flow-resistive properties of the airways, lungs, and chest wall (total respiratory system resistance) can be measured by the technique of forced oscillation.[31,32] The testing equipment consists of a sinusoidal small-volume pressure generator attached to one end of a pneumotachometer fitted with a transducer to measure proximal airway pressure (Fig. 7-11).

The subject breathes through the pneumotachometer from the end opposite the pressure generator. The generator is a large loudspeaker that can respond to

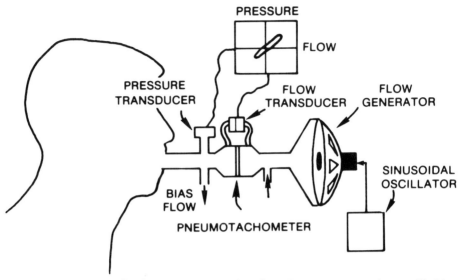

Fig. 7-11. Apparatus for the measurement of total respiratory system resistance (Rrs) by the forced oscillation method. The sinusoidal oscillator drives a flow generator at variable frequencies. The induced flow and pressure changes at the airway opening are monitored while the frequency is adjusted to the resonant frequency. Rrs is equal to the slope of the pressure-flow loop at resonance.

frequencies in the range of 5 to 10 Hz (oscillations per second). Each oscillation produces a volume displacement of 30 to 50 ml. The pneumotachometer has a continuous *bias flow* of air through it to prevent CO_2 buildup in the system.

The principle of resistance measurement by the forced oscillation technique is based on the relationship of the effects of externally applied forced oscillations on elasticity, inertia, and resistance of the lungs. When a sinusoidal flow is produced in the proximal airway by the oscillator, a back pressure develops in the airway. This pressure is the result of these three properties of the lung. The pressure response from *elasticity* is a property related to a change in lung volume. As applied frequency increases, the effect of elasticity decreases. The response to lung *inertia* is related to acceleration of gas in the respiratory system. As the frequency of applied oscillation increases (and hence the acceleration of injected volume), the effect of inertia increases. The pressure response to respiratory system *resistance* is largely independent of frequency in the ranges used for the test. The combined effect of these three factors in producing a back pressure in response to forced oscillation is termed *impedance*.

The pressure curve generated as a result of the flow produced by the oscillator lags behind the flow curve at lower frequencies (Fig. 7-12). When the frequency of applied oscillations is increased, the effect of elasticity decreases and that of inertia increases. At a certain frequency, termed the *resonant frequency,* the effects of these two cancel, leaving only the flow-resistive properties of the lung in effect. This is signaled by the loss of the lag between the flow and

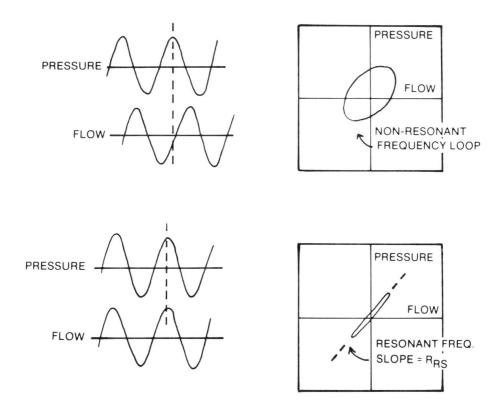

OSCILLOSCOPE TRACINGS

Fig. 7-12. Pressure and volume tracings obtained during the measurement of Rrs during forced oscillation. At frequencies below resonance (A) the pressure curve lags behind the flow curve, indicated by an open loop on the X-Y oscilloscope. As the frequency is increased and resonance is reached (B), the flow and pressure curves are in phase, indicated by the convergence of the open loop to a closed line on the oscilloscope. The slope of the line is equal to Rrs.

pressure curves. In normal subjects, this occurs at a resonant frequency of about 6 oscillations/sec, but may be altered in lung disease.

Traditionally, the forced oscillation method has been applied as the *resonant frequency technique*, in which the frequency of applied oscillations is increased to the point of resonance. The measurement of Rrs is made during spontaneous respiration with the forced oscillations imposed on the spontaneous activity. The phase lag between the pressure and flow waveforms are easily demonstrated by tracing flow versus pressure on an X-Y oscilloscope. At low starting frequencies the tracing will be an open loop. When the resonant frequency is reached by increasing the applied frequency, the loop will close into a line. At this point, the slope is measured during the end-expiratory pause. The calibrated slope is equal to Rrs.

Other methods have been developed to measure Rrs at any given frequency. The theory for these other methods is beyond the scope of this book, and the reader is referred to the literature.[33,34]

The value in normal individuals is approximately 1.5 cm H_2O/liter/sec greater than airway resistance. Most of this difference is caused by resistance to chest wall deformation, whereas the remainder is from lung tissue resistance.

ASSESSMENT OF BRONCHIAL RESPONSIVENESS

The response of the bronchi to certain inhaled substances can be important in the diagnosis and management of obstructive airway disease. The subject with obstructive airway disease may have a reversible component to his obstruction in addition to a fixed component. The ability to respond to bronchodilators can help assess the relative contributions of each, and to predict response to bronchodilator therapy. Bronchial provocation is useful in someone suspected of having reactive airway disease on the basis of the medical history who has no demonstrable abnormalities at the time of testing, or in someone known to have reactive airway disease in whom the degree of reactivity needs to be assessed.

Response to Bronchodilators

The response to bronchodilators is usually assessed in the pulmonary function laboratory whenever the diagnosis of obstructive airway disease is initially made.[35] Once baseline pulmonary function values are obtained, a bronchodilator is administered. The inhaled form is preferred to permit rapid onset of action and to decrease the incidence of side effects. The most commonly used drug has been isoproterenol, although isoetharine, metaproterenol, and albuterol are more specific. The drug may be administered by metered-dose inhaler (MDI), handheld nebulizer, or intermittent positive pressure breathing (IPPB) device. The latter two methods are more difficult to administer and have no advantage in most patients. They may be required, however, in children and patients who cannot use the MDI properly. Once administered, the subject waits 20 to 30 min for maximal drug effect before postbronchodilator tests are performed.

The tests used in the postbronchodilator period are forced expiratory mechanics, using spirometry with optional plethysmography. The most commonly performed tests are FEV_1, FVC, $FEF_{25-75\%}$, $FEF_{50\%}$, FEFmax, and specific airway conductance. Various combinations of these tests have been used to define reversibility. FEV_1 has been shown to be the best single discriminator of reversibility,[36] and is the test of choice if a single test is used. An increase in FEV_1 of 10% or greater is above the range expected from normal individuals and is indicative of reversibility.[35]

Bronchial Provocation Testing

Two nonantigenic substances are used to induce bronchospasm in the nonspecific assessment of hyperreactivity, methacholine chloride and histamine. Methacholine is the most widespread substance used for this purpose.

Baseline spirometry is obtained prior to the challenge. The challenge proceeds by having the subject inhale five standardized breaths of a 0.75 mg/ml solution of methacholine.[37] After 3 min, repeat spirometry is performed and checked for a response. If none is detected, the next higher concentration is used (approximately double the previous dose), and spirometry is again repeated after 3 min. This protocol is continued until a final concentration of 25 mg/ml is reached, or the subject shows a response.

The most commonly used index of response is a 15 percent decrease in FEV_1 or a 30 percent decrease in specific airway conductance. Any bronchospasm invoked by the test is then reversed with inhaled bronchodilators. Most normal individuals will not develop a response to the highest concentration. A significant number of individuals with immunologically mediated disease, such as hay fever, may demonstrate reactivity in the absence of manifest obstructive airway disease.

MAXIMAL RESPIRATORY PRESSURES

Diseases involving the respiratory muscles are not an uncommon cause of dyspnea and restrictive ventilatory dysfunction. When weakness of the respiratory muscles is suspected, the measurement of maximal inspiratory (MIP) and expiratory pressures (MEP) can provide an objective assessment of the degree of impairment.[38] Serial determinations of these pressures permit assessment of the progression of disease or the response to treatment. Because these are often measured at bedside in acutely ill patients, they are discussed in Chapter 13.

In the evaluation of neuromuscular disease the MIP is of most importance, since expiration is usually passive. Neuromuscular weakness is associated with a diminished MIP.[38] These pressures are usually increased in chronic obstructive airway disease,[39] and if low, may indicate neuromuscular weakness in the face of chronic obstructive pulmonary disease (COPD). In these patients, the presence of neuromuscular weakness cannot be detected by spirometry. The values of MIP and MEP are age- and sex-dependent, being lower in females and decreasing with age in the adult.[40]

TESTS OF SMALL AIRWAY FUNCTION

A number of disease processes affect small airways, defined as those 2 mm in diameter or less. Studies that correlate structure and function have revealed that airway disease can be extrinsic or intrinsic, yet result in similar changes in function. When small airway dysfunction is significant, its obstructive nature is easily detected on routine pulmonary function tests. However, early in the disease process small airway dysfunction may be undetectable. Because these airways contribute only 10 to 20 percent of total airway resistance, minimal small airway dysfunction may go unnoticed on most routine pulmonary function tests until it is advanced and contributes a significant fraction of total airway resistance. Although the relationship between minimal small airway disease and later development of chronic obstructive airway disease is unclear, detection of small airway disease may provide insight into this relationship and permit intervention. The following sections discuss various tests of small airway dysfunction, even though they are infrequently employed in the clinical setting.

Frequency Dependence of Compliance

When pulmonary compliance is measured during breathing it is termed *dynamic compliance* (Cdyn). Its measurement is identical to that of static compliance, with the exception that airflow is not interrupted and measurement occurs during active breathing. As opposed to static compliance, in which lung tissue elastic recoil provides the majority of the forces creating the pressure, dynamic compliance has several determinants, including airway resistance to flow and tissue resistance to deformation in addition to elastic recoil. This test is useful in the detection of small airway dysfunction.[41]

Preparation for the test is similar to that for static compliance. An esophageal balloon is placed to permit measurement of transpulmonary pressure. The subject begins breathing into the spirometer or pneumotachometer system at FRC and dynamic compliance is calculated by dividing the tidal volume by the pressure changes. Normal tidal volume is maintained. If volume and pressure are recorded using an X-Y oscilloscope to trace volume against pressure, then the slope of the resulting trace equals dynamic compliance. The subject is guided by a metronome to breathe at two frequencies, usually 20 and 80 breaths/min. Some laboratories record several frequencies, such as 20, 60, and 100.

The basis for frequency dependence of compliance in small airway disease is not entirely clear, but it is thought to be a result of asynchronous ventilation of lung units within small regions. In the normal lung there is no frequency dependence of compliance, that is, the compliance at the frequency of 80 is not significantly different from that recorded at the frequency of 20. In small airway disease, however, compliance decreases as frequency increases, so that $Cdyn_{80}$ is less than 90 percent of $Cdyn_{20}$ (Fig. 7-13).

The test is always abnormal in the presence of airway dysfunction severe enough to cause abnormal spirometry; therefore, the usefulness of the test is found in the individual with normal or slightly abnormal spirometry where early small airway disease is suspected. It has the capability of distinguishing smokers from nonsmokers with otherwise normal pulmonary function tests.[42] It is thought to be the most sensitive of the tests for early small airway dysfunction and is often used as the standard to which other small airway tests are compared.

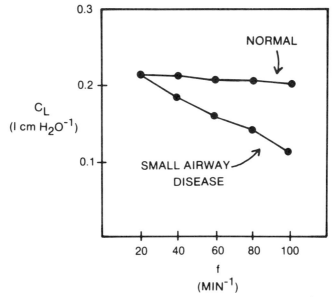

Fig. 7-13. Plot of dynamic compliance versus breathing frequency to demonstrate frequency dependence of compliance. The top tracing from a normal subject shows no significant change in Cdyn with increasing frequency. A subject with small airway disease (bottom tracing) demonstrates a decrease in Cdyn with increasing frequency.

Density-Dependent Gas Flow Studies

The maximal expiratory flow-volume curve can be performed with gas mixtures of two different densities to obtain more information about small airway function. The test is based on the relationship of gas flow to gas density, gas viscosity, and the presence of laminar or turbulent flow.

The test consists of performing two maximal expiratory flow-volume curves with gas mixtures of different densities but similar viscosities. The subject first performs a maximal expiration while breathing air and an expiratory flow-volume curve is recorded. The subject then breathes a gas mixture containing 20 percent oxygen and 80 percent helium for several minutes and repeats the expiratory flow-volume test. The two curves are aligned at residual volume for comparison. Unless the TLC points nearly coincide, a submaximal expiratory effort was performed and the test should be repeated.

The helium-oxygen curve shows greater flows over all the exhaled volume, except for the terminal portion of the curve near RV. These final 10 to 20 percent portions of the two curves have identical flow and volume over each other. The volume over which the two curves correspond is termed the *volume of isoflow* ($V_{iso}\dot{v}$). It is expressed as a percentage of the vital capacity rather than as an absolute volume ($V_{iso}\dot{v}/VC\%$). The second measurement is the increase in flow at 50% of vital capacity ($\Delta\dot{V}max_{50\%}$), expressed as a percent increase over the $\dot{V}max_{50\%}$ obtained on air. The physiological and physical basis of the test is introduced in Chapter 2 and will only be summarized here.

A gas mixture has two physical properties that are important in establishing whether turbulent or laminar flow will occur in a cylindrical conduit. Gas *density* is the ratio of mass to volume. Gas *viscosity* is a property related to the friction of the molecules of a fluid as they slide past each other. Both of these are determinants of the *Reynold's number* (see Eq. 2-9). A Reynold's number above 2,000 is associated with turbulent flow in a cylinder, whereas a number below is associated with laminar flow. It can be seen that a high Reynold's number results from gases of high density and low viscosity.

The rate of flow in fully developed laminar flow is dependent on gas viscosity but not density. In contrast, turbulent flow is dependent on density as well as viscosity. A helium-oxygen mixture is used in these tests because it has the same viscosity as air but a much lower density.

The small peripheral airways have been shown to have predominantly laminar flow whereas the larger airways are characterized by turbulent flow. During a forced expiration, flow limitation is initially in the larger (i.e., lobar) airways where turbulent flow is present. Since turbulent flow is dependent on gas density, the expiratory flow for the helium-oxygen mixture is significantly greater than for air. As lung volume approaches RV, the site of flow limitation may shift to smaller airways. If flow limitation is predominantly in the small peripheral airways at low lung volumes where laminar flow predominates, flow becomes independent of gas density. Because air and the helium-oxygen mixture have similar viscosities, the flows at this portion of the curve are identical and the curves develop identical characteristics (Fig. 7-14).

The volume of isoflow is normally 10 to 20 percent of vital capacity. However, in the presence of small airway disease, flow limitation occurs in the small airways at a higher than normal absolute lung volume, accounting for an increase in $V_{iso}\dot{v}$. This test may detect small airway disease before other sensitive spirometric tests become abnormal.

The $\Delta\dot{V}max_{50\%}$ is a test of the relative caliber of the small airways. As small airways develop increased resistance from a reduced diameter, their contribution to total resistance increases. Turbulent flow is less pronounced in the presence of this increased small airway resistance, so the effect of gas density is diminished, and $\Delta\dot{V}max_{50\%}$ is reduced from its normal value of about 50 percent. Because this takes place at 50 percent of vital capacity, loss of elastic recoil does not play a major role in reduction in $\Delta\dot{V}max_{50\%}$; thus, the test primarily reflects increased small airway resistance from reduced airway diameter.

Closing Volume

The single-breath nitrogen test is used to assess three different aspects of pulmonary function: the calculation of residual and dead space volume, the

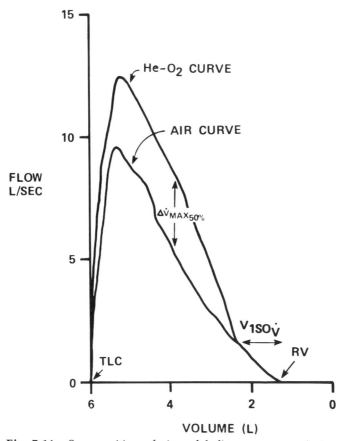

Fig. 7-14. Superposition of air and helium-oxygen expiratory flow-volume curves in the volume of isoflow test. The volume of isoflow ($V_{iso}\dot{v}$) is the volume above RV in which flow patterns become nearly identical, representing laminar flow limitation in the small airways. $\Delta\dot{V}max_{50\%}$ is the percent increase in flow at 50 percent of vital capacity when breathing the helium-oxygen mixture. [Reproduced from Conrad SA, George RB: Clinical pulmonary function testing. p. 161. In George, RB, Light RW, Matthay RA (eds): Chest Medicine. Churchill Livingstone, New York, 1983]

assessment of gas distribution, and the assessment of small airway function using the closing volume measurement.[43] It is the last feature that is discussed in this chapter. Closing volume is the volume above residual volume at which airway closure starts to occur, and provides information on loss of elastic recoil, a major determinant of premature airway closure.

The subject is seated in the upright position. The subject exhales to residual volume, at which point the breathing circuit is switched to admit 100 percent oxygen, which is then inhaled fully to TLC. The subject then exhales again completely to residual volume. The nitrogen concentration of the expired gas

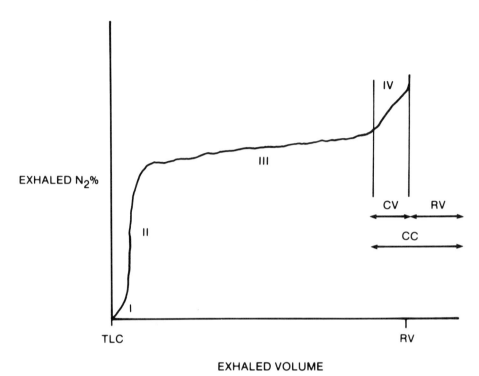

EXHALED N$_2$%

EXHALED VOLUME

Fig. 7-15. Graph of nitrogen concentration versus volume exhaled in the single-breath nitrogen test. The closing volume is the volume of phase IV, indicated by the abrupt increase in nitrogen concentration near the tail end of the curve. The closing capacity is the sum of the closing volume and the residual volume. [Modified from Conrad SA, George RB: Clinical pulmonary function testing. p. 161. In George RB, Light RW, Matthay RA (eds): Chest Medicine. Churchill Livingstone, New York, 1983]

during this last exhalation is continuously monitored and plotted as a function of the volume exhaled. A typical curve is given in Figure 7-15. Phase IV is the section of the curve near residual volume where the nitrogen concentration shows an abrupt increase. The volume of phase IV is the *closing volume* (CV), expressed as a fraction of vital capacity in percent (CV/VC%). The sum of the closing volume and the residual volume is the *closing capacity* (CC), expressed as a fraction of total lung capacity (CC/TLC%).

The closing volume test is dependent on the differential distribution of inspired air. With the subject breathing atmospheric air, nitrogen concentration in the alveoli is nearly constant throughout the lungs. Because of the effects of gravity on pleural pressure in the upright subject, the apical alveoli are subject to a greater distending pressure at rest. As the subject takes a breath of 100 percent oxygen, expansion of the apical regions is more pronounced initially. The dead space gas in the tracheobronchial tree, which is largely nitrogen, is distributed preferentially to the upper regions of the lung. As inspiration continues, when the apical alveoli are distended, inspired oxygen is then preferentially distributed to the bases. When total lung capacity is reached the apexes have a higher concentration of nitrogen because they preferentially received dead space gas. The subject is then instructed to exhale to RV. When lung volume approaches residual volume, small airway closure begins. This closure starts to take place in the bases from the effect of gravity on pleural pressure. Near the end of expiration apical gas becomes the predominant component of the expirate. Because nitrogen concentration is greater in the apexes, it results in a sudden increase in nitrogen concentration. The inflection point is the volume at which airway closure in the bases is presumed to occur.

An increase in closing volume is sensitive for detecting early airway closure, but not specific as to its etiology, that is, whether caused by loss of elastic recoil or decreased airway caliber. Closing volume increases with advancing age, and values up to 30 percent are to be expected.[44] Smokers with normal spirometry and airway resistance measurements may have an abnormal closing volume, but whether this represents reversible changes or early (preclinical) obstructive airway disease is unknown.[43]

In some patients, the slope of the entire alveolar plateau is increased and no easily discernible inflection point is able to be recorded. This is because of the presence of inhomogeneous distribution of ventilation, as may occur in emphysema. The closing volume cannot be reported for these individuals.

REFERENCES

1. Mead J, McIlroy MB, Selverstone NJ, and Kriete BC: Measurement of intraesophageal pressure. J Appl Physiol 7:491, 1955
2. Milic-Emili J, Mead J, Turner JM, et al: Improved technique for estimating pleural pressure from esophageal balloons. J Appl Physiol 19:207, 1964
3. Lemen R, Benson M, Jones JG: Absolute pressure measurements with hand-dipped and manufactured esophageal balloons. J Appl Physiol 37:600, 1974
4. Mead J, Whittenberger JL, Radford EP: Surface tension as a factor in pulmonary volume-pressure hysteresis. J Appl Physiol 10:191, 1957
5. Ferris BG, Mead J, Frank NR: Effect of body position on esophageal pressure and measurement of pulmonary compliance. J Appl Physiol 14:521, 1959
6. Lim TPK, Luft VC: Alterations in lung compliance and functional residual capacity with posture. J Appl Physiol 14:164, 1959
7. Marshall R: The physical properties of the lungs in relation to the subdivisions of lung volume. Clin Sci 16:507, 1957
8. Permutt S, Martin HB: Static pressure-volume characteristics of lungs in normal males. J Appl Physiol 15:819, 1960
9. Begin R, Renzetti AD Jr, Bigler AH, et al: Flow and age dependence of airway closure and dynamic compliance. J Appl Physiol 38:199, 1975
10. Pierson DJ, Dick NP, Petty TL: A comparison of spirometric values with subjects in sitting and standing positions. Chest 70:17, 1976
11. Smith AA, Gaensler EA: Timing of the forced expiratory volume in one second. Am Rev Resp Dis 112:882, 1975
12. Ferris BG: Epidemiology standardization project. III. Recommended standardized procedures for pulmonary function testing. Am Rev Resp Dis, part 2, 118:55, 1978

13. Gardner RM (chairman): Snowbird workshop on standardization of spirometry. ATS statement. Am Rev Resp Dis 119:831, 1979
14. Nathan SP, Lebowitz MD, Knudson RJ: Spirometric testing: Number of tests required and selection of data. Chest 76:384, 1979
15. Kanner RE, Morris AH: Clinical Pulmonary Function Testing. Intermountain Thoracic Society, Salt Lake City, Utah, 1975
16. Sorensen JB, Morris AH, Crapo RO, Gardner RM: Selection of the best spirometric values for interpretation. Am Rev Resp Dis 122:802, 1980
17. Miller WF, Johnson RL Jr, Wu N: Relationships between fast vital capacity and various timed expiratory capacities. J Appl Physiol 14:157, 1959
18. Johnson RL Jr, Miller WF, Wu N: Timed forced expiratory volumes and pulmonary conductance. Am Rev Resp Dis 86:228, 1962
19. Leueallen EC, Fowler WS: Maximal midexpiratory flow. Am Rev Tuberc 72:783, 1955
20. McFadden ER, Linden RA: A reduction in maximal end-expiratory flow rate. A spirographic manifestation of small airway disease. Am J Med 52:725, 1972
21. Morris JF, Koski A, Breese JD: Normal values and evaluation of forced end-expiratory flow. Am Rev Resp Dis 111:755, 1975
22. Olsen CR, Hale FC, Newman M: Decreases of forced expiratory flow after a bronchodilator aerosol. Physiologist 9:257, 1966
23. Olsen RR, Hale FC: A method for interpreting acute response to bronchodilators from the spirogram. Am Rev Resp Dis 98:301, 1967
24. Cockcroft DW, Berscheid BA: Volume adjustment of maximal mid-expiratory flow. Chest 78:595, 1980
25. Hyatt RE, Schilder DP, Fry DL: Relationship between maximum expiratory flow and degree of lung inflation. J Appl Physiol 13:331, 1958
26. Hyatt RE, Black LF: The flow-volume curve. Am Rev Resp Dis 107:191, 1973
27. Miller RD, Hyatt RE: Evaluation of obstructing lesions of the trachea and larynx by flow-volume loops. Am Rev Resp Dis 108:475, 1973
28. Lord PW, Edwards JM: Variation in airway resistance when defined over different ranges of airflow. Thorax 33:401, 1978
29. Briscoe WA, DuBois AB: The relationship between airway resistance, airway conductance, and lung volume in subjects of different age and body size. J Clin Invest 37:1279, 1958
30. Skough BE: Normal airways conductance at different lung volumes. Scand J Clin Lab Invest 31:429, 1973
31. DuBois AB, Brody AW, Lewis DH, Burges BF: Oscillation mechanics of lungs and chest in man. J Appl Physiol 8:587, 1956
32. Fisher AB, DuBois AB, Hyde RW: Evaluation of the forced oscillation technique for the determination of resistance to breathing. J Clin Invest 47:2045, 1968
33. Grimby G, Takishima T, Graham W, et al: Frequency dependence of flow resistance in patients with obstructive lung disease. J Clin Invest 47:1455, 1968
34. Goldman M, Knudson RJ, Mead J, et al: A simplified measurement of respiratory resistance by forced oscillation. J Appl Physiol 28:113, 1970
35. Light RW: Use of the pulmonary function laboratory in the treatment of obstructive airway disease. Adv Asthma Allergy, 5:suppl. 2, 10, 1978
36. Light RW, Conrad SA, George RB: The one best test for evaluating the effects of bronchodilator therapy. Chest 72:512, 1977
37. Chai H, Farr RS, Froehlich LA, et al: Standardization of bronchial inhalation challenge procedures. J Allergy Clin Immunol 56:323, 1975
38. Black LF, Hyatt RE Maximal respiratory pressures in generalized neuromuscular disease. Am Rev Resp Dis 103:641, 1971
39. Byrd RB, Hyatt RE: Maximal respiratory pressures in chronic obstructive lung disease. Am Rev Resp Dis 98:848, 1968

40. Black LF, Hyatt RE: Maximal respiratory pressures: Normal values and relationship to age and sex. Am Rev Resp Dis 99:696, 1969
41. Woolcock AJ, Vincent NJ, Macklem PT: Frequency dependence of compliance as a test for obstruction in the small airways. J Clin Invest 48:1099, 1969
42. McFadden ER, Kiker R, Holmes B, deGrott WT: Small airway disease: An assessment of the tests of peripheral airway function. Am J Med 57:171, 1974
43. McCarthy DS, Spencer R, Greene R, Milic-Emili J: Measurement of "closing volume" as a single and sensitive test for early detection of small airway disease. Am J Med 52:747, 1972
44. LeBlanc P, Ruff F, Milic-Emili J: Effects of age and body position on "airway closure" in man. J Appl Physiol 28:448, 1970

8

Distribution of Ventilation and Perfusion

Steven A. Conrad, M.D.

Optimal transfer of oxygen and carbon dioxide across the alveolar-capillary membrane requires adequate ventilation of the alveoli as well as a proper matching of alveolar ventilation to capillary perfusion. Diseases of the lungs can affect the distribution of ventilation, perfusion, or both, resulting in poor matching of ventilation to perfusion and less efficient gas exchange.

Abnormalities of ventilation and perfusion may be localized or widespread and diffuse. Localized ventilation abnormalities include lobar collapse or bronchial obstruction. An example of a localized perfusion abnormality is a lobar pulmonary embolus. Diffuse diseases include emphysema and chronic bronchitis, and these affect both ventilation and perfusion.

Each of these abnormalities can be assessed in pulmonary function or related laboratories. Table 8-1 outlines the tests used to evaluate these abnormalities, which are discussed in more detail in the following sections.

OVERALL DISTRIBUTION OF ALVEOLAR VENTILATION

To achieve adequate alveolar ventilation for proper gas exchange the inspired gas must be distributed to the alveoli with a high degree of efficiency and homogeneity. There may be slight variation in ventilation-perfusion relationships between regions of the lung, but within each region distribution to the alveoli must be fairly uniform to permit maximal utilization of the alveolar-capillary membrane. Assessment of alveolar gas distribution is useful in supporting diagnoses suggested by other tests and in defining the degree of impairment.

The tests described in this section provide an index of overall homogeneity of alveolar gas distribution, but provide little anatomic information about regional differences. Techniques to delineate abnormalities of distribution on a regional or lobar basis are discussed later in the chapter.

Table 8-1 Tests Used to Assess Distribution and Matching of Ventilation and Perfusion

Physiological Variable	Tests
Overall distribution of ventilation	Multibreath N_2 washout Single-breath N_2 test Helium mixing time
Localized distribution of ventilation	^{133}Xe ventilation scan Lateral position test Bronchospirometry
Distribution of perfusion	[^{99m}Tc]HAM perfusion scan
Relationship of ventilation to perfusion	^{133}Xe $\dot{V}/\dot{Q}$ scan Physiological dead space Physiological shunt Single-breath CO_2 test

Open-Circuit Multibreath Nitrogen Washout

In a person with normal lungs, gas is distributed rapidly to all lung regions and the alveoli promptly fill with the inspired gas. By the same principle, a tracer gas in the alveoli is eliminated (i.e., it is "washed out" of the alveoli by the process of ventilation) rapidly during repeated inhalations of a tracer-free gas. In lungs that have slowly ventilating regions as a result of airway obstruction, an alveolar tracer gas is eliminated more slowly as the tracer gas continues to leak from poorly ventilated regions for an extended period of time. An overall index of the efficiency of gas distribution to the alveoli can be obtained from analysis of the washout curve of a tracer gas. Because alveoli contain a near-constant fractional concentration of nitrogen while breathing ambient air (about 80 percent), the resident nitrogen is used as the tracer gas in the multibreath nitrogen elimination (or washout) test. The testing method is possible because nitrogen is inert, is in equilibrium with the blood, and diffuses only very slowly from the blood across the alveolar-capillary membrane. Alveolar concentration is estimated by measuring end-tidal nitrogen concentration.

A normal lung has ventilatory capabilities that can approach but not attain those of the ideal physiological lung model consisting of a single alveolar compartment. During washout of an ideal lung the nitrogen concentration of the alveolar compartment drops exponentially. When end-tidal nitrogen concentration is plotted on a logarithmic scale the result is a decline that is a straight line (Fig. 8-1A). The slope of the line is dependent on the ratio of tidal volume to functional residual capacity (FRC), but the linearity on the log scale is characteristic of ideal nitrogen washout. Because of its complexity, ventilation of a normal lung is slightly inhomogeneous, which results in a slight curvilinear plot of end-tidal nitrogen concentration on a logarithmic scale (Fig. 8-1B). As washout of the lungs becomes less homogeneous, as occurs in certain diseases, the curve takes on an increasingly curvilinear characteristic with a prolongation of the tail of the curve (Fig. 8-1C).

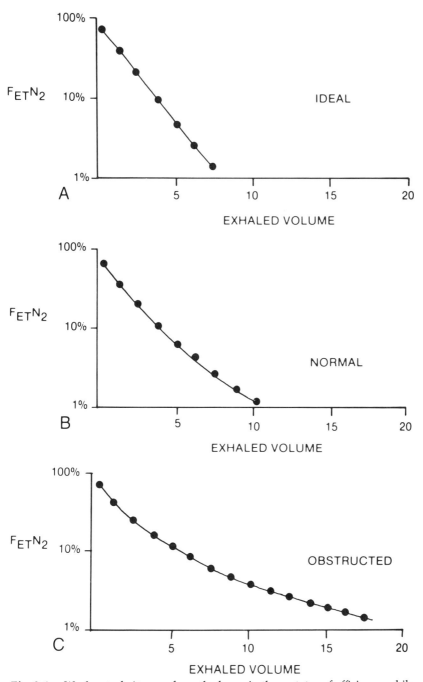

Fig. 8-1. Washout of nitrogen from the lungs in three states of efficiency while breathing oxygen. (A) In the ideal lung, composed of a single alveolar compartment, the alveolar nitrogen concentration (approximated by the end-tidal concentration) falls in a true exponential fashion. On a semilog plot this type of washout is a straight line. (B) The normal lung has a mild degree of ventilation inhomogeneity because of its complex structure. Nitrogen washout is slightly prolonged over the ideal lung and is represented by a slight curvilinear washout curve. (C) With severe inhomogeneity washout is greatly prolonged, and the washout curve is significantly extended.

Although the multibreath nitrogen elimination curve may be analyzed in many ways, the technique of performing the test is common to all. The testing equipment employed is identical to that used for the FRC open-circuit method described in Chapter 6. The nitrogen concentration of expired air is measured at the mouth by a rapid-response nitrogen analyzer, most commonly an ionizing emission spectroscopy unit (see Chapter 5). The analyzer must be able to record nitrogen concentration on a breath-by-breath basis, with a response time on the order of milliseconds. The analyzer output is converted to fractional concentration of nitrogen and plotted against the cumulative expired volume. The intake manifold of the mouthpiece can be switched from air to oxygen by the technician to start the testing process.

The patient is seated in front of the equipment. The nitrogen analyzer is turned on and permitted to stabilize, then calibrated just prior to use. The subject then begins breathing through the mouthpiece, which is initially open to the atmosphere. After the subject relaxes into a stable breathing pattern, the mouthpiece is switched to admit 100 percent oxygen on inspiration, and the X-Y recorder is activated. The switch should take place at end-expiration (FRC). The subject is encouraged to maintain a normal breathing pattern throughout the testing period, which usually continues until end-tidal nitrogen concentration is seen to drop below 1 percent.

The resulting graph consists of the logarithm of the nitrogen concentration on the y axis of the plot and the cumulative expired volume on the x axis (Fig. 8-2). The end-tidal points, identified as the maximal nitrogen concentration for each breath, are connected by a curve. This curve approximates the decline in mean alveolar nitrogen concentration. Analysis of the curve is based on one of two approaches. The first approach is to calculate an index based on one point or characteristic of the curve, such as the nitrogen concentration remaining after 7 min. The second approach is to use a series of points from the entire curve in the analysis, through the use of mathematical approximations or descriptions of the curve. The latter approach uses information from the entire curve, but is more time consuming and has not been routinely used in the clinical setting. The following sections will describe in brief five single-point methods and two multipoint methods. Although only the first is in common use, the others are often referred to in the medical literature.

Timed Nitrogen Washout Test   Patients with normal lungs breathing with a normal respiratory pattern can reduce alveolar nitrogen concentration to less than 2.5 percent by breathing oxygen for 7 min. Young subjects often reduce the concentration to under 1.5 percent in this time interval. Ventilation inhomogeneities induced by disease increase end-tidal nitrogen concentration to greater than 2.5 percent after 7 min. An end-tidal N_2 concentration greater than 2.5 percent after 7 min is considered abnormal, and is an index of inhomogeneity of ventilation.[1]

The index is dependent on the pattern of breathing as well as ventilation inhomogeneity because increases in tidal volume and raising of the TV/FRC ratio increase the dilution of FRC, resulting in a quicker elimination of nitrogen from the alveoli. There is a great deal of variability in the test because of this

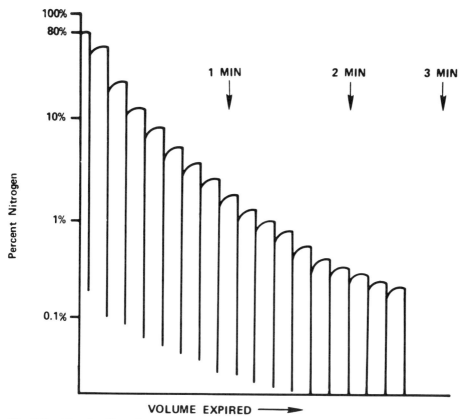

Fig. 8-2. Graph of log nitrogen concentration versus cumulative volume exhaled in the multibreath nitrogen washout test. The peak of the curve for each breath represents the end-tidal N_2 concentration. Analysis of the curve generated by the peak concentrations enables assessment of the homogeneity of gas distribution by one of the methods described in the text. [Reproduced with permission from Conrad SA: Clinical pulmonary function testing. p. 161. In George RB, Light RW, Matthay RA (eds): Chest Medicine. Churchill Livingstone, New York, 1983]

dependence on tidal volume. Some individuals will reduce their nitrogen concentration to 2.5 percent in less than 2 min. Thus, the 7-min N_2 concentration is not a sensitive index of distribution inhomogeneities, but is the most commonly used because of its simplicity.

Becklake Index and the Lung Clearance Index (LCI) The lung clearance index is an index of nitrogen washout that attempts to correct for the TV/FRC ratio dependence of washout dynamics. Introduced by Becklake,[2] the original LCI (now called the *Becklake index*) was originally calculated as the ratio of the volume of gas required to clear 90 percent of alveolar nitrogen and the volume comprising 90 percent of FRC:

$$\text{Becklake index} = \frac{\text{volume to clear 90\% FRC of } N_2}{90\% \text{ FRC}} \qquad \text{(Eq. 8-1)}$$

As currently used, however, the lung clearance index is the ratio of the volume of oxygen required to reduce end-tidal N_2 concentration to 2 percent and FRC[3]:

$$LCI = \frac{\text{volume to reduce } N_2 \text{ to } 2\%}{\text{FRC}} \qquad \text{(Eq. 8-2)}$$

The value in normal individuals ranges from about 6 to 9, and may be increased as much as threefold in chronic obstructive lung disease. Its major disadvantage is large intrasubject variability.

Mixing Ratio   The mixing ratio is the ratio of the actual number (n) and the ideal number (n') of breaths required to reduce end-tidal nitrogen concentration to 2 percent.[4] The ideal number of breaths is based on an ideal lung with a single alveolar compartment. The ideal number of breaths is calculated by

$$n' = \frac{ln(.025)}{ln[\text{FRC}/(\text{FRC} + V_T - V_D)]} \qquad \text{(Eq. 8-3)}$$

where FRC, V_T, and V_D are the values of the patient during the test. The mixing ratio (MR) is then:

$$MR = \frac{n}{n'} \qquad \text{(Eq. 8-4)}$$

Since V_T, V_D, and FRC are taken into account, the pattern of breathing theoretically does not significantly affect the results as long as the pattern is consistent. In practice, however, the MR is not entirely independent of these factors.[4] Normal subjects have a MR ranging from about 1.3 to 1.7 with an average value of 1.5.

Index of Efficiency   The index of ventilation efficiency $(E_{90\%})$ is the ratio of the ideal turnover value to the turnover value of the subject required to reduce lung nitrogen volume by 90 percent of its initial value. Turnover (TO) is the subject's cumulative exhaled volume expressed as the number of times the FRC was diluted[5]:

$$E_{90\%} = \frac{\text{ideal TO}}{\text{measured TO}}$$

$$\text{(Eqs. 8-5)}$$

$$TO = \frac{V_E}{\text{FRC}}$$

The index has been shown to be readily repeatable and to be relatively independent of the pattern of ventilation. The average value is between 75 and 80 percent.

Five-Breath Index (FBI)   The FBI is the ratio of the amount of nitrogen eliminated in the first five breaths and the amount that could be eliminated if no impairment of ventilation were present.[6] The tidal volume is held constant at 1 liter to remove the effect of its variation and the exhaled gas over the first five breaths is collected in a Douglas bag and analyzed. The ideal amount is calculated from the patient's FRC, an estimation of his dead space, his actual V_T of each of the first five breaths, and an assumed initial value of alveolar nitrogen concentration of 0.75. Each exhalation results in the elimination of the following volume of nitrogen:

$$V_{E_{N_2}} = V_T(F_{A_{N_2}}) \qquad \text{(Eq. 8-6)}$$

After each breath the $F_{A_{N_2}}$ is reduced by the factor:

$$\frac{FRC}{FRC + (V_T - V_D)} \qquad \text{(Eq. 8-7)}$$

The calculation of exhaled nitrogen volume is repeated in this manner on a breath-by-breath basis until five breaths have been reached. The five-breath index is then calculated:

$$FBI = \frac{\text{actual } N_2 \text{ volume of 5 breaths}}{\text{ideal } N_2 \text{ volume of 5 breaths}} \times 100 \qquad \text{(Eq. 8-8)}$$

The normal range of the FBI is 90 to 100 percent and falls to as low as 50 percent in subjects with chronic obstructive pulmonary disease.

Moment Analysis Although the washout curve is the result of a complex property of the lung, it may be treated as a distribution (comparable to a statistical distribution) of nitrogen concentration over volume, independent of any assumed underlying processes. Moments can be obtained from this distribution and used to characterize the curve.[7] The moments are sums of nitrogen concentration over the washout volume, weighted to a certain degree by the volume. For analysis, the curve is first rendered dimensionless to remove dependencies on the breathing pattern. The nitrogen concentration is expressed as fractional concentration and the volume exhaled is converted to *dilution number* by dividing by FRC. The first moment is calculated over the first 10 dilution numbers and normalized by dividing by the zero'th moment. The resulting ratio (M_1/M_0) is the index used to characterize the curve. Moment analysis takes the entire curve into account, unlike most of the other indexes described which use a single point or characteristic of the curve on which to base calculations. Details of the calculations are available in the literature.[7]

Index of Uniformity A mathematical equation was derived that described nitrogen washout dynamics as a form of an exponential equation[8]:

$$\frac{F_iN_2 - F_{eq}N_2}{F_{ET_{N_2}} - F_{eq}N_2} = e^{k(V/FRC)^B} \qquad \text{(Eq. 8-9)}$$

in which the decreasing end-tidal nitrogen concentration ($F_{ET_{N_2}}$), a function of cumulative exhaled volume (V), depends on the FRC, the initial and equilibrium nitrogen concentrations (F_iN_2 and $F_{eq}N_2$) as well as parameters k and B. The parameter B, termed the index of uniformity, is the index used to describe the degree of inhomogeneity of alveolar ventilation. It is a sensitive measurement but requires extensive calculating ability. Details of the calculations are available in ref. 8.

Comparison of Methods Because no standardization of multibreath nitrogen elimination test procedures has been made and washout dynamics depend on a large number of variables, no recommendation of a particular method can be made. The choice of method is left to the individual laboratory. In general, the two indexes that use information from the entire curve (moment analysis and index of uniformity) may be more sensitive to abnormalities and are relatively independent of patient variables, but their routine calculation is beyond the resources of most laboratories and they have not been extensively evaluated or accepted for routine use. The other methods are easier to calculate, but suffer from a relative lack of sensitivity. As a result, most laboratories use the simplest of those described, which is alveolar nitrogen concentration after 7 min of washout (timed N_2-washout test).

Helium Equilibrium Time

Assessment of the distribution of inspired gas can be made with the multibreath helium equilibration method when this method is used for the measurement of FRC. The test is performed in the same fashion as that used for FRC measurement, and the two may be done simultaneously. The measurement used is the *helium equilibrium* or *mixing time*, introduced by Meneely and Kaltreider.[9] The helium mixing time is measured as the time from the start of breathing in the helium circuit to the point at which the helium concentration of the circuit remains unchanged for 1 min.

The helium mixing time correlates fairly well with the single-breath nitrogen test[10] and the multibreath nitrogen washout test[11] in identifying abnormal function. The helium mixing time is less than 3 min in normal individuals,[10] and is increased in diseases producing ventilation inhomogeneity, especially airway diseases.

Single-Breath Nitrogen Elimination

The *single-breath nitrogen elimination test,* also known as the single-breath oxygen test, was also discussed in Chapter 7 with reference to its use in assessment of small airway dysfunction by the measurement of closing volume. It is useful in the assessment of gas distribution during ventilation.[12]

The equipment required to perform the test is similar to that for the multibreath N_2 test and consists of a mouthpiece with one-way valves. The inspired gas can be switched from environmental air to oxygen. A rapid-response nitrogen analyzer is attached to the exhalation port near the mouth for the continuous monitoring of nitrogen concentration in the expired gas. The expired volume is recorded with a spirometer. An X-Y recorder plots exhaled N_2 concentration on the y axis and expired volume on the x axis.

In the upright position while breathing room air, the subject is asked to make

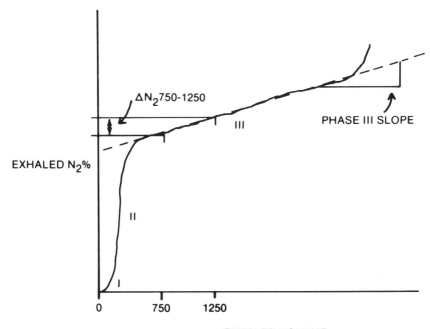

Fig. 8-3. Graph of nitrogen concentration versus volume exhaled in the single-breath nitrogen test. The $\Delta N_2 750-1250$ is the change in nitrogen concentration over the curve from 750 to 1,250 ml exhaled volume. The phase III slope is the change in nitrogen concentration per liter of the plateau, based on a line of best fit through the latter two-thirds of phase III. Both are indexes of the homogeneity of ventilation. [Modified from Conrad SA: Clinical pulmonary function testing. p. 161. In George RB, Light RW, Matthay RA (eds): Chest Medicine. Churchill Livingstone, New York, 1983]

a full expiration to residual volume, then inhale a full vital capacity with oxygen. Without breathholding, the subject then exhales fully to residual volume at a slow, constant rate of about 0.5 liter/sec while nitrogen concentration in the expired gas is continuously monitored with the nitrogen analyzer. The concentration of nitrogen is plotted against the volume exhaled (Fig. 8-3).

The inhalation of a full breath of oxygen from residual volume permits distribution of oxygen to all regions of the lung. The first gas to be distributed to the alveoli is the anatomic dead space gas, followed by inhaled oxygen. There is a gradient of distribution of gas between the upper and lower regions of the lungs, which is important in the measurement of closing volume as presented in Chapter 7. Within a small region of the lung, however, alveoli should inflate and deflate with a fairly high degree of homogeneity, and inspired gas should be distributed uniformly into and out of the alveoli. Ventilation may become inhomogeneous in a variety of disease states. There may be small airway disease, which slows ventilation to some alveolar groups, or a partial atelectasis and surfactant deficiencies, which alter the relative degree of expansion of some alveoli. Inspiration of oxygen in these cases results in varying concentrations of alveolar oxygen concentration, with poorly ventilating alveoli having lower concentrations of oxygen and greater concentrations of nitrogen.

During expiration four phases of nitrogen concentration can be identified (Fig. 8-3). Phase I is the initial phase in which dead space oxygen is expired and nitrogen concentration is zero. At the end of anatomic dead space expiration an abrupt increase in nitrogen concentration occurs; this is called phase II. It is the transition between airway and alveolar gas. Phase III is the alveolar phase during which alveolar gas is exhaled, and phase IV is the final increase in nitrogen concentration. Nitrogen concentration during phase III reaches a plateau, and the slope of this plateau is related to the homogeneity of alveolar filling and emptying. In an ideal lung in which all alveoli ventilate synchronously the nitrogen concentration would be constant and phase III would be strictly horizontal. As a result of mild inhomogeneities in the normal lung there is a small gradual rise to this phase, whereas in disease states with abnormalities in alveolar gas distribution the slope increases.

Anatomic Dead Space   The volume of anatomic dead space (VD_{anat}) is obtained from the graph by measuring the volume between the initiation of the test and phase II. Since phase II is not a perfect transition, its midpoint is used as the limiting value. VD_{anat} is therefore the volume of phase I and one-half of the volume of phase II (Fig. 8-4). Its predicted value for a given subject is the weight

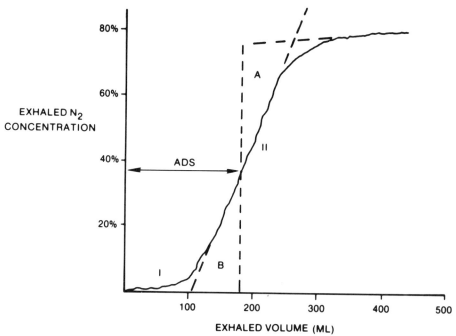

Fig. 8-4.   Measurement of anatomic dead space from the single-breath nitrogen washout curve. Phase II is divided into two segments at a point in which triangle A has an area equal to triangle B. The volume of phase I plus the volume of the initial portion of phase II up to the point of division is the anatomic dead space.

of the subject in pounds, that is, 150 ml in the average adult. It is increased in any disease-producing dilation of the nonrespiratory tracheobronchial tree, such as bronchiectasis, and it is decreased by loss of bronchial volume, such as plugging of the larger airways.

Phase III Slope The relationship between the *slope of the alveolar plateau* (phase III slope) and the distribution of ventilation permits the use of this slope as an index of ventilation homogeneity. A line is drawn through the latter two-thirds of the plateau, primarily to remove unevenness from cardiac oscillations. The change in nitrogen concentration over 1 liter of the plateau is the phase III slope (ΔN_2/liter). It is normally under 1 percent/liter in healthy young adults, and may increase to 1.5 or 2 percent/liter with normal aging. Its value is increased in any lung disease resulting in ventilation inhomogeneities. Subjects with chronic obstructive pulmonary disease may have values of up to 20 percent/liter or higher. Purely restrictive diseases generally do not produce abnormalities in the phase III slope.

Related to the phase III slope is the $\Delta N_2 750 - 1250$, or change in N_2 concentration over the 0.5-liter interval between 750 and 1,250 ml of expired air. It is approximately half the value of the phase III slope, but may differ slightly if the phase III plateau is not linear. The $\Delta N_2 750 - 1250$ value is set at the initial portion of the plateau to standardize the measurement, offset by 750 ml to ensure full dead space exhalation.

LOCALIZED DISTRIBUTION OF VENTILATION

The tests described in the previous section give an index of overall assessment of gas distribution in the lungs. They are useful in assessing the severity of lung dysfunction in a variety of disease states, but do not provide specific anatomic information about distribution of pulmonary ventilation. More selective tests are required to obtain this type of information. Bronchospirometry involves selective intubation of the bronchi, but its use has been largely supplanted by radionuclide imaging and the use of simpler, although less sensitive tests, such as the lateral position test.

Radionuclide Ventilation Imaging

The use of a radioactive tracer gas to study relative distribution of ventilation was developed over 20 years ago.[13,14] The initial systems utilized several scintillation counters that could discriminate only large regions, typically three fields per lung. Xenon-133 (^{133}Xe) gas was rebreathed for ventilation studies, and counts made over the posterior thorax. Modern nuclear medicine imaging systems permit static and dynamic imaging of the distribution of gas in the lungs on a regional basis, with image resolution at the level of the bronchopulmonary segments or better. Dynamic studies permit wash-in and washout analysis on a regional basis as well.

In order to study ventilation by radionuclide imaging, a tracer is inhaled and rebreathed. The tracer emits low-level radiation which can be detected at the surface of the body by instruments that can produce an image of the density of radioactivity (gamma camera). The density of radioactivity is a result of the concentration of the tracer gas in a particular region. Gamma cameras are large enough to permit both lungs to be imaged simultaneously.

To study ventilation a radionuclide tracer should have the following characteristics:

1. Exist solely in the gas phase
2. Have a low solubility in aqueous or lipid substances
3. Exhibit biochemical inertness
4. Not be involved in uptake or production by the body
5. Have a radionuclide half-life only long enough to permit a single series of scans
6. Produce sufficient radiation for imaging, yet remain at a "safe" level

The radionuclide most commonly employed for ventilation imaging in practice today is still ^{133}Xe. It is an inert gas with a half-life of 5.27 days and a low solubility in water, and is not significantly taken up by the body. Krypton-81m is an alternate gas, with a half-life of only 13 sec. Because its half-life is so brief, only limited scanning can be performed.

Pulmonary imaging is performed in three phases.[15-17] In the first phase, a single postinspirational image gives information on areas readily ventilated. The second phase involves imaging after a period of rebreathing to allow more time for slowly ventilating areas to appear. In the final phase, a series of washout or elimination images permit dynamic viewing of gas elimination to demonstrate areas of trapping and slow ventilation. This is the most useful phase.

The subject is usually placed in a sitting position for imaging, unless his condition requires the horizontal position. The imaging camera is placed against the posterior thorax. The subject exhales to residual volume, then inhales a breath of the ^{133}Xe mixture containing 5 mCi of the radionuclide per liter and holds his breath. During the breathhold an initial scan is made *(single-breath image)*. Each image requires at least 50,000 scintillation counts. The subject then rebreathes the ^{133}Xe gas mixture in a closed system to permit equilibrium of ventilation. After 3 to 6 min a second scan is made *(equilibrium image)* (Fig. 8-5). The subject then begins breathing environmental air and the xenon is collected by a disposal system. Serial scans are made at intervals of 30 to 60 sec until all residual activity is gone. This series of scans constitutes the *elimination* or *washout image* phase (Fig. 8-6).

For the inspiration and elimination scans the anterior or posterior view is imaged. Although it is standard practice to image the posterior view during the equilibrium phase, it is possible for other projections to be imaged, such as the anterior, posterior, right and left lateral, and right and left posterior obliques.

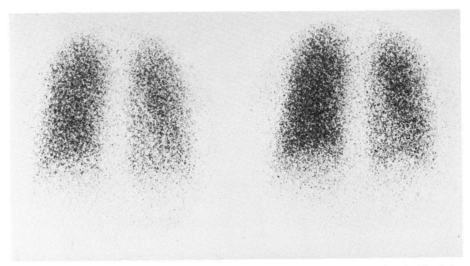

Fig. 8-5.   Equilibrium images from a ^{133}Xe ventilation scan in a normal individual, in which the gas is rebreathed from a closed system. (Courtesy of Mary J. Wood, M.D., Shreveport, Louisiana.)

Xenon-133 ventilation scans allow assessment of regional ventilation. Qualitative assessment is made on the basis of visual examination of the images. Quantitative assessment is performed by comparing radionuclide scintigraphic counts from individual regions. Ventilation scanning is most commonly performed in conjunction with a perfusion scan (to be discussed later) to identify regional perfusion defects in the presence of normal ventilation for the diagnosis of pulmonary embolization. Another use is to determine differences in ventilation as a preoperative method of predicting retained ventilation capacity after pneumonectomy; this use is largely replacing bronchospirometry for regional ventilation assessment. Details on the interpretation of ventilation scans requires knowledge and expertise in nuclear medicine procedures and is beyond the scope of this book. For further information, the reader is referred to the references cited.[15-17]

Lateral Position Test

A simple, noninvasive means of assessing the relative ventilatory function of each lung is the lateral position test.[18,19] This test estimates the relative contribution of each lung to total ventilation and correlates well with oxygen consumption. It also compares favorably with radionuclide ventilation scanning.[20]

The test is based on the relative change in FRC produced by changing from the supine to each of the lateral positions. The subject begins rebreathing in the supine position from an oxygen-filled closed-circuit spirometer system with a CO_2 absorber. After a stable decreasing baseline is reached, the subject is turned onto one side, and rebreathing continues for several breaths. The supine position

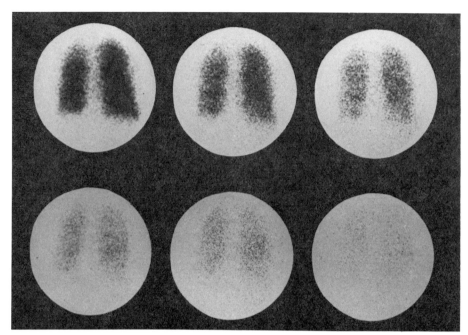

Fig. 8-6. Washout image series from a ^{133}Xe ventilation scan in a normal individual. These images, approximately 1 to 2 min apart, demonstrate the decrease in radioactivity with time. (Courtesy of Mary J. Wood, M.D., Shreveport, Louisiana.)

is repeated, then the subject is turned onto the other side, and the test is repeated again. The subject then turns again to the supine position to complete the test. A tracing is depicted in Figure 8-7. The relative distance from the baseline represents the relative degree of function.

Bronchospirometry

When accurate assessment of ventilation and gas exchange of the individual lungs is required, bronchospirometry can be employed.[21] This method is invasive and requires anesthesia with a significant risk of complications. Bronchospirometry is performed by selective intubation of the bronchi with a double-lumen, double-cuff tube. Ventilation and other indexes of pulmonary function, such as oxygen consumption (indicative of $\dot{V}/\dot{Q}$ matching) and carbon monoxide diffusion, can be made from each lung through the mainstem bronchi. This method requires special resources not available in most hospitals. Comparable information about individual lung function can be obtained by radionuclide imaging or noninvasive tests, such as the lateral position test. Bronchospirometry therefore is rarely indicated.

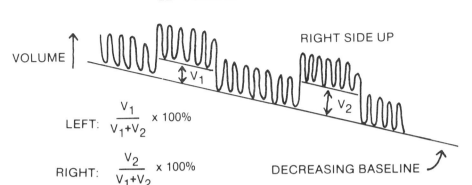

Fig. 8-7. Graph of spirometer volume change as a function of time in the lateral position test. As the subject is turned from supine to the left or right lateral position, a change in the FRC baseline occurs. The relative degree of change between the right and left sides reflects the relative contributions of the right and left lungs, respectively, to overall pulmonary function. The test is detailed in text.

DISTRIBUTION OF PULMONARY BLOOD FLOW

Assessment of pulmonary perfusion is not routinely performed in the evaluation of pulmonary function. Because of the equipment resources involved and the invasiveness of the procedure, total pulmonary blood flow (cardiac output) is measured only in specially indicated circumstances (see Chapter 13). Imaging of the distribution of pulmonary perfusion, however, is performed noninvasively by radionuclide techniques.

Radionuclide Perfusion Imaging

The regional distribution of pulmonary blood flow may be obtained by the injection of a radioactive substance that collects in the pulmonary capillary bed in proportion to the amount of blood flow in a given region.[15-17] Imaging of the radionuclide results in an image in which activity in a given region is proportional to the perfusion in that region.

The subject receives an intravenous injection of 2 to 4 mCi of technetium-99m-labeled human albumin microspheres, or [99mTc]HAM. The microspheres, 20 to 50 μm in diameter, pass through the right heart and lodge in a relatively uniform pattern in the pulmonary capillary bed. The number of capillaries occluded is small and there is a rich vascular bed, so no adverse effects occur on pulmonary tissues. Shortly after injection a series of scintigraphic images is made. The gamma camera is positioned over the surface of the body overlying the area to be imaged. A total of 300,000 to 500,000 counts is required

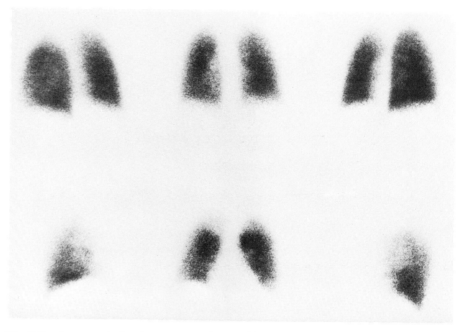

Fig. 8-8.   Lung perfusion image series from a [^{99m}Tc]HAM perfusion scan, with images made in several orientations. The projections in the figure are, clockwise from the top left, left posterior oblique, posterior, right posterior oblique, left lateral, anterior, and right lateral. (Courtesy of Mary J. Wood, M.D., Shreveport, Louisiana.)

in each view for a satisfactory image. Views are routinely made in the anterior, posterior, right and left lateral, and right and left posterior oblique positions (Fig. 8-8).

The primary objective of perfusion radionuclide imaging is to locate perfusion defects, usually for the purpose of screening for pulmonary embolization. It will image areas of the lung with a functioning capillary bed; however, it will not image areas occluded by thromboembolism or in which lung capillary beds have been destroyed, such as bullae. Bullae and related anatomic changes must be distinguished by comparing perfusion images with ventilation images. The technique also will not image vascular lesions free of capillaries, such as arteriovenous malformations. Further details on interpretation are beyond the scope of this book; the reader is referred to the cited references.[15-17,22]

RELATIONSHIP OF VENTILATION TO PERFUSION

The physiological basis of the interface between ventilation and perfusion is given in Chapter 3. Mismatching of ventilation and perfusion for the purposes of this section can be considered to occur by two mechanisms. The first is when gas exchange units have a relative *hypoperfusion*. The second is when gas exchange units have a relative *hypoventilation.* Both of these mechanisms reduce the effectiveness of the alveolar-capillary interface. Mismatch results in a diminished capability for gas exchange.

Alveoli that are ventilated but not perfused contribute to *alveolar dead space.* The *anatomic dead space* created by conducting airways also contributes to ineffective ventilation. The sum of alveolar and anatomic dead spaces constitutes the *physiological dead space.* In the pulmonary function laboratory physiological and not alveolar dead space is measured; the latter may be derived by subsequent measurement of anatomic dead space.

Capillaries not in contact with functioning alveoli contribute to the *alveolar* or *relative shunt. Anatomic shunt* is that which bypasses the lungs completely through the heart or arterio-venous (A-V) communications. The combination of alveolar and anatomic shunts comprises the *physiological shunt* or total venous admixture.

These are the two extreme examples of $\dot{V}/\dot{Q}$ mismatch. True dead space does not cause hypoxemia or hypercarbia if ventilation is increased to maintain a normal level of ventilation in properly functioning respiratory units. Shunting, however, does produce hypoxemia, usually without hypercarbia. In actual lungs there is a combination and continuum of these two processes. Techniques are available, discussed in the next section, for assessing physiological dead space and shunt. Although these indexes do not give any anatomic information about ventilation-perfusion matching in the lungs, they do give overall indexes of function that are useful in assessing disorders of gas exchange.

Physiological Dead Space

The measurement of physiological dead space is based on the simple principle of gas dilution, and is derived in the appendix. The Bohr equation for the determination of the *physiological dead space fraction* (V_D/V_T) is obtained from these principles:

$$\frac{V_D}{V_T} = \frac{P_{A_{CO_2}} - P_{E_{CO_2}}}{P_{A_{CO_2}}} \qquad \text{(Eq. 8-10)}$$

Because the alveolar-arterial gradient for CO_2, or $P(A-a)_{CO_2}$, is negligible and alveolar P_{CO_2} is not easily measured, arterial P_{CO_2} is used in place of alveolar P_{CO_2}.

The test is performed by collecting expired gas into a Douglas bag for 1 to 5 min. During collection an arterial blood sample is obtained and analyzed for P_{CO_2}. The mixed expired gas is also analyzed for CO_2 tension.

To calculate the *physiological dead space volume* (V_D), the expired gas volume is measured and average tidal volume calculated from the total volume and respiratory frequency. The dead space fraction equation is rearranged to the following:

$$V_D = \frac{\dot{V}_E}{F} \left(\frac{P_{A_{CO_2}} - P_{E_{CO_2}}}{P_{A_{CO_2}}} \right) \qquad \text{(Eq. 8-11)}$$

Alveolar dead space volume is the difference between physiological and anatomic dead space:

$$V_{D_A} = V_D - V_{D_{anat}}$$ (Eq. 8-12)

Anatomic dead space may be measured by the single-breath nitrogen elimination test or estimated as 1 ml/lb body weight.

Physiological Shunt

The principle underlying the determination of physiological shunt (total venous admixture) is analogous to that for physiological dead space, that is, the principle of dilution of concentration of a substance, in this case, oxygen. The equation for the physiological shunt fraction, derived in Appendix C, is

$$\frac{\dot{Q}s_{phys}}{\dot{Q}_T} = \frac{Cc'_{O_2} - Ca_{O_2}}{Cc'_{O_2} - C\bar{v}_{O_2}}$$ (Eq. 8-13)

The content of oxygen must be measured at three points. The *mixed venous* content of oxygen ($C\bar{v}$) is the amount of oxygen entering both normal and shunt paths. The *arterial* content is the mixture of both shunt and nonshunt fractions. The *pulmonary end-capillary* content (Cc') is ideally measured at the exitus of the functioning capillary bed. This measurement is obviously not possible because of the microscopic and inhomogeneous nature of the capillary bed, so an estimate must be made. It is assumed for purposes of this calculation that complete equilibrium of oxygen tensions has taken place between the alveolar spaces and capillaries within functioning respiratory units. By use of the alveolar gas equation one may estimate alveolar oxygen tension, and hence, end-capillary oxygen tension. Applying the oxyhemoglobin dissociation relationship permits estimation of the blood oxygen content. If one assumes further that the hemoglobin of blood at all three points is equal and $F_{I_{O_2}}$ is low, such that the volume of physically dissolved oxygen is negligible, then saturation may be used in place of oxygen content:

$$\frac{\dot{Q}s_{phys}}{\dot{Q}_T} = \frac{Sc'_{O_2} - Sa_{O_2}}{Sc'_{O_2} - S\bar{v}_{O_2}}$$ (Eq. 8-14)

The physiological shunt is the sum of two components, a right-to-left *anatomic shunt* ($\dot{Q}s_{anat}$) in which no blood is in contact with alveoli, as in intracardiac defects, and a less well-defined alveolar or *relative shunt* ($\dot{Q}s_{rel}$) because of poor ventilation-perfusion matching. The two may be separated by repeating the shunt calculation after 20 to 30 min of breathing oxygen to remove all nitrogen from the alveoli. The alveoli are then filled with carbon dioxide and a high concentration of oxygen. This process ensures high alveolar oxygen tensions in the face of $\dot{V}/\dot{Q}$ disturbance and effectively eliminates the relative shunt. Any shunt fraction remaining constitutes anatomic shunt.

In this measurement of shunt while breathing 100 percent oxygen there are two additional considerations. First, high oxygen tensions in blood produce a nonnegligible volume of oxygen dissolved in plasma (up to approximately 1.5 ml/dl blood), so that saturation measurements must be replaced by content measurements in which the volume of oxygen physically dissolved must be added. The second consideration permits simplification of shunt calculation when the inspired gas is oxygen. In this case the end-capillary blood can be assumed to be completely saturated, and therefore Cc' becomes equal to Ca. The resulting equation is:

$$\frac{\dot{Q}s_{anat}}{\dot{Q}_T} = \frac{0.0031[P(A\text{-}a)_{O_2}]}{C(a\text{-}\bar{v})_{O_2} + 0.0031[P(A\text{-}a)_{O_2}]} \qquad \text{(Eq. 8-15)}$$

Details of the derivation are available in Appendix C. This equation requires only measurements of arterial and mixed venous blood and calculation of $P(A\text{-}a)_{O_2}$, the A-a gradient for oxygen. Mixed venous blood is preferably obtained from the pulmonary artery because right atrial blood may not be well mixed. If mixed venous blood is not available, the normal value for the arteriovenous content difference of 5 ml/dl may be substituted. If the patient is critically ill the difference is frequently altered, requiring measurement of the difference. In many critically ill patients in the intensive care unit mixed venous and arterial blood are readily available.

Single-Breath CO_2 Elimination

By using a gas that resides in the pulmonary blood and rapidly diffuses into the alveoli, the matching of ventilation and perfusion as well as the distribution of ventilation can be assessed. Carbon dioxide has these properties and does not need to be introduced into the body.

The subject is seated and initially breathes environmental air. After a full inspiration to total lung capacity the subject exhales slowly but completely and steadily into a rapid-response carbon dioxide analyzer. The expiratory flow rate is maintained at about 0.5 liter/sec. The concentration of exhaled CO_2 is plotted against the volume exhaled.

The resulting curve is similar to that of the single-breath nitrogen elimination test with three phases corresponding to the first three phases of the nitrogen test (Fig. 8-9). The principles underlying these phases are identical to those for nitrogen except that the CO_2 eliminated is only from functioning respiratory units with intact perfusion *and* gas exchange, since nonperfused alveoli will be relatively free of CO_2. In the nitrogen test the results depended only on functioning ventilation, as N_2 is present in both perfused and nonperfused alveoli.

Interpretation of the results involves determination of the slope of the alveolar plateau. Increases in the slope result from abnormal matching of ventilation and perfusion as well as abnormal distribution of ventilation in the lungs.

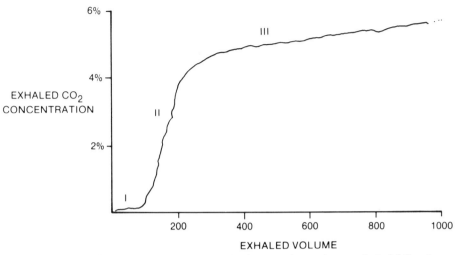

Fig. 8-9. Graph of CO_2 concentration in expired gas against volume exhaled following a full inspiration of oxygen in the single-breath CO_2 test. The slope of phase III is representative of the matching of ventilation and perfusion as well as the homogeneity of ventilation, with an increased slope indicative of poor $\dot{V}/\dot{Q}$ matching and poor ventilation.

Radionuclide Ventilation/Perfusion Imaging

Regional differences in $\dot{V}/\dot{Q}$ matching can be assessed by radionuclide imaging of a radioactive substance that traverses from the bloodstream into the alveoli in functioning respiratory units.[22] Imaging in various projections of the lungs permit regional assessment of $\dot{V}/\dot{Q}$ matching. The basic principle is to inject a radionuclide tracer gas in aqueous solution into the circulation that will diffuse from the blood into the alveoli. The tracer gas used should be completely removed from the circulation with a single pass so that residual radionuclide activity comes from the alveoli and not from recirculation. A suitable tracer is xenon-133, an inert gas of very low solubility in aqueous solutions. Essentially all of the gas diffuses into the lungs during the first pass after an intravenous injection of the gas in solution.

Five to 10 mCi of ^{133}Xe gas are dissolved in a sterile aqueous solution. The solution is injected intravenously during a breathhold. As the gas passes through the pulmonary capillaries, over 95 percent leaves solution in the gas phase of the alveoli. It is transferred only into those alveoli that are perfused. A single posterior image is made during the breathhold. The subject then breathes environmental air to wash out the [133]Xe. Further images may be made during washout to identify areas with functional perfusion but poor ventilation, which show up as slowly diminishing areas of radioactivity.

The [133]Xe $\dot{V}/\dot{Q}$ scan reveals regions of the lungs with intact alveolar-capillary interfaces. Areas of perfusion with no alveoli (shunt) are not imaged because there is no gas phase to trap the [133]Xe. Areas of ventilation without perfusion are not imaged as there is no perfusion to deliver ^{133}Xe to the alveoli. Areas of relative hypoperfusion will be imaged with lesser intensity because gas exchange is impaired. The images obtained after several breaths will reveal areas of poor ventilation.

The test is difficult to perform because the gas is difficult to handle and only limited scans can be obtained at a time. It is infrequently utilized. A more common approach to assess matching of ventilation to perfusion is performed by separately imaging ventilation and perfusion with inhaled xenon and tagged human albumin microspheres, respectively, and comparing the two sets of images.

REFERENCES

1. Cournand A, Baldwin E, Darling RC, Richards RW: Studies of the intrapulmonary mixture of gases. IV. The significance of the pulmonary emptying rate and a simplified open circuit measurement of residual air. J Clin Invest 20:681, 1941
2. Becklake M: A new index of the intrapulmonary mixture of inspired air. Thorax 7:111, 1952
3. Bouhuys A: Pulmonary nitrogen clearance in relation to age in healthy males. J Appl Physiol 18:297, 1963
4. Edelman NH, Mittman C, Norris AH, Shock NW: Effects of respiratory pattern and age differences in ventilatory uniformity. J Appl Physiol 24:49, 1967
5. Prowse K, Cumming G: Effects of lung volume and disease on the lung nitrogen decay curve. J Appl Physiol 34:23, 1973
6. Weygandt GR: A sensitive five-breath N_2 washout test of distribution of ventilation. J Appl Physiol 40:464, 1976
7. Saidel GM, Salmon RB, Chester EH: Moment analysis of multibreath lung washout. J Appl Physiol 38:328, 1975
8. Light RW, George RB, Meneely GR, et al: A new method for analyzing multiple breath nitrogen washout curves. J Appl Physiol 48:265, 1980
9. Meneely GR, Kaltreider NL: The volume of the lung determined by helium dilution: Description of the method and comparison with other procedures. J Clin Invest 28:129, 1949
10. Hathirat S, Renzetti AD Jr, Mitchell M: Intrapulmonary gas distribution: A comparison of the helium mixing time and nitrogen single breath test in normal and diseased subjects. Am Rev Resp Dis 102:750, 1970
11. Motley HL: Comparison of a simple helium closed with the oxygen open-circuit method for measuring residual air. Am Rev Tuberc 76:601, 1957
12. Comroe JH, Fowler WS: Lung function studies. VI. Detection of uneven alveolar ventilation during a single breath of oxygen. Am J Med 10:408, 1951
13. Ball WC Jr, Stewart PB, Newsham LGS, Bates DV: Regional pulmonary function studied with xenon[133]. J Clin Invest 41:519, 1962
14. Dollery CT, Hugh-Jones P, Matthews CME: Use of radioactive xenon for studies of regional lung function. Br Med J 2:1006, 1962
15. Sodee DB, Early PJ: *Mosby's Manual of Nuclear Medicine Procedures.* 3rd Ed. C.V. Mosby, St. Louis, Mo, 1981
16. Keyes JW Jr, Carey JE, Moses DC, Beierwaltes WH: Manual of Nuclear Medicine Procedures. 2nd Ed. CRC Press, Cleveland, Ohio, 1973

17. Sodee DB, Early PJ: Technology and Interpretation of Nuclear Medicine Procedures. 2nd Ed. C.V. Mosby, St. Louis, Mo, 1975
18. Bergan F: A simple method for determination of the relative function of the right and left lung. Acta Chir Scand, suppl., 253:58, 1960
19. Hazlett DR, Watson RL: Lateral position test: A simple, inexpensive, yet accurate method of studying the separate functions of the lungs. Chest 59:276, 1971
20. Marion JM, Alderson PO, Lefrak SS, et al: Unilateral lung function: Comparison of the lateral position test with radionuclide ventilation-perfusion studies. Chest 69:5, 1976
21. Svanberg L: Bronchospirometry in the study of regional lung function. Scand J Resp Dis, suppl., 62:91, 1966
22. Early PJ, Razzak MA, Sodee DB: Textbook of Nuclear Medicine Technology. 3rd Ed. C.V. Mosby, St. Louis, Mo, 1979

9

Gas Diffusion

Steven A. Conrad, M.D.

The interface between alveolar gas and pulmonary capillary blood is complex, and a number of factors are involved in the exchange of gases. A brief review of the principles involved in pulmonary gas diffusion are given here as a foundation for an understanding of the tests used in the assessment of diffusion. For further discussion of gas exchange, refer to Chapter 3.

Diffusion of a substance in fluids (liquids and gases) is a passive process occurring between regions of differing concentration. If a constant-thickness membrane permeable to a particular gas is placed between two fluid compartments, the diffusion of a gas across the membrane is described by Fick's law of diffusion:

$$\dot{V} = k\left(\frac{A}{L}\right) \times (P_1 - P_2) \qquad \text{(Eq. 9-1)}$$

The driving force for the rate of gas diffusion ($\dot{V}$) is the difference in partial pressure of the gas between the two compartments ($P_1 - P_2$). For a given driving force the membrane characteristics determine the rate of gas transfer. These characteristics include: (1) the *coefficient of diffusion* (k) determined by the solubility and interactions of the gas and the membrane, (2) the *area* of the membrane (*A*), and (3) its *thickness* (*L*). These three characteristics are not directly applicable to the lungs because of the complex morphology and dynamic state of the lungs. They are lumped into a single coefficient, termed the *diffusing capacity* of the lungs (DL):

$$\dot{V} = D_L(P_1 - P_2) \qquad \text{(Eq. 9-2)}$$

DL is also called the *transfer factor* (TL), a more appropriate term because the tests employed in the clinical laboratory measure more than membrane diffusion alone, and the term *capacity* is an imprecise description of this type of measurement.

Because diffusion of a gas in a fluid depends on the concentration of the gas in the fluid, the principles of Fick's law apply to the alveolar-capillary interface. A

185

gas will diffuse until the concentration gradient is reduced to zero. In a closed system, equilibrium will occur after a period of time and gas diffusion will cease. The pulmonary system, however, is an open system in that the alveolar and capillary blood compartments are continually replenished, thereby maintaining a concentration gradient across the alveolar-capillary membrane and permitting diffusion to continue. Marked changes of the gradient from tidal ventilation and pulsatile blood flow are buffered by the residual air in the lungs and rapid capillary blood flow. Thus, the gradients of oxygen and carbon dioxide are nearly constant in steady-state breathing.

DIFFUSING CAPACITY FOR CARBON MONOXIDE

The measurement of diffusing capacity for oxygen (DL_{O_2}) is possible but not technically feasible for routine use and has been limited to research applications. Measurement of the diffusing capacity for carbon monoxide (DL_{CO}) is a commonly performed method of assessment of gas diffusion. Carbon monoxide has several characteristics that make it a useful gas in place of oxygen for the measurement of DL:

1. Carbon monoxide has a membrane diffusion coefficient and a rate of reaction with hemoglobin, which are similar to and linearly related to that of oxygen. Essentially the same information on diffusion can therefore be obtained with CO as with oxygen.
2. Carbon monoxide is not normally present in the blood in appreciable amounts, facilitating the calculation of carbon monoxide uptake.
3. The carboxyhemoglobin dissociation curve is such that very low partial pressures of CO result after even large amounts of CO have combined with hemoglobin. This feature permits assumptions to be made about the capillary partial pressure of CO, eliminating the need for this difficult measurement in most instances.
4. The affinity of hemoglobin for CO is much greater than for oxygen (approximately 210 times), so that a partial pressure of oxygen that remains in the physiological range is not a major interfering factor.
5. Low concentrations of the gas are easily measured in the laboratory and do not result in any harm to the subject.

The methods used in the routine measurement of diffusion are incapable of separating the diffusion of CO across the membrane from its diffusion through the red cells and combination with hemoglobin. Intracapillary diffusion of CO and its combination with hemoglobin has been shown to be slow enough to constitute a significant fraction of the total diffusion, as measured in the laboratory, and cannot be neglected. Methods are described in this chapter that differentiate between the two components (membrane diffusion and combina-

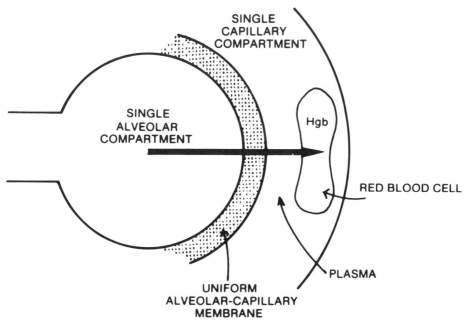

Fig. 9-1. Diagram of a model for the clinical measurement of gas diffusion in the lungs. This model consists of a single alveolar compartment, a uniform alveolar-capillary membrane, and a capillary compartment. In addition to the diffusion across the alveolar-capillary membrane, the measurement made in the laboratory includes diffusion across the plasma, the red cell membrane, and the rate of reaction with the intracellular hemoglobin. Although the lungs are morphologically more complex than this model, all components of the diffusing capacity are present.

tion with hemoglobin in the red cell). As rountinely measured, D_L gives only an overall value for diffusion and is related primarily to the alveolar-capillary surface area available for gas exchange. The model for gas diffusion in the lungs as measured clinically is diagrammed in Figure 9-1.

There are four approaches to the measurement of carbon monoxide diffusing capacity: the single-breath, steady-state, rebreathing, and equilibrium wash-out methods. Each has advantages and disadvantages that make it appropriate for a particular situation. All four methods are based on the common underlying principle given in Equation 9-2. Diffusing capacity is reported as the milli-liters of gas transferred per minute per torr of gas partial pressure gradient [ml/min/torr]. The equation representing this concept is

$$D_{L_{CO}} = \frac{\text{volume of CO uptake by lungs}}{\text{alveolar-capillary } P_{CO} \text{ difference}} = \frac{\dot{V}_{CO}}{P_{A_{CO}} - P_{C_{CO}}} \quad \text{(Eq. 9-3)}$$

The actual equations and techniques of measurement are somewhat more complex than this equation but are based on this concept.

Single-Breath Method (DLsb$_{CO}$)

The single-breath method for diffusing capacity is the most commonly used means of assessing carbon monoxide transfer, primarily because of the ease and noninvasiveness of the test. The test is also known as the modified Krogh method because it was developed by Marie Krogh[1] as a research tool and modified by Forster, Olgilvie, and others for clinical use.[2-4] The test is performed by having the subject exhale to residual volume, then inhale a gas mixture containing 0.3 percent carbon monoxide, 10 percent helium, 20 percent oxygen, and the remainder nitrogen. The subject inhales the gas mixture to total lung capacity and holds his breath for 10 sec, then exhales. During exhalation the gas is dried and the concentrations of CO and He are continuously measured. A graph of volume versus time permits timing of the breathhold interval (Fig. 9-2).

In order to determine the amount of CO transferred across the membrane, the concentration of alveolar CO must be determined at the beginning and at the end of the 10-sec breathhold. The concentration at the end is measured by monitoring the expired CO concentration and taking a value near the end of expiration, assumed to represent alveolar gas. The concentration at the beginning of the breathhold period must be determined indirectly, as the concentration of inhaled CO is diluted by the residual volume in the lungs and cannot be measured directly. Calculation of this dilution is performed by measuring the concentration of helium at the beginning and end of the breathhold. Because

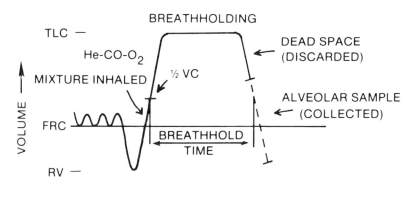

Fig. 9-2. Kymograph tracing during the single-breath DL$_{CO}$ maneuver. The patient first exhales to residual volume, then takes a full breath of a known mixture of oxygen, helium, and carbon monoxide. The breath is held at full inspiration for 10 sec to allow gas transfer, then the subject exhales. After the initial dead space is exhaled, a sample of alveolar gas is collected and analyzed, and used in the calculation of DL$_{CO}$. The graph permits determination of the actual breathhold time, which is the time interval between the midpoint of vital capacity during inspiration and the point of sample collection during exhalation. [Modified from Conrad SA, George RB: Clinical pulmonary function testing. p. 161. In George RB, Light RW, Matthay RA (eds): Chest Medicine. Churchill Livingstone, New York, 1983]

helium is not transferred across the alveolar-capillary interface to any significant degree, any decrease in concentration in helium is caused by dilution in the lungs. Since helium is transported along with CO, the concentration of carbon monoxide after dilution in the residual gas may be calculated by the formula:

$$F_iA_{CO} = F_{I_{CO}}\left(\frac{F_{A_{He}}}{F_{I_{He}}}\right) \qquad \text{(Eq. 9-4)}$$

where $F_{I_{CO}}$ is the concentration of inhaled CO and $F_{I_{He}}$ and $F_{A_{He}}$ are the initial and final (end-tidal or alveolar) concentrations of He. The end-inspiratory alveolar volume is computed from the helium dilution in a manner similar to that used for the helium dilution for functional residual capacity:

$$V_A = V_I\left(\frac{F_{I_{He}}}{F_{A_{He}}}\right) \qquad \text{(Eq. 9-5)}$$

where V_I is the inspired volume, and $F_{I_{He}}$ and $F_{A_{He}}$ are the inspired and measured alveolar (end-tidal) concentrations of helium.

With this information DL_{CO} may be determined by the following formula:

$$DL_{CO} = \frac{V_A}{(P_B - P_{H_2O})} \times \frac{60}{BH_t} \times ln\left(\frac{F_iA_{CO}}{F_fA_{CO}}\right) \qquad \text{(Eq. 9-6)}$$

where V_A is equal to the calculated end-inspiratory alveolar volume in milliliters, 60 is the conversion factor from seconds to minutes, P_B is the measured barometric pressure, BH_t is the actual breathhold interval, and F_iA_{CO} and F_fA_{CO} are the fractional concentrations of carbon monoxide at the beginning and at the end of the breathhold period.

Although the technique requires more equipment and more calculation than some of the other methods, the single-breath method is quick to perform and noninvasive. The single-breath test should be performed when the subject is at rest, therefore precluding the use of this test for exercise studies. The vital capacity should exceed 1.5 liters for results to be acceptable. The breathholding interval is usually 10 sec, and should be a minimum of 5 sec. The disadvantages of the single-breath method include the fact that the measurement of diffusing capacity is made during a single breathhold. Breathholding, especially in poorly ventilating lungs, probably does not represent conditions during steady tidal breathing. In addition, the measurement of helium concentration for estimating alveolar volume and initial CO concentration is required.

Rebreathing Method ($DLrb_{CO}$)

A method similar in principle to the single-breath method for measurement of carbon monoxide diffusing capacity is the rebreathing method.[5] In place of measuring the change in CO concentration during a breathhold, the subject rebreathes a test gas from a closed system and the concentration of CO in the system is monitored over a period of several minutes. The change in concentration of CO over this time period (after an initial 10-sec phase of equilibrium with te alveolar volume) represents the amount of CO transferred across the membrane. Using this technique, diffusing capacity is measured during spontaneous respiration, which more closely approximates the normal conditions of gas exchange than that obtained by the breathholding method. The method yields results that correlate with the single-breath method in most instances.

The test is performed by filling a reservoir bag with a gas mixture containing 0.1 percent CO, 10 percent helium, 20 percent oxygen, and the remainder nitrogen. The volume in the reservoir bag is adjusted to equal the patient's vital capacity. The patient then exhales to residual volume, is attached to the reservoir bag, and begins rebreathing into the bag for a period of 30 to 60 sec. The respiratory frequency is maintained at about 30 breaths/min to help assure mixing of gas in the bag with alveolar gas. The depth of respiration is full vital capacity so that the subject empties the bag with each breath. The concentration of CO in the bag is sampled continuously and plotted as a function of time on a semilog scale. The resulting curve is one in which there is an immediate small drop in concentration followed by an exponential decrease that appears as a straight line on the semilog plot (Fig. 9-3). This line represents the change in CO concentration in the lungs as a result of CO transfer across the alveolar-capillary

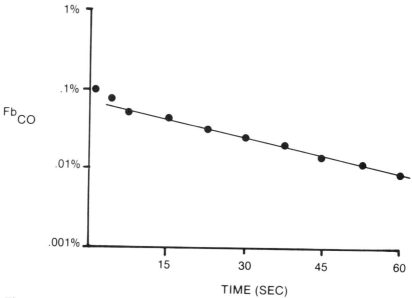

Fig. 9-3. Graph of CO concentration in the rebreathing system (Fb_{CO}) as a function of time. The subject rebreathes the gas mixture containing CO. The initial drop in CO concentration is caused by equilibrium of the gas with the alveolar volume. The subsequent drop over the testing interval is from diffusion of CO out of the alveolar volume. By measuring CO concentration at two points on the graph, $D_{L_{CO}}$ by the rebreathing method can be calculated.

interface. By choosing two concentrations on the line and the corresponding time interval between these two points, one may calculate the amount of CO transferred in a manner analogous to that of the single-breath method by the following formula:

$$D_{L_{CO}} = \frac{V_S}{(P_B - P_{H_2O})} \times \frac{60}{(t_2 - t_1)} \times \ln\left(\frac{Fb_{CO(1)}}{Fb_{CO(2)}}\right) \qquad \text{(Eq. 9-7)}$$

where V_S represents the total system volume of the lungs, which is defined as the residual lung volume and the volume of the reservoir bag. The concentrations subscripted 1 and 2 represent two concentrations of CO in the rebreathing bag plotted on the linear section of the curve, and t_1 and t_2 are the corresponding times. The total system volume is calculated from the dilution of helium that is present in the test gas mixture according to the following formula (derived from the helium dilution method for FRC):

$$V_S = V_{bag}\left(\frac{F_i b_{He}}{F_f b_{He}}\right) \qquad \text{(Eq. 9-8)}$$

where $F_i b_{He}$ and $F_f b_{He}$ are the initial and final fractional concentrations of helium in the bag. Correction must be made for volume loss because of exchange of oxygen and carbon dioxide as well as the loss of volume from CO transfer.

There are two main differences between this method and the single-breath method. First, the measurement is made after equilibrium during active breathing over about 60 sec, which may represent more physiological conditions for gas transfer. In the event there are slowly ventilating spaces, the single-breath method may not permit gas to distribute adequately. Second, the average volume at which transfer takes place with the rebreathing method is lower than that of the breathholding method. The latter is at TLC whereas the former is some value between TLC and RV. As a result of the lower volume, diffusing capacity as measured by the rebreathing technique is generally lower than that of the single-breath technique. Nonetheless, the two methods correlated well. After correction for the lung volume at which the measurements are made, there is no significant difference between the two unless significant ventilation-perfusion disturbances are present, to which the rebreathing method is less sensitive. The rebreathing method is not commonly employed in the clinical laboratory because it is more difficult to perform.

Steady-State Methods (D$L_{SS_{CO}}$)

$D_{L_{CO}}$ may be determined under steady-state conditions by measuring the uptake of carbon monoxide during breathing of a mixture of constant CO concentration and dividing by the alveolar-capillary CO gradient. Three steady-state techniques are available. The means for measuring the CO uptake is common to all three techniques; the difference between the three techniques is in the measurement or estimation of alveolar CO concentration.

The test is performed by having the subject breathe a gas mixture containing 0.1 percent CO ($F_{I_{CO}}$), 20 percent O_2 ($F_{I_{O_2}}$), and the remainder nitrogen for several minutes. The expired gases are released to the atmosphere. After several minutes a steady state is assumed, and the expired gas is collected into a reservoir system for a 1-min period. The gas is analyzed for fractional concentration of CO ($F_{E_{CO}}$), CO_2 ($F_{E_{CO_2}}$), and O_2 ($F_{E_{O_2}}$).

The volume of CO transferred is calculated as the difference between fractional concentrations of inhaled and exhaled CO *times* the volume measured during the 1-min gas collection period:

$$\dot{V}_{CO} = \dot{V}_E \left[F_{I_{CO}} \left(\frac{F_{E_{N_2}}}{F_{I_{N_2}}} \right) - F_{E_{CO}} \right] \tag{Eq. 9-9}$$

where $\dot{V}_{CO}$ is the volume of CO diffused and $\dot{V}_E$ is the exhaled volume during the 1-minute period corrected to STPD. The nitrogen dilution factor (ratio of $F_{E_{N_2}}$ to $F_{I_{N_2}}$) is needed to correct the inspired CO for the change in concentration from the O_2 and CO_2 exchange. Because nitrogen is not measured, the following calculations are used:

$$\begin{aligned} F_{I_{N_2}} &= 1.000 - F_{I_{O_2}} - F_{I_{CO_2}} \\ F_{E_{N_2}} &= 1.000 - F_{E_{O_2}} - F_{E_{CO_2}} \end{aligned} \tag{Eq. 9-10}$$

The next step is to determine alveolar CO concentration ($P_{A_{CO}}$). This is difficult because the tension fluctuates throughout the respiratory cycle and cannot be measured directly. The three methods described in the following sections are used to calculate $P_{A_{CO}}$. Once obtained, the diffusing capacity is calculated as:

$$D_{L_{CO}} = \frac{\dot{V}_{CO}}{P_{A_{CO}}} \tag{Eq. 9-11}$$

since the partial pressure of capillary CO is assumed to be negligible.

Filley Method   Because the expired gas that is analyzed contains contributions from both the alveolar volume and physiological dead space, the concentration of CO thus measured represents dilution of the alveolar gas into the sum of the alveolar and dead spaces. $P_{A_{CO}}$ may therefore be determined by the following formula, in a manner similar to that of the Bohr equation[5]:

$$P_{A_{CO}} = P_{I_{CO}} - \frac{P_{a_{CO_2}}}{P_{E_{CO_2}}} (P_{I_{CO}} - P_{E_{CO}}) \tag{Eq. 9-12}$$

An arterial blood sample is required to obtain $P_{a_{CO_2}}$, which estimates $P_{A_{CO_2}}$. $P_{E_{CO}}$ and $P_{E_{CO_2}}$ are obtained from analysis of the collected expired gas. $P_{I_{CO}}$ is the partial pressure of CO in the inspired gas mixture.

End-tidal CO Determination   In this technique CO tension is monitored during an exhalation. End-tidal CO tension is averaged over multiple breaths and assumed to be equal to alveolar CO tension. The method makes assumptions about end-tidal CO concentration and is not as accurate as the Filley method, but is quicker and useful for screening purposes.

Assumed Dead Space Method In this method the subject is assumed to have a physiological dead space comprised of anatomic dead space only. Under this assumption alveolar volume may be estimated and the following formula is used:

$$P_{A_{CO}} = \frac{V_T(P_{E_{CO}}) - V_D(P_{I_{CO}})}{V_T - V_D} \qquad \text{(Eq. 9-13)}$$

V_T represents tidal volume, which is averaged over multiple breaths. V_D is the anatomic dead space, which is either estimated (one milliliter per pound of body weight) or measured with the single-breath nitrogen test. $P_{I_{CO}}$ and $P_{E_{CO}}$ are the inspired and expired CO partial pressures. Because this method does not require arterial puncture and is quickly calculated, it is often used during exercise testing. It makes an important assumption that total physiological dead space is equal to anatomic dead space, which is invalid in the presence of significant lung disease; therefore it is not the method of choice.

Equilibrium Washout Method (DLeq$_{co}$)

Another alternate but infrequently employed technique of measuring CO uptake is to introduce a gas mixture into the lungs containing two gas species. One species is CO, which is transferred across the alveolar-capillary interface. The second species is an inert gas, which does not cross the interface in any appreciable amount. The gases will show identical washout dynamics if no CO is taken up by the capillary blood. In practice, however, washout dynamics of CO will differ from that of the inert gas; the difference is caused by CO diffusion across the alveolar-capillary membrane. This difference can be quantitated to give a measure of $D_{L_{CO}}$.[6,7]

The subject rebreathes a gas mixture containing 0.1 percent CO and 10 percent He for several minutes, until an equilibrium is reached. At this point the subject is switched to breathing room air and the CO and helium concentrations in the expired gas are monitored continuously or at frequent intervals during the washout. The end-tidal concentrations are plotted on a semilog scale (Fig. 9-4). The exponential constant is calculated for CO based on the fractional concentration at two points on the washout curve:

$$K_{CO} = \frac{-\ln(F_{A_{CO(2)}}/F_{A_{CO(1)}})}{t_2 - t_1} \qquad \text{(Eq. 9-14)}$$

where $F_{A_{CO(1)}}$ and $F_{A_{CO(2)}}$ concentrations of CO at times t_1, and t_2, respectively. An identical calculation is performed for K_{He} using two fractional concentrations of helium.

$D_{L_{CO}}$ is calculated from the two exponential constants:

$$D_{L_{CO}} = \frac{V_A}{(P_B - P_{H_2O})}(K_{CO} - K_{He}) \qquad \text{(Eq. 9-15)}$$

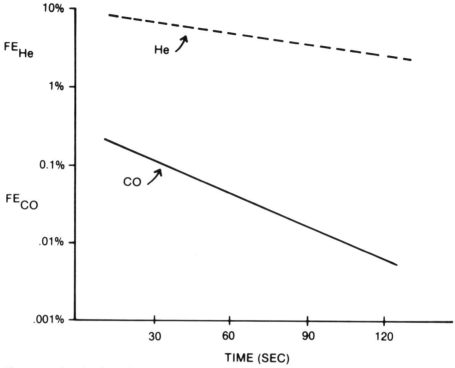

Fig. 9-4. Graph of the decline in concentrations of helium and carbon monoxide in the equilibrium washout method for $D_{L_{CO}}$. The decline in helium is caused solely by the washout of gas during repeated inhalations of air. The decline in CO is from both washout and diffusion into the pulmonary capillary blood. The difference in the two washout curves is related to the diffusion of CO alone, permitting calculation of $D_{L_{CO}}$ (see text).

The lung volume V_A must be determined separately by measuring FRC and recording the average tidal volume during the tests and using the following equation:

$$V_A = FRC + \frac{V_T}{2} \qquad \text{(Eq. 9-16)}$$

V_A represents the average volume of gas in the lungs during the test. Nitrogen present in room air may be used in place of helium as the inert gas and oxygen may be used to wash out the CO and N_2; however, high O_2 concentrations may decrease CO binding with hemoglobin and falsely decrease $D_{L_{CO}}$.

The technique is easily applied if equipment for end-tidal sampling of CO and He is available. It does not require much patient cooperation and is relatively independent of ventilation-perfusion abnormalities. The results should be slightly lower than that of the single-breath method because it is measured at an average alveolar volume smaller than that of the single-breath method. However, because it is independent of ventilation-perfusion mismatch it may be equal.

SPECIFIC DIFFUSING CAPACITY

The major determinant of diffusing capacity when measured by the single-breath ($DLsb_{CO}$) method is the alveolar volume at which the measurement is made.[8,9] For example, following pneumonectomy $DLsb_{CO}$ will decrease by about half. Thus, the ratio DL_{CO}/VA, the *specific diffusing capacity* or *diffusion constant*, remains relatively constant in a given individual, and may be a more sensitive indicator of changes in an individual over time. The correction for alveolar volume essentially eliminates the effects of lung volume. Thus, if DL_{CO} decreases more rapidly than lung volumes in diseases such as diffuse interstitial fibrosis, this suggests that additional factors, like lower capillary blood volume, decreased membrane diffusion, or increased ventilation-perfusion mismatch, are causing the fall in DL_{CO}.

MEMBRANE AND INTRACAPILLARY COMPONENTS OF DL_{CO}

The diffusing capacity measured by carbon monoxide methods in the pulmonary function laboratory has two discernible components that contribute to the overall value of DL_{CO}. The first component, *membrane diffusion*, consists of the processes involving transfer across the alveolar cells, the interstitial tissue, the capillary basement membrane and endothelium, and into the plasma of the capillary. The second component is the combination of CO with hemoglobin, and consists of both the *reaction rate* of hemoglobin with carbon monoxide and the *capillary blood volume*. This second component of the DL_{CO} is sufficiently slow to contribute significantly to the rate of gas diffusion. It comprises one-third to one-half of the total resistance to diffusion at physiological levels of alveolar oxygen tension. It is possible to measure the individual components of DL_{CO} in the clinical laboratory, but because this involves repeated determinations of diffusing capacity with varying FI_{O_2}'s and a multitude of calculations, it is not performed in the routine assessment of patients with lung disease.

To facilitate the understanding of the relationship of these two components, gas diffusion may be thought of in terms of *resistance* to diffusion. Diffusing capacity itself is analogous to *conductance*, but it is helpful to use the resistance form because the resistances offered by the two components of DL_{CO} are additive. The total resistance to diffusion ($1/DL$) is equal to the sum of the component resistances. In these terms, the relationship among components is

$$\frac{1}{DL} = \frac{1}{DM} + \frac{1}{\theta(Qc)}$$
(Eq. 9-17)

where DM is the *membrane diffusing capacity*, θ is the *reaction rate* of CO with hemoglobin, and Qc is the *capillary blood volume* available for carboxyhemoglobin formation.*

---

* For consistency in nomenclature, Qc is used in place of the more common term Vc.

The method for obtaining the two individual components of $D_{L_{CO}}$ is based on the ability to alter the value of θ.[10] Membrane diffusion and pulmonary capillary blood volume are relatively constant in steady-state conditions. The reaction rate of CO with hemoglobin can be altered by widely varying capillary oxygen tension. Under these conditions, Equation 9-17 may be viewed as a linear equation of the form:

$$y = b + m(x) \qquad \text{(Eq. 9-18)}$$

with y, b, m, and x representing $1/D_L$, $1/D_M$, $1/Q_c$, and $1/\theta$, respectively. By making a series of measurements of $D_{Lsb_{CO}}$ at different values of θ and extrapolating $1/\theta$ to zero, $D_{L_{CO}}$ at this extrapolated value is equal to D_M. A value of zero for $1/\theta$ corresponds to a reaction rate of CO with hemoglobin, which is uninhibited by oxygen.

The measurements are made in two steps. In the first step, the back pressure of CO in the pulmonary capillary blood and the oxygen consumption are measured. The second step consists of measurement of the single-breath diffusing capacity at different capillary oxygen tensions. The methods for making the diffusing capacity measurements are identical to the standard single-breath method with the exception that the oxygen concentration of the test gases varies.

The subject initially breathes oxygen to saturate his bloodstream and alveoli with a high oxygen tension. The subject is then switched to and rebreathes from a reservoir bag containing only oxygen with a CO_2 absorbent. After 5 min the CO present in the bloodstream has equilibrated with the alveoli. The partial pressure of CO in the gas after equilibrium is considered equal to pulmonary capillary P_{CO} ($P_{C_{CO}}$). Oxygen consumption may likewise be determined from the volume of oxygen lost from the reservoir bag.

Diffusing capacity is measured using the single-breath method and an initial test gas comprised of 0.3 percent CO, 10 percent He, and the remainder oxygen. The measurement and calculation of $D_{L_{CO}}$ proceeds as for the standard single-breath method with the $P_{C_{CO}}$ used to calculate the CO gradient if it is significant. The subject is switched to room air for 20 min, after which $D_{L_{CO}}$ is repeated using a test gas of 0.3 percent CO, 10 percent He, and 21 percent oxygen.

Once the two measurements are complete, a graph of $1/D_{L_{CO}}$ versus $1/\theta$ is constructed and used for the analysis. Capillary P_{O_2} ($P_{C_{O_2}}$) must first be estimated to calculate $1/\theta$. The membrane diffusion equation for oxygen is:

$$D_{M_{O_2}} = \frac{\dot{V}_{O_2}}{P_{A_{O2}} - P_{C_{O_2}}} \qquad \text{(Eq. 9-19)}$$

is rearranged to solve for $P_{C_{O_2}}$, with $D_{M_{O_2}}$ estimated as 1.23 times $D_{M_{CO}}$. $D_{M_{CO}}$, in turn, is estimated as 1.5 times $D_{L_{CO}}$ using the 21 percent oxygen test gas. The resulting equation is

$$P_{C_{O_2}} = P_{A_{O_2}} - 0.542\left(\frac{\dot{V}_{O_2}}{D_{L_{CO}}}\right) \qquad \text{(Eq. 9-20)}$$

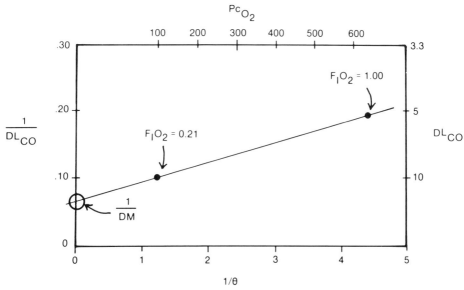

Fig. 9-5. Graph of DL_{CO} as a function of pulmonary capillary oxygen tension (Pc_{O_2}). By measuring DL_{CO} at two different values of Pc_{O_2} and extrapolating this to a point where the reaction rate is uninhibited by oxygen ($1/\theta = 0$), membrane-diffusing capacity (DM) and pulmonary capillary blood volume can be calculated. The details of this technique are in the text.

The inverse reaction rate is determined according to the following formula obtained from experimental data[11]:

$$\frac{1}{\theta} = 0.0057(Pc_{O_2} + 0.75) \qquad \text{(Eq. 9-21)}$$

These calculations are repeated for both determinations of DL_{CO} and the values of $1/DL_{CO}$ and $1/\theta$ are plotted (Fig. 9-5). A line drawn between the two points is extrapolated to the ordinate corresponding to an inverse reaction rate of zero. The value on the ordinate at the intercept is the inverse membrane diffusion coefficient. Once DM is obtained, Qc is calculated by

$$Qc = \frac{DL(DM)}{\theta(DM - DL)} \qquad \text{(Eq. 9-22)}$$

where DM and DL are obtained at the same value of θ.

DETERMINANTS OF CARBON MONOXIDE DIFFUSING CAPACITY

The processes involved in diffusion are complex and cannot be completely characterized. Measurements of CO diffusion can be altered by both physiological and technical factors. Physiological factors are either the result of normal physiological mechanisms or changes induced by disease. Technical problems generally vary, depending on the type of test performed (single breath, rebreathing, steady state, or equilibrium) and the conditions under which the measurements are made.

Physiological Determinants of CO Diffusion

Diseases of the pulmonary parenchyma with a loss of functioning alveolar-capillary units, and consequently, a decrease in the total membrane surface area available for gas exchange may result in a decreased diffusing capacity. Parenchyma can be lost in destructive diseases such as emphysema. Interstitial lung diseases also alter the parenchymal structure and result in a decreased surface area for diffusion and an increased thickness of the alveolar-capillary membrane. The relative contribution of increased membrane thickness produced by interstitial lung disease is thought to be less significant than the loss of a functioning alveolar-capillary membrane in reducing $D_{L_{CO}}$.

The combination of carbon monoxide with hemoglobin is a process that contributes to the overall value of diffusing capacity as usually measured. The amount of hemoglobin available to take up CO, determined by both *hemoglobin concentration* and *pulmonary capillary blood volume,* is a factor affecting diffusing capacity, an effect often overlooked in some pulmonary function labs. It is useful to determine hemoglobin levels if an unexpected increase or a decrease in $D_{L_{CO}}$ is found. Correction factors for anemia and polycythemia are available.[12] In contrast, a change in cardiac output in the absence of changes in blood volume will not significantly alter $D_{L_{CO}}$. Carbon monoxide binds with hemoglobin at the same site as oxygen, so large variations in oxygen partial pressure can also affect the capillary blood component of $D_{L_{CO}}$.

Normal function of the alveolar-capillary membrane in gas diffusion depends on normal distribution of ventilation and perfusion to the functioning respiratory units. Poor matching of ventilation and perfusion can result in diminished gas diffusion, but the mechanism is not exactly clear. Examples of pulmonary factors that affect $D_{L_{CO}}$ are given in Table 9-1.

Technical Factors

Regardless of the method used, the measurement of $D_{L_{CO}}$ is subject to error for several reasons. Each of the methods requires the determination of CO uptake by the lungs, involving measurements of very low concentrations of CO, with or without the estimation of CO partial pressure based on several assumptions. The determination of alveolar P_{CO} is critical, yet cannot be measured directly. A variety of methods for estimating $P_{A_{CO}}$ indirectly during the process of diffusion are used. Likewise, $P_{c_{CO}}$ either is assumed to be zero or measured separately from the diffusion test itself.

Table 9-1 Causes of Changes in Diffusing Capacity

Physiological Basis	Clinical State
Decreased $D_{L_{CO}}$	
Ventilation-perfusion relationships	
Ventilation-perfusion mismatching	Many diseases
Membrane factors	
Loss of surface area	Emphysema
Increased thickness	Interstitial disease
Alveolar filling	Pneumonia
Blood factors	
Decreased pulmonary capillary blood volume	Pulmonary vascular occlusion
Increased $D_{L_{CO}}$	
Ventilation-perfusion relationships	
Improved ventilation-perfusion matching	Exercise
	Asthma
Blood factors	
Increased pulmonary capillary blood volume	Left-to-right intracardiac shunt

Source: Adapted with permission from Conrad SA, George RB: Clinical pulmonary function testing. p. 161. In George RB, Light RW, Matthay RA (eds): Chest Medicine. Churchill Livingstone, New York, 1983

A significant factor in some testing techniques is the effect of alveolar volume at the time diffusing capacity is measured. It has been shown that $D_{Lsb_{CO}}$ varies with alveolar volume above FRC, thought initially to be a result of changes in surface area, but recent evidence has suggested that it is a result of changes in capillary blood volume.[13] To account for this factor, alveolar volume is simultaneously measured in the single-breath and rebreathing methods.

Improper calibration of the meters, incomplete flushing of the breathing circuit with the test gas, and poor effort or misunderstanding by the subject can contribute to the overall error. Because prolonged inspiratory or expiratory time can alter diffusion dynamics, it is important to time these maneuvers precisely to avoid errors. In spite of these potential sources of error, however, the results of these methods are fairly reproducible and have become an established part of routine pulmonary function testing.

Comparison of Methods

The four methods for measuring diffusing capacity are compared in Table 9-2. The single-breath method is the easiest to perform, especially with automated equipment. It is noninvasive, entails only a modest amount of error, and is the most commonly used method for measuring $D_{L_{CO}}$. It is one of the recommended screening tests for interstitial lung disease.[14] Its principal disadvantages

Table 9-2 Comparison of the Four Methods for Measurement of Carbon Monoxide Diffusing Capacity

	Single Breath	Rebreathing	Steady State	Equilibrium Washout
Principal clinical utility	Routine and screening	Little	Exercise studies	Little
Ease of performance	Simple	Complex	Moderate	Complex
Overall accuracy	Moderate	Great	Least	Great
Invasiveness	None	None	Yes[a]	None
$\dot{V}/\dot{Q}$ sensitivity	Yes	Some	Yes	None
V_A sensitivity	Yes	Some	Yes	None
CO_{hgb} sensitivity	Little	Yes	Yes	Little
D_M calculation	Yes	No	No	No
V_A calculation	Yes	Yes	No	Yes

[a] Depends on technique used.

are that it is not practical for use in exercise studies and requires the largest investment in instrumentation. It may be impractical in subjects with severe dyspnea because prolonged breathholding is required. Although this method is subject to the criticism that breathholding is not "physiological," this does not detract from its clinical usefulness as an indicator of disease.

The steady-state methods are best suited for exercise studies, but are subject to more error than the single-breath method, especially from ventilation-perfusion abnormalities. A sample of arterial blood or an assumption about the value of Pc_{CO} is required. Because it requires the least patient cooperation, it is useful for patients who cannot perform the single-breath test, including those who cannot hold their breath for the recommended 10 sec.

The rebreathing method may have less overall error, and is less sensitive to distribution of ventilation and alveolar volume, but these factors are not of clinical significance. As this test is more difficult to perform, it is not commonly employed. The equilibrium washout method is the least sensitive to alveolar volume, ventilation-perfusion mismatch, and abnormalities in the distribution of ventilation, but requires complex data collection, necessitating a computer system for effective analysis. It is therefore not routinely employed, except in research.

REFERENCES

1. Krogh M: The diffusion of gases through the lungs of man. J Physiol 49:271, 1915
2. Forster RE, Fowler WS, Bates DV, Van Lingen B: The absorption of carbon monoxide by the lungs during breathholding. J Clin Invest 33:1135, 1954
3. Forster RE, Cohn JE, Briscoe WA, et al: A modification of the Krogh carbon monoxide breathholding technique for estimating the diffusing capacity of the lung; a comparison with three other methods. J Clin Invest 34:1417, 1955

4. Ogilvie CM, Forster RE, Blakemore WS, Morton JW: A standardized breathholding technique for the clinical measurement of the diffusing capacity of the lung for carbon monoxide. J Clin Invest 36:1, 1957
5. Filley GF, MacIntosh DJ, Wright GW: Carbon monoxide uptake and pulmonary diffusing capacity in normal subjects at rest and during exericise. J Clin Invest 33:530, 1954
6. Burrows B, Harper PV Jr.: Determination of pulmonary diffusing capacity for carbon monoxide equilibrium curves. J Appl Physiol 12:283, 1958
7. Burrows B, Niden AH, Harper PV Jr., Barclay WR: Non-uniform pulmonary diffusion as demonstrated by the carbon monoxide equilibration technique: mathematical considerations. J Clin Invest 39:795, 1960
8. McGrath MW, Thomson ML: The effect of age, body size and lung volume change on alveolar-capillary permeability and diffusing capacity in man. J Physiol 146:572, 1959
9. Mittman G, Burrows B: Uniformity of pulmonary diffusion: Effect of lung volume. J Appl Physiol 14:496, 1959
10. Roughton FJW, Forster RE: Relative importance of diffusion and chemical reaction rates in determining the rate of exchange of gases in the human lung, with special reference to the true diffusing capacity of the pulmonary membrane and volume of blood in the lung capillaries. J Appl Physiol 11:290, 1957
11. Bates DV, Varvis CJ, Donovan RE, Christie RV: Variations in the pulmonary capillary blood volume and membrane diffusion component in health and disease. J Clin Invest 39:1401, 1960
12. Dinakara P, Blumenthal WS, Johnson RF et al: The effect of anemia on pulmonary diffusing capacity with derivation of a correction equation. Am Rev Respir Dis 102:965, 1970
13. Cadigan JB, Marks A, Ellicott MF et al: An analysis of factors affecting the measurement of pulmonary diffusing capacity by the single breath method. J Clin Invest 40:1495, 1961
14. Ferris BG, et al: Epidemiology standardization project: Recommended standardized procedures for pulmonary function testing. Am Rev Resp Dis 118:part 2, 62, 1978

Section III

CLINICAL APPLICATION
AND INTERPRETATION

10

Interpretation of Pulmonary Function Tests

Stephen G. Jenkinson, M.D.

The lung represents a fascinating organ for the study of function and physiology because of its unique ability to inflate and deflate inside the human chest. From 12 to 15 times/min, this organ enlarges by approximately 500 ml and then returns to its original size. The lungs and chest wall act together as a pump where pressure differences between alveoli and the atmosphere are produced, resulting in airflow, and ultimately, gas exchange. Although hundreds of different types of diseases can affect the lungs, only a few measurable pulmonary function derangements are found. Identifying the type of physiological abnormality present by using pulmonary function tests narrows the list of possible causes of lung disease and allows the health care professional to determine accurately the degree of impairment present and assess the response to therapy.

Physiological abnormalities that can be measured by pulmonary function testing include restriction of lung size, obstruction of airflow, and decreases in transfer of gases. By combining a number of different pulmonary function tests, the abnormality present in a particular patient can be defined and the list of diagnostic possibilities can often be narrowed. Abnormal values of pulmonary function tests are those outside the mean value obtained from a group of normal individuals matched according to age, height, and sex. These normal "predicted values" are calculated from specific prediction equations. The equations give a mean value for the group of normals and usually a range defined by confidence limits that include 95 percent of the variation of the normal group. Before a pulmonary function test is labeled abnormal, the results should fall outside the range in which 95 percent of people the same age, height, and sex would be found. All lung volumes obtained by spirometry or gas dilution studies should be corrected to body temperature saturated with water vapor (BTPS) in order to produce uniformity of interpretation from one pulmonary function laboratory to another.

Pulmonary function testing equipment continues to become increasingly complex as the technology surrounding these machines becomes more sophisticated. A major problem that occurs in teaching the interpretation of pulmonary function testing is the endless new analyses being applied to these very simple curves. Although complicated mathematical analyses of pulmonary function tests play a role in the continuing research and understanding of pulmonary physiology, they are often not very useful in the day-to-day management of patients with lung diseases. This chapter concentrates on the basic clinical interpretation of routine pulmonary function tests to diagnose and treat patients with lung disorders. More sophisticated interpretations of newer testing techniques and their role in understanding early small airway dysfunction are also briefly discussed.

RESTRICTION OF LUNG SIZE

Restrictive lung disease results in decreased lung volumes without reduction of airflow. This abnormality can be measured using static lung volumes. In Figure 10-1 the subdivisions of lung volumes are seen from a normal patient and a patient with restrictive lung disease. Restrictive disease reduces all the various subdivisions of lung volume. These patients have normal airway resistance, and their *forced expiratory volume in 1 sec* (FEV_1) is greater than 75 percent of their forced vital capacity ($FEV_1/FVC > 75\%$).

Total lung capacity (TLC) is the volume of gas in the lungs and airways after a maximum inspiration. A general classification of the severity of restrictive lung dysfunction can be produced by grouping patients with a decrease in TLC into mild, moderate, or severe categories. Reduction of TLC to less than 80 percent of the predicted value is interpreted as mild restrictive lung dysfunction. Reduction to less than 60 percent is moderate restriction, and reduction to less than 40 percent is severe restriction.[1] This is the most important single test of lung volume to determine whether a patient has restrictive lung disease and serves as the

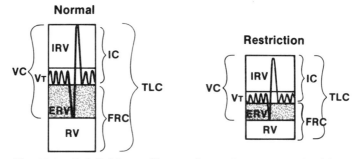

Fig. 10-1. Subdivisions of lung volumes from a normal subject and from a patient with restrictive lung disease. All subdivisions of lung volume are reduced with restrictive lung disease.

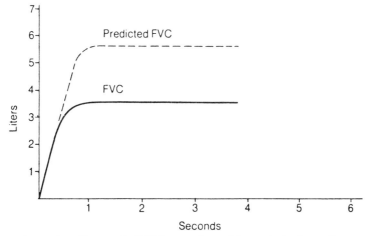

Fig. 10-2. Changes in FVC in a patient with restrictive lung disease.

"gold standard" for measuring restrictive dysfunction. TLC can be measured by closed-circuit helium dilution, open-circuit nitrogen washout, or body plethysmography. As explained in Chapter 6, all of these methods determine *functional residual capacity* (FRC) and then TLC is calculated from this value. When the body plethysmograph is used to determine TLC, the volume measured is termed the *thoracic gas volume* (VTG) and usually equals FRC. TLC is then calculated as the sum of VTG and the inspiratory capacity (IC). TLC determined by this method measures the total amount of gas in the chest, including gas that is trapped and not communicating with a bronchus. A patient with gas trapped in large cysts or bullae in the lungs will have a much larger TLC measured by plethysmography than that measured by dilution or washout techniques.

Evidence of restrictive disease found on spirometry includes a decreased two-stage *vital capacity* (VC) or a decreased *forced vital capacity* (FVC) with normal expiratory flow rates. The FVC measurement is useful in quantitating restriction if a patient has no obstructive abnormality (Fig. 10-2). In the presence of obstructive disease, however, the FVC measurement depends on the time in which the patient is able to perform the maneuver and the amount of increase in *residual volume* (RV) (Fig. 10-3). For this reason, the diagnosis of restrictive ventilatory dysfunction in patients who also exhibit airway obstruction should always be confirmed by measurement of TLC. Race must also be considered in the diagnosis of restrictive lung disease because black subjects have been shown to have a VC approximately 12 percent lower than that of whites of the same age and height.[2] Restriction of lung function can be produced either by diseases that affect the lungs themselves or decrease the ability of the chest to perform as a bellows. A list of the common causes of restrictive lung disease is given in Table 10-1.

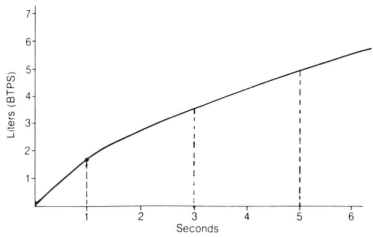

Fig. 10-3. Dependence of the FVC on time of exhalation in a patient with obstructive lung disease. If the patient stops exhaling at 1 sec, FVC = 1.8 liters; if the same patient stops exhaling at 3 sec, FVC = 3.2 liters; and if the patient stops exhaling at 5 sec, FVC = 5 liters.

Mechanical Inhibition of Chest Bellows

Diseases that mechanically inhibit the chest bellows mechanism include deformity of the chest wall and skeleton, loss of neuromuscular function to perform inspiration, abnormalities of the pleural space, and abdominal overdistention causing upward displacement of the diaphragm and decreased diaphragm movement. The lung parenchyma itself remains normal in these disorders. The most common pulmonary function pattern seen with mechanically deforming diseases is a decrease in TLC and VC with only a slight decrease in RV. This situation produces an increased ratio of RV to TLC. RV is maintained in these diseases because lung compliance remains normal.

The specific *diffusing capacity* (DL_{CO} corrected for lung volume) is also normal because no intrinsic lung disease exists. (In patients with long-standing deformities of the chest bellows mechanism, lung compliance measurements and DL_{CO} can become abnormal because of retained secretions and pulmonary parenchymal changes associated with recurrent infections.) With chest wall deformities, ventilation can usually be increased in these patients by increasing the respiratory rate; therefore, the measurement of *maximum voluntary ventilation* (MVV) is not affected unless the restrictive dysfunction is extremely severe (Table 10-2).[3]

Various types of diseases causing inhibition of the chest bellows mechanism sometimes do produce subtle differences in pulmonary function testing that may indicate a particular diagnosis. Obesity and abdominal distention from pregnancy or ascitic fluid produce a decrease in both functional residual capacity (FRC) and the *expiratory reserve volume* (ERV). (Doubling a patient's predictive

Table 10-1 Common Etiologies of Restrictive Lung Disease

I. Interstitial lung diseases
   A. Collagen vascular disease
   B. Interstitial pneumonitis
   C. Hypersensitivity pneumonitis
   D. Pneumoconiosis
   E. Pulmonary fibrosis
   F. Pulmonary edema
II. Infiltrative lung disease
   A. Granulomatosis
   B. Tumor
III. Pleural disease
   A. Fibrothorax
   B. Pleural effusion
   C. Pneumothorax
IV. Chest wall disease
   A. Kyphoscoliosis
   B. Ankylosing spondylitis
   C. Neuromuscular disease
V. Other causes
   A. Obesity
   B. Paralyzed diaphragm
   C. Ascites
   D. Pregnancy
   E. Flail chest
   F. Resectional surgery

body weight decreases FRC by 25 percent and ERV by 40 percent.) The *closing capacity* (CC) can rise above FRC in these patients and airway closure will consequently occur, resulting in hypoxemia. With massive obesity, chest wall compliance also decreases and MVV falls, probably because of the increase in oxygen demand required per unit of work done by the respiratory muscles.

Patients with deforming skeletal abnormalities, such as kyphoscoliosis or ankylosing spondylitis, also have characteristic pulmonary function abnormalities associated with their restrictive lung dysfunction. Mild-to-moderate kyphoscoliosis causes a slightly decreased VC with no change in FRC or RV. Severe kyphoscoliosis produces a marked decrease in VC and TLC with only a slight

Table 10-2 Pulmonary Function in a 53-Year-Old Man with Mechanical Inhibition of the Chest Bellows Mechanism

Function	Observed	% Predicted
FEV_1	2.67 liters	68
FVC	3.21 liters	69
TLC	4.64 liters	71
RV	1.70 liters	92
RV/TLC	37%	146
MVV	135 liters/min	88
$D_{L_{CO}}$	24 ml/min/torr	92

decrease in FRC. This produces an increased ratio of RV to TLC because RV will remain normal. Ankylosing spondylitis also produces a decrease in VC and TLC, but FRC and RV are *increased* above normal values. This increase is caused by a decrease in chest wall compliance. Because of these findings, patients with ankylosing spondylitis usually do not experience problems with arterial hypoxemia from increased $\dot{V}/\dot{Q}$ mismatching due to airway closure.

Neuromuscular diseases produce decreases in VC, TLC, and MVV and increases in RV as chest wall compliance falls. Flow rates during the early part of a forced expiration (effort-dependent flows) are reduced because these patients cannot generate the amount of force necessary to greatly distend the lung above its mechanical resting point. Because the flow rates are reduced more during the effort-dependent portion of exhalation in the forced expiratory spirogram, the *maximum expiratory flow rate* (forced expiratory flow measured between 200 and 1,200 ml of the FVC maneuver, $FEF_{0.2-1.2}$) will be more affected than the *maximum midexpiratory flow rate* (flow between 25 percent and 75 percent of the forced expiratory volume, $FEF_{25-75\%}$) since $FEF_{0.2-1.2}$ is measured earlier during expiration.[4]

Restrictive Parenchymal Diseases

Diseases that cause pathological changes in the lungs, resulting in restriction of lung function, can usually be differentiated from those causing mechanical restriction because of chest bellows malfunction. These diseases are caused by intrinsic restriction of lung function that occurs when the lung parenchyma becomes involved with a disease process. Restrictive parenchymal diseases are associated with a reduction in alveolar volume or an increase in lung elastic recoil. Pulmonary function testing reveals decreased lung volumes, decreased static compliance, increased lung elastic recoil, and decreased DL_{CO} (Table 10-3). The measurement of static lung compliance is the single best test for determining whether restriction is caused by parenchymal disease.[3] These patients also exhibit mild resting hypoxemia that worsens with exercise. Monitoring gas exchange during exercise is the most sensitive test for detecting worsening interstitial disease in patients with restrictive parenchymal diseases.[5] DL_{CO} can

Table 10-3 Pulmonary Functions in a 31-Year-Old Man with Restrictive Parenchymal Disease

Function	Observed	% Predicted
FEV_1	3.04 liters	66
FVC	3.37 liters	68
TLC	4.74 liters	66
RV	1.54 liters	72
RV/TLC	32%	102
MVV	147 liters/min	94
DL_{CO}	16 ml/min/torr	68

Table 10-4 Classification of Restrictive Dysfunction

↓ Lung Volumes $FEV_1/FVC \geq 75\%$ Normal Airway Resistance	
Restrictive Parenchymal Disease	Restrictive Chest Bellows Disease
↓ Static compliance ↓ Diffusing capacity	↑ RV/TLC ratio Normal compliance Normal specific diffusing capacity

also be abnormal in patients with restrictive parenchymal disease, even with a normal chest radiograph.

Patients with advanced pulmonary fibrosis may also have evidence of obstructive airway disease caused by peribronchiolar fibrosis. More sensitive tests of small airway function, such as *frequency dependence of dynamic lung compliance, slope of phase III* on the *single-breath nitrogen washout test,* and *closing volume* (CV) expressed as a percentage of the VC, are often abnormal in patients with pulmonary fibrosis or sarcoidosis. Other tests of obstructive airway disease, such as the absolute value of FEV_1, the FEV_1/FVC ratio, and airway resistance, are usually normal in these patients. A summary of changes in restrictive pulmonary dysfunction caused by parenchymal disease is given in Table 10-4.

OBSTRUCTION OF AIRFLOW

Obstructive ventilatory diseases are manifested by a reduction of airflow through the conducting airways caused by a decrease in their diameter or loss of their integrity. This situation has a variety of causes, including bronchial smooth muscle contraction (asthma), airway collapse from loss of radial traction (emphysema), anatomic thickening of bronchial walls (chronic bronchitis), infiltration of the bronchial wall (tumor or granuloma), or aspiration of objects that mechanically obstruct bronchi (foreign bodies). The standard pulmonary function test used to measure airway obstruction is the forced expiratory spirogram. This maneuver allows an assessment of the rate of change in volume that occurs as a function of time.

The forced expiratory spirogram can be analyzed several ways to decide whether obstructive lung disease is present. One of the simplest and most commonly used analyses is measurement of the forced expiratory volume exhaled after 1 sec (FEV_1). A single value of this measurement can be compared with normal predicted values adjusted for age, height, and sex, and different degrees of obstruction can be documented (Fig. 10-4). The most widely used general classification for interpretation of obstructive lung dysfunction states that decreases in FEV_1 to less than 75 percent of predicted is mild obstruction, less than 60 percent of predicted is moderate obstruction, and less than 40 percent of predicted is severe obstruction. Measurement of $FEF_{0.2-1.2}$ and $FEF_{25-75\%}$ will also be abnormal in patients with obstructive airway disease. Neither of these two

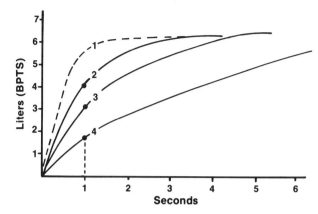

Fig. 10-4. The measurement of forced expiratory volume in 1 sec (FEV$_1$) in a normal subject (1); a patient with mild airway obstruction (2); a patient with moderate airway obstruction (3); and a patient with severe airway obstruction (4).

tests adds any more clinical information about an obstructed patient than FEV$_1$ and both are more variable.

FEV$_1$ measured as a percent of predicted cannot be used to assess airway obstruction if a patient also has restrictive lung disease because all lung volumes are reduced. A better measurement in these patients is the percentage of total forced vital capacity exhaled in the first second (FEV$_1$/FVC%) and the first 3 sec (FEV$_3$/FVC%). These measurements are called *timed vital capacities.* A normal FEV$_1$/FVC% is 75 percent and a normal FEV$_3$/FVC% is 92 percent. (The ratios are age-dependent and lower values may be normal in older patients.) These ratios remain normal even in the presence of severe restrictive lung disease. The values also usually remain normal in patients with small airway disease. Measurement of FEV$_1$/FVC% is very useful at the bedside because it can be interpreted rapidly without having to consult a table of normal values. There is some decline of these ratios with increasing age, but even in the elderly the decline is very modest. Mild obstruction is represented by an FEV$_1$/FVC% ratio between 70 and 60 percent. Moderate obstruction produces an FEV$_1$/FVC% ratio between 60 and 40 percent, and severe obstruction produces an FEV$_1$/FVC% ratio of < 40 percent. When an FEV$_1$ measurement and the FEV$_1$/FVC% ratio are found to differ in evaluating the degree of obstruction in a single patient (e.g., FEV$_1$ equals 58 percent of predicted and FEV$_1$/FVC% ratio equals 62 percent), then the FEV$_1$/FVC% ratio measurement should be used for the interpretation because FEV$_1$ can be decreased by concomitant restrictive disease. (The patient in the example has *mild* obstructive ventilatory dysfunction.)

Forced expiratory flow can also be measured by plotting instantaneous airflow against lung volume during a maximum forced expiration. This is called a *maximum expiratory flow volume curve* (MEFV) (Fig. 10-5). As discussed in Chapter 2, the early portion of this maneuver is effort-dependent and flow will increase in proportion to the intensity of effort. The latter portion is effort-independent and flow depends on the resistance of the peripheral bronchi and the recoil pressure of the lung in the mid-vital capacity range. A number of different

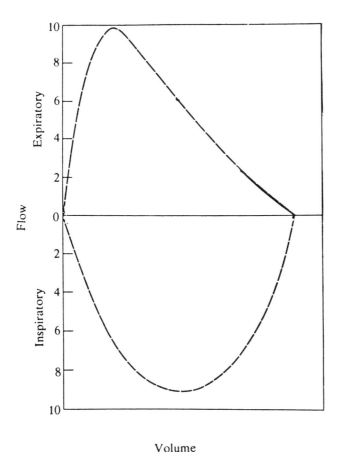

Volume

Fig. 10-5. A maximum expiratory flow volume curve from a normal subject.

patterns occur in the MEFV curve in patients with obstructive lung disease, and specific patterns can often be used to help identify the site of obstruction (see Fig. 7-7).

Upper Airway Obstruction

Patients with obstructing lesions of the upper airway can go unrecognized and misdiagnosed if pulmonary function testing is not closely examined. They have the same physiological derangements as patients with asthma or chronic obstructive pulmonary diseases (COPD) and are often seen with wheezing, shortness of breath, and severe hypoxemia. The type of upper airway obstruction in these patients can be either fixed or variable.[6] Fixed lesions do not allow the

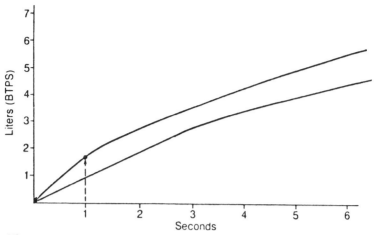

Fig. 10-6. Forced expiratory spirogram from a patient with asthma (top curve) and from a patient with upper airway obstruction (bottom curve). The patient with upper airway obstruction shows a "straightening" of the early portion of the forced expiratory spirogram.

airway to change cross-sectional area regardless of the changes in transmural pressure. With variable lesions, however, the size of the airway does respond to changes in transmural pressure. Variable lesions are subclassified as intrathoracic or extrathoracic because of their location and response to changes in transmural pressure.[7] Pulmonary function testing can usually distinguish among these various types of upper airway obstruction. It should be noted, however, that patients with bilateral obstruction of both main bronchi can have pulmonary function changes identical to patients with intrathoracic upper airway obstruction.

Pulmonary function tests used to diagnose and classify upper airway obstruction include spirometry and MEFV curves. In normal individuals, the maximum airflow achieved during the first 25 percent of a FVC maneuver is directly dependent on effort. With upper airway obstruction, flow at high lung volumes becomes limited much earlier by the obstruction and produces changes in the early portion of the forced expiratory spirogram. Rotman et al.[8] have defined variables that can be used to distinguish patients with upper airway obstruction from those with COPD or asthma. With spirometry alone, the $FEV_1/FEV_{0.5}$ (forced expiratory volume in 1 sec/forced expiratory volume in 0.5 sec) ratio in patients with upper airway obstruction is greater than or equal to 1.5. This is because $FEV_{0.5}$ is proportionately more reduced by obstruction of the upper airway because it occurs at higher lung volumes than FEV_1 (Fig. 10-6). This abnormality in the forced expiratory spirogram seen with upper airway obstruction has been referred to as "straightening" of the curve during the early portion of this test.

Spirometry can sometimes be misleading in patients with variable extrathoracic obstruction. With this type of lesion, intraluminal pressure during expiration is much higher than pressure outside the lumen (atmospheric pressure). This

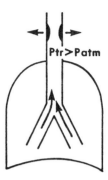

Fig. 10-7. Changes in flow during expiration in a patient with a variable extrathoracic obstruction. The airway tends to dilate in the area of the obstruction because intraluminal pressure (Ptr) is much higher than extraluminal pressure (Patm).

actually causes the airway to dilate in the area of the obstruction during an expiratory maneuver (Fig. 10-7).

MEFV curves are the pulmonary function tests of choice in diagnosing upper airway obstruction because they define the site of obstruction as well as document its presence. The various changes in MEFV curves from upper airway obstruction can be seen in Figure 10-8. With fixed obstruction, the plateau and limitation of flow is seen both during inspiration and expiration. Variable extrathoracic obstruction produces flow limitation and a plateau only on inspiration for the reasons mentioned previously. Variable intrathoracic obstruction causes flow limitation and a plateau only on expiration because the pressure outside the lumen (pleural pressure) becomes much greater than intraluminal pressure.

Differentiating Among Causes of Chronic Obstructive Pulmonary Diseases

Although all patients with obstructive lung disease of any etiology have reduced flow rates on forced exhalation, the use of pulmonary function testing can sometimes be helpful in differentiating among the various causes. The

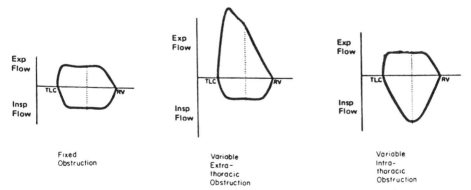

Fig. 10-8.   Maximum expiratory flow volume curves from patients with fixed obstruction, variable extrathoracic obstruction, and variable intrathoracic obstruction.

Table 10-5 Specific Response of Patients with COPD

	Causes of COPD		
	Asthma	Chronic Bronchitis	Emphysema
Decreased FEV_1	++++	++++	++++
Decreased FEV_1/FVC ratio	++++	++++	++++
Increased airway resistance	++++	++++	+
Decreased specific airway conductance	++++	++++	+
Decreased DL_{CO}	−	−	++++
Response to bronchodilators	++++	+	−

different responses these patients show to selected pulmonary function tests are illustrated in Table 10-5. Patients with asthma usually exhibit decreased specific airway conductance, a significant improvement in airflow in response to bronchodilators, and normal DL_{CO} because asthma causes reversible *bronchial* obstruction. Patients with chronic bronchitis also have a decreased specific airway conductance and a normal DL_{CO}, but they usually have only a slight increase in flow after bronchodilators. Patients with emphysema exhibit little (if any) decrease in specific airway conductance, no response to bronchodilators, and a marked decrease in DL_{CO} because emphysema is a disease of the terminal respiratory units characterized by loss of *alveoli*. A near-normal specific airway conductance in the face of decreased forced expiratory flow is characteristic of emphysema, as specific airway conductance is measured in the absence of dynamic airway compression. The use of these pulmonary function tests combined with the clinical assessment of a patient can often reveal which cause of obstructive lung disease is most prevalent in a given subject.

Reversibility of Obstructive Dysfunction

When patients are found to have obstructive lung disease from causes other than upper airway obstruction, they should then be evaluated for their response to bronchodilators. If a patient improves after the use of a bronchodilator at the time of their pulmonary function testing, they are more likely to benefit from long-term administration of these drugs.[9] The interpretation of bronchodilator studies is often difficult because even small changes in reversibility of airway obstruction could be significant in a given patient if his obstruction is severe enough.

Studies in which bronchodilators were administered to normal persons have shown a mean increase in FEV_1 of 2.5 percent with a standard deviation of 3.9 percent.[7] If a positive response to bronchodilators is defined as a response of at least 2 standard deviations (s.d.) above the mean response in normal individuals, then the FEV_1 must improve by at least 10 percent after bronchodilators to be considered significant. Other spirometric parameters, such as the FVC or $FEF_{25-75\%}$, have also been used by some to detect reversibility, but FEV_1 remains the best test for evaluating bronchodilator response. This is because increases in FEV_1, although not large, have a very small variability, which makes it a good discriminating test.[10] Some patients will not respond to a single inhalation from an aerosolized bronchodilator, but may still have reversible bronchospasm. These subjects may have used a bronchodilator prior to their arrival at the pulmonary function laboratory, or they may have an acute exacerbation of some other pulmonary disease that does not allow them to respond to the inhaled aerosols (such as bronchitis). Although their pulmonary function tests are interpreted as "no significant response to bronchodilators," the health care professional who ordered the tests may decide to administer bronchodilators for a period of days to weeks and then repeat pulmonary function tests to assess any "long-term" effects. Delayed improvement has been reported in some patients with "irreversible" airway obstruction after corticosteroid therapy.

Obstruction of the Small Airways

A number of pulmonary function tests have been developed to detect early obstructive disease in the small airways of the lung. Most of these tests have been used in an attempt to show a difference between smokers and nonsmokers as a means of proving their value in detecting early small airway dysfunction. Early small airway obstruction is not detected in routine tests used to diagnose obstructive dysfunction because small airways contribute less than 20 percent of total airway resistance and early changes will not produce enough increase in airway resistance to be detectable. These tests should not be performed in patients that already have evidence of obstructive ventilatory dysfunction with an abnormal FEV_1 or $FEV_1/FVC\%$ ratio. Spirometric evidence of small airway disease has been reported to be characterized by a reduced $FEF_{25-75\%}$ with a normal $FEF_{0.2-1.2}$, a normal FEV_1, and a normal $FEV_1/FVC\%$ ratio.

Difficulties that arise in using these new tests to examine the "quiet zones" of the lung stem from problems related to their reproducibility, sensitivity, and specificity. An important lesson learned thus far about the use of tests for small airway dysfunction is that abnormalities of the small airways are not necessarily indicative of progressive obstructive lung disease, although there has been some support for this hypothesis from structural studies of the lung.[11]

One of the earliest tests used to detect small airway disease and nonuniformity of lung function is the *frequency dependence of compliance.* When regional differences in airflow resistance or compliance exist in the lung, some areas will receive a disproportionate amount of air during inspiration. This nonuniformity of ventilation progresses with increasing rates of breathing.[12] The increase is caused by differences in the time constants of the various areas and results in a decreased compliance as respiratory frequency increases. This test is considered positive if compliance falls to 80 percent of the static value at the highest

Normal

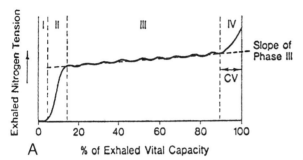

A

Fig. 10-9. The single-breath nitrogen washout test from a normal subject (A) and from a patient with obstructive airway disease (B).

Obstructive Airway Disease

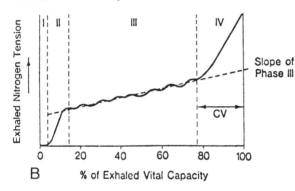

B

respiratory rate. Because this test is complex and requires the use of an esophageal balloon, it is not routinely used in most hospitals.

The single-breath nitrogen washout test is another test of small airway dysfunction (Fig. 10-9). In this test, the more obstructed regions of the lung tend to receive less of the 100 percent O_2 that is inspired and therefore have higher nitrogen concentrations. These obstructive areas also tend to empty late in expiration. The result of these physiological events is a gradually increasing nitrogen concentration throughout exhalation. This can be found by measuring the *slope of phase III. Closing volume* (CV) can also be measured from this test and when this volume is added to the residual volume, it is referred to as the *closing capacity* (CC). Dosman and Cotton have shown that using both the slope of phase III and CV to determine small airway dysfunction increases the sensitivity and specificity of the test.[13] Normally, CV is less than 25 percent of VC and the slope of phase III increases 2.5 percent from beginning to end. Predicted normal values for the slope of phase III, CV, and CC can be found in the work reported by Buist and Ross[14] and other references given in Appendix B.

Another test being investigated as a measurement of small airway dysfunction is the air-helium flow-volume curve (Fig. 10-10).[15] A MEFV curve is done,

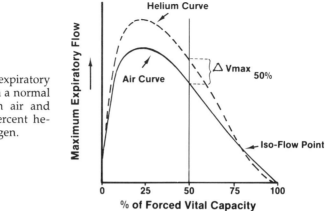

Fig. 10-10. Maximum expiratory flow volume curves from a normal subject first using room air and then a mixture of 80 percent helium and 20 percent oxygen.

first using room air and then again using a mixture of 80 percent helium and 20 percent O_2. Normally, helium increases forced expiratory flow in the early portion of the curve (where flow is turbulent and limitation is in the large airways), but not during the latter part (where flow is laminar and limitation is in the small airways). A response to helium can be assessed by measuring an increase in flow with helium when 50 percent of FVC has been exhaled ($\Delta \dot{V}max_{50\%}$) or by measuring the remaining volume to be exhaled when flow becomes identical on air and helium (the isoflow volume). With small airway disease, the value of $\Delta \dot{V}max_{50\%}$ will decrease and the isoflow volume will increase. This is because flow limitation occurs in the small airways at abnormally large lung volumes and helium fails to have an effect over a larger portion of the flow-volume curve. The $\Delta \dot{V}max_{50\%}$ and isoflow volume improve more evenly following smoking cessation than any other test of small airway dysfunction.[16] The normal value for $\Delta \dot{V}max_{50\%}$ is 47.3 ± 25% (2 s.d.). Isoflow volume is age-dependent and the upper limit is approximately 25 percent of VC at age 20 rising to 35 percent of VC by age 60.

ABNORMALITIES OF GAS TRANSFER

Measurement of diffusing capacity allows an evaluation of lung alveolar membranes and the pulmonary vascular bed. A reduction in diffusing capacity occurs with loss of alveolar surface area, thickening of alveolar membranes, loss of pulmonary capillary bed, increases in $\dot{V}/\dot{Q}$ mismatch, or decreases in the amount of hemoglobin in the lung capillaries. *Single-breath diffusing capacity for carbon monoxide* (DL_{CO}) is the most common measurement of diffusing capacity performed in pulmonary function laboratories, although a number of steady-state tests can also be performed. When the measurement of diffusing capacity is corrected for alveolar volume, it is referred to as the "specific" DL_{CO} (DL_{CO}/V_A). A decrease in DL_{CO} is most commonly seen with emphysema, loss of parenchymal tissue from surgery, interstitial lung disease, or pulmonary vascular disease. DL_{CO} should be less than 80 percent of predicted value to be considered abnormal because of the marked variability of the test.

Increased DL_{CO} can also occur and has been reported in patients with polycythemia, high-altitude dwellers, patients with intracardiac shunts, patients with congestive heart failure, and in some patients with asthma (thought to be caused by redistribution of perfusion). Increased DL_{CO} is normally seen during exercise because of an increase in blood flow into the lung with a resultant increase in blood-filled capillaries in the lung apexes. This same mechanism causes a slight increase in DL_{CO} when one assumes the supine position. All of the changes that cause an increase in DL_{CO} do so by increasing the amount of blood available in the pulmonary capillaries to take up carbon monoxide.

PULMONARY FUNCTION TESTING FOR PREOPERATIVE EVALUATION

Pulmonary problems continue to represent the most frequent postoperative complications in surgical patients. The complication rate is especially high in those surgical patients with obstructive lung disease. Elective surgery procedures may even be prohibitive in a large number of COPD patients because of the severity of their lung disease. These patients must be identified preoperatively to avoid pulmonary complications in the postoperative period. Their evaluation should include an estimation of the amount of lung function to be lost or gained as a result of the surgery, and a measure of the patient's pulmonary reserve. Patients who are smokers, obese, elderly (over age 60), and those with a past history of pulmonary symptomatology or lung disease are examples of surgical candidates who should receive a preoperative pulmonary evaluation (Table 10-6).

Pulmonary function testing is the most important laboratory test series for predicting postoperative complications. Following surgery of the upper abdomen, FVC has been found to decrease to 35 percent of normal on the first postoperative day, gradually returning to normal within approximately 1 week following surgery.[17] A smaller decrease in FVC is found in patients undergoing lower abdominal surgery. The decrease in vital capacity postoperatively has been related to decreased diaphragmatic excursion, most prominent in the upper abdominal group.[18]

Table 10-6 Indications for Preoperative
Pulmonary Evaluation
1. Thoracic surgery and/or lung resection
2. Upper abdominal surgery
3. Cigarette smoking
4. Obesity
5. Old age (60 years and older)
6. History of prior pulmonary diseases or COPD

Vital capacity can actually increase after some types of pulmonary surgery. This is seen when bullae that have been compressing normal lung tissue are removed or patients undergo decortication of a trapped lung. Improvement in function occurs gradually over a period of several weeks; this means that these patients may have decreased vital capacities immediately after their surgery.

Spirometry is the simplest pulmonary function test to perform preoperatively. If a forced expiratory spirogram is normal, then no further pulmonary function testing is necessary. High-risk patients are identified as those undergoing abdominal surgery who have an FEV_1 of $\leq$ 1 liter. Patients undergoing thoracic surgery are at increased risk if their FEV_1 is $\leq$ 2 liters.[19] When obstructive lung disease is found in a preoperative patient, bronchodilator studies should also be performed to identify those patients who might benefit from bronchodilator therapy.

Prediction of postoperative pulmonary function in patients undergoing lung resectional surgery has been attempted by the use of a number of techniques. One of the most commonly used tests is *quantitative macroaggregate lung scanning*. Overall lung function is multiplied by the right-left fractional perfusion estimated from the lung scan. The calculated function of the lung to be resected is then subtracted from the overall preoperative pulmonary function to obtain the postoperative predicted function. Good correlation has been found with this method in predicting the postoperative values of FEV_1, FVC, MVV, and $D_{L_{CO}}$.[20] A predicted postoperative FEV_1 of less than 800 ml is believed to be associated with a significant risk of respiratory failure or death.

Special emphasis was once placed on the MVV as a preoperative predictor of lung complications because this maneuver tests all components of the respiratory pump, including the respiratory center, respiratory muscles, thoracic cage, and lungs. The MVV was correlated with mortality in patients undergoing thoracic surgery by Gaensler,[21] and a mortality rate of 50 percent was found when MVV was less than 50 percent of predicted. This test is still used to evaluate COPD patients who are candidates for lung resection in many institutions, but the correlation is not as good as that found with macroaggregate lung scanning.

Another pulmonary function test currently being assessed to predict postoperative pulmonary function is the *lateral position test* developed by Bergan.[22] This test has gained popularity because it is noninvasive and safe. It can also be performed inexpensively with basic pulmonary function testing equipment using a spirometer filled with oxygen. The test is performed by first establishing a ventilatory baseline during tidal ventilation while the patient lies supine and breathes from the spirometer. The patient then rolls over on one side and the baseline rises proportionately to the function of the uppermost lung. This procedure is repeated for the other lung by again establishing a baseline while supine and then rolling over on the other side. The baseline will rise in the uppermost lung during the test because of increases in lung volume caused by shifting of the diaphragm and mediastinum. The test is used to assess unilateral pulmonary function and has been reported to correlate well with postoperative function predictions obtained from perfusion lung scanning techniques. Jay et al.,[23] however, have reported the variability of repeated measurements obtained from the lateral position test and concluded that several tests must be performed on a single patient before meaningful data can be gathered.

Basic exercise tolerance has also been used to attempt to predict postoperative outcome in patients who must undergo pneumonectomy. Reichel[24] used a standardized treadmill-walking test to evaluate 75 patients prior to pneumonectomy. The test was performed in stages with a maximum speed obtained of 3 mi/hr with a slope of 10 percent and a cumulative time of 14 min. No patient completing all six stages of the test had any cardiorespiratory complications postoperatively. Of those patients that were unable to complete the test, 57 percent had postoperative ventilatory failure, cardiac arrhythmias, or pulmonary embolism. Data on the use of more sophisticated exercise testing for preoperative evaluation are presently being collected.

MISINTERPRETATION OF PULMONARY FUNCTION TESTS

The information obtained from pulmonary function tests must be carefully assessed to avoid any misinterpretation of a patient's functional status. The manner in which a patient performs each test is very important in interpreting the results. Numbers generated on a data sheet summarizing pulmonary function tests can be misleading if the tests are not performed properly. The actual curves that produced these numbers must also be examined to obtain a meaningful interpretation of pulmonary function data. Abnormalities like coughing, inconsistent effort, or mechanical malfunctions can easily be identified by direct examination of the tracings. Interpretations of lung function from only a list of numbers produced by a computer should be avoided if an accurate assessment of a patient's pulmonary function status is to be made.

Other mistakes that can be made in test interpretation include changes in function caused by variability in patients themselves. A normal diurnal rhythm is now recognized that produces the worst function in the early morning, improves during the day, and again falls during the evening.[25] Large variations can also occur on a day-to-day basis in a single patient, especially if he has reversible obstructive airway disease. Patients may also inadvertently change their test results by doing such things as smoking immediately before the tests or using bronchodilator medications prior to arrival at the laboratory. This type of information must be made available to the health care professional interpreting the pulmonary function tests before a patient can be labeled as abnormal or unresponsive to bronchodilators.

Finally, an abnormal finding on a single pulmonary function test should always be confirmed at another time in order to avoid overinterpretation of the data and mislabeling of a normal person. Single determinations of bronchodilator studies should also be repeated serially before a patient with obstructive lung disease is denied the use of these drugs. The performance of pulmonary function tests requires the interaction of a machine, a technician, a patient, and the interpreter.[25] On a given day, problems pertaining to any of these four components can arise and produce data that do not truly represent a patient's baseline pulmonary status.

To avoid any problems with misinterpretation,

1. Pulmonary function equipment should be calibrated regularly.
2. Volumes should be corrected for BTPS.
3. Patients should be instructed not to smoke or use inhaled bronchodilators within 4 hr of testing, or use oral bronchodilators within 12 hr of testing.
4. Testing should be performed according to strict protocol.
5. Repeat tests should be performed at the same time of day.
6. Patient effort should be recorded.
7. Copies of pulmonary function tracings should be provided to the interpreter along with the computerized data printout sheets.

By following these simple steps, misinterpretation of pulmonary function testing can be minimized and maximum information from the tests can be obtained. Because of the psychological, financial, and legal implications of interpreting a patient's pulmonary function as being abnormal, any tests that are not clearly abnormal should be repeated before a final interpretation is made.

REFERENCES

1. Scheinhorn DJ, Emory WB: Putting spirometry to use in your practice. J Resp Dis 2(8):8, 1981
2. Lapp NL, Amandus HE, Hall R, Morgan WKC: Lung volumes and flow rates in black and white subjects. Thorax 29:185, 1974
3. Wanner A: Interpretation of pulmonary function tests. p. 353. In Sackner MA (ed): Diagnostic Techniques in Pulmonary Disease. Marcel Dekker, New York, 1980
4. McFadden ER Jr, Linden DA: A reduction in maximum mid-expiratory flow rate. A spirographic manifestation of small airway disease. Am J Med 52:725, 1972
5. Keogh BA, Crystal RG: Pulmonary function testing in interstitial pulmonary disease. Chest 78:856, 1980
6. Acres JC, Kryger MH: Upper airway obstruction. Chest 80:207, 1981
7. Lazarus A: Pulmonary function tests in upper airway obstruction. Basics RD 8:1, 1980
8. Rotman HH, Liss HP, Weg JG: Diagnosis of upper airway obstruction by pulmonary function testing. Chest 68:796, 1975
9. Light RW: Use of the pulmonary function laboratory in the treatment of obstructive airway disease. Adv Asthma Allergy 5:10, 1978
10. Light RW, Conrad SA, George RB: The one best test for evaluating the effects of bronchodilator therapy. Chest 72:512, 1977
11. Berend N, Wright JL, Thurlbeck WM, Marlin GE, Woolcock AJ: Small airways disease—Reproducibility of measurements and correlation with lung function. Chest 79:263, 1981
12. Woolcock AJ, Vincent NJ, Macklem PT: Frequency dependence of compliance as a test for obstruction in the small airways. Clin Invest 48:1097, 1969
13. Dosman JA, Cotton DJ: Interpretation of tests of early lung dysfunction. Chest 79:261, 1981
14. Buist AS, Ross B: Predicted values for closing volumes using a modified single breath nitrogen test. Am Rev Resp Dis 107:744, 1973

15. Dosman JA, Bode F, Urbanetti J, et al: The use of helium-oxygen mixtures during maximum expiratory flow to demonstrate obstruction in small airways in smokers. J Clin Invest 55:1090, 1975
16. Bode FR, Dosman JA, Martin RR, Macklem PT: Reversibility of pulmonary function abnormalities in smokers. Am J Med 59:43, 1975
17. Jenkinson SG, Light R: Management of surgical patients with chronic obstructive lung disease. p. 1. In Spittell JA Jr (ed): Clinical Medicine. Vol. 5. Harper & Row, Hagerstown, Md, 1980
18. Tahir A, George R, Weill H: Effects of abdominal surgery upon diaphragmatic function and regional ventilation. Int Surg 58:337, 1973
19. Boushy SF, Billig DM, North LB, et al: Clinical course related to preoperative postoperative pulmonary function in patients with bronchogenic carcinoma. Chest 59:383, 1971
20. Olsen GN, Block AJ, Tobias JA: Prediction of postpneumonectomy pulmonary function using quantitative macroaggregate lung scanning. Chest 66:13, 1974
21. Gaensler EA: Preoperative evaluation of lung function. Int Anesthesiol Clin 3:249, 1965
22. Bergan F: A simple method for the determination of the relative function of the right and left lung. Acta Chir Scand, suppl., 253:58, 1960
23. Jay SJ, Stonehill RB, Kiblowi SO, Norton J: Variability of the lateral position test in normal subjects. Am Rev Resp Dis 121:165, 1980
24. Reichel J: Assessment of operative risk of pneumonectomy. Chest 62:570, 1972
25. Butler J: The pulmonary function test, cautious overinterpretation. Chest 79:498, 1981

11

Interpretation of Lung Function in Children

Howard Eigen, M.D.

This chapter demonstrates the differences between pulmonary function testing in children and adults. It is assumed the reader has a grasp of the basic concepts of normal physiology and the techniques of pulmonary function testing in the adult, so that special considerations in children can be discussed without reference to testing methodology and rationale in older patients.

Several basic premises underlie the discussion:

1. The difference between children and adults is not one of scale but of basic physiology.
2. Pulmonary function testing is useful in children and is generally underutilized.
3. Whenever possible, pulmonary function testing in children should be performed and interpreted by persons specializing in and knowledgeable about the care of children.

The anatomic and physiological differences between the respiratory system of the child and that of the adult, and how these differences must be accounted for when administering and interpreting lung function studies in children, is a main concern. In testing children we must consider (1) changes in baseline or normal values because of growth and development of the respiratory system, (2) technical factors based on the size of the patient and his ability or willingness to cooperate, and (3) different indications for pulmonary function testing in children and adults based on the relative likelihood of specific disease entities.

It is also important to have a feel for the general pattern of changes that occur as a child grows from infancy to adolescence, and to consider the differences that exist physiologically betwen the child and the adult. As the child develops, the structures of the respiratory system grow and mature at different rates, so that at any given age the interplay among these factors results in a different sum of forces and an ever-changing physiological baseline. These differences in physiology also result in a difference in susceptibility to pathological states among children of different ages and between children and adults.

There is a significant gap in knowledge due to our inability to routinely measure lung function between ages 1 and 6. Unfortunately, this coincides with a period of active growth and development of the respiratory system. During the time from birth to 6 years, lung volume increases about 13-fold but cannot be satisfactorily measured, whereas from 6 years to adulthood it rises only threefold. This leaves us with a "blind spot" in the development of the adult respiratory system. With these changes comes the problem of comparing pulmonary function and physiological data at different ages. Because of differential growth in the respiratory system, comparing absolute values among children often leads to confusion so that methods for meaningful comparison must be established and proven physiologically valid. As an example, the elastic recoil of the lungs has been extensively studied; it is low in infants and increases with age.

Low elastic recoil in the infant is relatively unopposed because the bony thorax is soft and pliable, resulting in an end-expiratory resting point that tends to be at a low lung volume close to residual volume (RV). The high respiratory rate of infants compensates, in part, for the low volume at which this balance point occurs by causing the initiation of each subsequent breath before the exhalation from the previous breath allows the chest to come to its mechanical balance point, thus elevating functional residual capacity (FRC). As expected, FRC of an apneic infant is less than that of one breathing at a normal rate. There is a progressive increase in elastic recoil with growth as elastic tissue increases in amount and the pulmonary architecture becomes more complex. Mansell et al.,[1] when comparing the values for elastic recoil at a pressure of 25 cm H_2O (irrespective of what lung volume results), found a 6 cm H_2O increase in elastic recoil from birth to teen years. The changes in chest wall compliance are also dramatic. The outward recoil of the chest wall in the mature fetus is zero and increases with growth, having a profound effect on resting lung volume (Fig. 11-1). These changes in mechanics, in addition to true growth of airspaces, lead to an increase in functional residual capacity.[2]

Total lung capacity, being an effort-dependent measurement, has different determinants in children and adults. The child has weaker musculature with which to expand his thoracic cage and has less outward recoil to assist him in attaining high lung volume. Compensation for this comes from the shape of the child's chest, which is round in young children and slowly flattens in anterior-posterior diameter as the child matures (Fig. 11-2). The round chest shape provides the chest muscles and diaphragm with a smaller radius of curvature, and enhances the increase in thoracic volume as the ribs lift with inspiration (the so-called bucket handle effect), creating a greater change in pressure for a given change in tension. This does not apply to the accessory muscles of inspiration, however, which rely only on contractile strength for achieving high lung volume. The combination of these two factors results in a total lung capacity that increases with increasing muscular strength (and age), but is never as low in the infant as would be predicted on the basis of muscle strength alone.

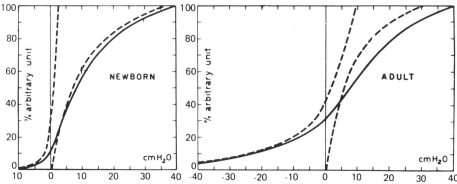

Fig. 11-1. Static pressure-volume relationships of the lung, chest wall, and total respiratory system of the newborn compared with the adult. The highly compliant chest wall provides little outward force, resulting in a passive FRC (balance point) very close to RV. The infant must expend energy to maintain FRC at higher volumes. [Reproduced with permission from Bryan AC, Mansell AL, Levison H: Development of the mechanical properties of the respiratory system. p. 445. In Hodson WA (ed): Development of the Lung. Marcel Dekker, New York, 1977. Courtesy of Marcel Dekker Inc. Masson Publishing USA Inc. © 1977 Masson Publishing USA Inc., New York]

Residual volume in the older adult is determined in great part by airway closure resulting from the loss of elastic recoil at low lung volumes. In young men, Leith and Mead[3] found that external pressure applied to the chest wall at RV could force out additional gas, reducing the naturally attained RV. This indicates that strength of the expiratory muscles and not airway closure determined RV in this experimental population. Mansell et al.[4] showed an increase in closing capacity with decreasing age, concluding that airway closure begins above RV in younger children and by inference must contribute to residual volume.

PULMONARY FUNCTION TESTING IN INFANTS

The infant, although unable to cooperate, generally will take a passive role during pulmonary function testing; thus, it has been possible to measure FRC and thoracic gas volume.

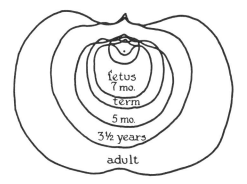

Fig. 11-2. The chest flattens in the anterior-posterior diameter as the child grows. The loss of mechanical advantage of a round chest is compensated by an increase in muscle strength. [Modified with permission from Waring WW: The history and physical examination. p. 77. In Kendig EL, Chernick V (eds): Disorders of the respiratory tract in children. 3rd Ed. W.B. Saunders, Philadelphia, 1977]

Estimates of vital capacity have been made using the *crying vital capacity* obtained with a face mask and a pediatric wedge spirometer. Employing this method, Krauss et al.[5] demonstrated good correlation with FRC in premature newborns and that infants with hyaline membrane disease had a reduction in crying vital capacity compared to normal prematures. However, the physiological relationships between true vital capacity and crying vital capacity is not understood, as there is no way of knowing whether these breaths are maximal. Crying vital capacity is measured during phonation, so expiratory flow must be limited; no measurement comparable to forced expiratory volume in 1 sec (FEV_1) is obtained while measuring a crying vital capacity.

Respiratory induction plethysmography (Respitrace; Ambulatory Monitoring Inc., Ardsley, N.Y.) has been used by Duffty and colleagues[6] to measure tidal volume and minute ventilation in infants weighing 1.3 to 5.4 kg and of varying postconceptional ages. A time-consuming calibration is required, but the device appears to be reliable in measuring tidal volume and long-term minute ventilation.

PULMONARY FUNCTION TESTING IN YOUNG CHILDREN (AGES 4 TO 6)

A test that can be used in young children (ages 4 to 6) is measurement of maximal expiratory flow at FRC. After FRC has been established by recording tidal breathing, the child is encouraged to exhale forcefully. In the group of children reported by Taussig,[7] flows at FRC of normal children differed from those of children with known obstructive disease. Although the test has not been widely adopted, it may be useful in following small children with lung disease. The variation within the normal population appears too wide for single values to be helpfully compared to a reference population.

An excellent clinical test of lung function in the infant and young child is the sleeping respiratory rate. In addition to offering an accurate assessment of respiratory system compliance, it is easy, inexpensive, and can be used at home for repeated testing during the course of an illness or to monitor response to therapy. Parents are taught to count respirations over a full minute without touching the child. They record three separate readings each night, the mean of which can be graphed by the physician for easier identification of trends. Monitoring sleeping respiratory rate is helpful in many conditions in which respiratory system compliance is reduced, such as pulmonary edema, pleural effusions, and pneumonia. We have used the technique to monitor infants and young children with interstitial pneumonitis, pulmonary hemosiderosis, and those who are at risk for opportunistic infections. The span of normal respiratory rates at a give age is wide and rates also vary considerably between sleep and wakefulness (Table 11-1).[8,9]

At this age too, many children are able to perform a satisfactory peak flow

Table 11-1 Normal Sleeping and Awake Respiratory Rates in Children

Age	Sleeping	Awake	Mean Difference
6–12 months	27 (22–31)ᵃ	64 (58–75)	37
1–2 years	19 (17–23)	35 (30–40)	16
2–4 years	19 (16–25)	31 (23–42)	12
4–6 years	18 (14–23)	26 (19–36)	8
6–8 years	17 (13–23)	23 (15–30)	6
8–10 years	18 (14–23)	21 (15–31)	3
10–12 years	16 (13–19)	21 (15–28)	5
12–14 years	16 ((15–18)	22 (18–26)	6

ᵃ Values expressed as mean with range in parentheses.
Source: Modified from Waring WW: The history and physical examination. p. 77. In Kendig EL, Chernick V (eds): Disorders of the Respiratory Tract in Children. 3rd Ed. W.B. Saunders, Philadelphia, 1977

maneuver. The test can provide useful information, particularly when serial measurements are compared.

PULMONARY FUNCTION TESTING IN OLDER CHILDREN

By the time a child reaches age 6, most of the pulmonary function tests used to assess lung function in adults can be employed successfully. There are, of course, many special considerations as to technique, reference populations, and test performance that are special to children. To produce reliable data, the laboratory personnel must have a major commitment to pulmonary function testing in children, have special training and experience, devote considerable time and effort to each child, and create an appropriate atmosphere for testing.

Choice of Equipment

The room itself should be attractively decorated for children and free from distractions. Instruments associated with painful procedures should be kept out of sight. The report of the Cystic Fibrosis Foundation Committee on the Standardization of Lung Function Testing in Children offers guidelines for choosing equipment to be used in testing children.[10] It is preferable to use a system that displays the volume of the inspiratory breath taken prior to the forced vital capacity (FVC) maneuver being recorded, such as a closed spirometer or a pneumotachographic system. The child should place the mouthpiece in his mouth at FRC and inspire from FRC to total lung capacity (TLC), drawing air from the spirometer as part of the recorded maneuver. One must be sure that the inertia of the system is not so great as to impart a respiratory load on small or weak patients. In addition, some systems have dead space that is considerable in relation to the child's lung volume. In such a case, having the child breathe

Table 11-2 Recommended Specifications for Pulmonary Equipment

Flow	
Accuracy	±5% or ±0.1 liter/sec, whichever is greater
Response	±5% to 8 Hz
Volume	
Accuracy	±3% of reading or 30 ml, whichever is greater
Sensitivity	20–40 mm of chart equals 1 liter
Response	±5% to 5 Hz
Time	
Discrimination	0.05 sec/mm
Timer threshold	50 ml/sec
Dynamic calibration	
Inertia	Low
Amplitude response	±5% to 15 Hz
Other considerations	
Ability to assess adequacy of inspiration effort (closed circuit or a pneumotachograph)	
Should produce a hard copy of curve	

Source: Data from Taussig LM, Chernick V, Wood R, et al: Standardization of lung function testing in children. J Pediatr 97:668, 1980; and Lemen RJ: Pulmonary function testing in the office and clinic. p. 166. In Kendig EL, Chernick V (eds): Disorders of the Respiratory Tract in Children. 3rd Ed. W.B. Saunders, Philadephia, 1977

through the circuit for a prolonged period of time prior to performing the measured maneuver will cause rebreathing of carbon dioxide which may result in or exacerbate hypoxemia or hypercarbia. Recommendations for equipment specifications are summarized in Table 11-2.[10,11]

Preparing the Child for the Test

Most tests require a similar respiratory maneuver: a full inspiration and a forced or controlled expiration. Acceptable measurements in children depend on a maximal effort in attaining TLC and RV, and in producing maximum flows. Most children entering a pulmonary function test laboratory for the first time will be curious, slightly timid, very willing to cooperate, and anxious to please the technician, physician, and parents by performing well. The laboratory and its staff should realize this and be careful not to alter this positive attitude by their actions (Table 11-3).

Children are generally very responsive to explanations, even of technical material, and enjoy the chance to ask questions. Those who do not deal with children daily tend to underestimate the child's ability to understand and his eagerness to do a good job. They often talk down to the child, or misinterpret his tentative actions or genuine fear as lack of cooperation. Brough et al.[12] have shown that performance can be improved if children ages 5 to 7 are given 15 min of instruction that explain the test and how it works, give a demonstration of the respiratory maneuvers, and provide a chance to practice. A formal instruction

Table 11-3 Techniques for Improving Performance in Children

1. The technician should blow against the child's hand so the breath can be felt as well as seen.
2. Practice by having the child and technician blow against each other's hands, making a contest of who can blow longer. Let the child win a few times to build confidence.
3. Demonstrate that the mouthpiece goes between the teeth.
4. Show that the noseclips do not hurt by placing them on the child's finger.
5. Be positive and give praise. Even if an effort is not perfect, give encouragement by saying it is "A good try" or "You're really good at blowing hard" *not* "Let's blow long, too."
6. In answer to how many times they will have to blow, say: "It depends on you. We need four good curves, so let's see how many times you need."

period improved performance on FVC and FEV_1 by about 10 percent compared to a group given routine instruction just prior to testing. It is also helpful if a goal or element of competition is introduced to the test.

Obtaining an adequate expiratory curve may require a great deal of coaching. Children often cannot grasp the idea of blowing out with maximum force *and* for as long as possible. Children that blow out very hard, giving a good peak flow, often stop short of RV. Those that blow a long time, obtaining a true vital capacity, will try to "save some air" and not blow out forcefully at the beginning of the effort.

All breathing maneuvers should be done wearing noseclips. Although the child may sit or stand for the test with no effect on its result, the technician should be certain that the trunk is held upright and the head erect during the maneuver.

After the child has performed the test comes the problem of selecting the appropriate tracing for analysis. To get a curve representative of a child's actual lung function may require the performance and evaluation of many curves, since effort may vary greatly with each try. Although learning takes place in some cases, making later curves better than earlier ones, we have also experienced just the opposite where the early efforts were the best, presumably because the test procedure exceeded the child's attention span or fatigue set in. In any case, a large set of curves must be generated and saved before a "best effort" can be chosen. This severely limits the usefulness of computer-based systems that store only three to five curves and those in which each effort must be rejected before the next attempt is made. The best-effort curve is selected as the one having the greatest sum of FEV_1 and FVC. Any calculated values, such as the ratio of FEV_1 and FVC, should come from the same curve.[13] Peak flow is usually measured separately as the best effort from three to five efforts using a peak flowmeter or from the best-effort flow-volume curve, which is reported as maximum forced expiratory flow (FEFmax).

An incomplete effort is especially difficult to judge using a standard spirogram, yet in obtaining valuable data it is crucial to know the effort is a true vital capacity maneuver. We find that it is easier to identify an effort in which the child has stopped short of RV using a flow-volume plot rather than a standard

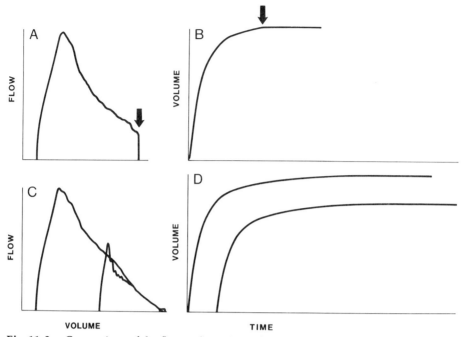

Fig. 11-3.   Comparison of the flow-volume (A and C) and volume-time (B and D) plots of FVC maneuvers. The point where flow ceases (arrow in A and B) is more easily identified in the flow-volume plot, permitting rejection of the effort as submaximal. Parts C and D illustrate curves blown from a volume less than TLC. The submaximal curves appear normal until compared with those representing a better effort.

volume-time tracing. More difficult still is judging whether the child has inspired to TLC at the start of the test, as curves blown from a lower lung volume will have the same shape as those blown from TLC using either graphic format (Fig. 11-3).

STATIC LUNG VOLUME

Plethysmography

Using a constant-volume, variable-pressure plethysmograph with a large, clear Plexiglas door we have had only rare instances when a child would not enter the instrument. The panting maneuver is easily understood and does not require the sustained cooperation of the FVC effort. Thus, FRC and airway resistance (Raw) can be measured in young school-age children with few problems. Lindemann[14] has demonstrated that an adult may accompany the child into the box as a helper without affecting the results. To prevent distortion of the child's signal, the adult must hold his breath at the time of measurement. There is no difference in Raw and thoracic gas volume (VTG) measured with and without a companion, but one must be certain to account for the added displacement of box volume by the adult.

The calculations of RV and TLC by adding and subtracting spirometric volumes to FRC assumes that the child's breathing pattern does not vary significantly while using the two pieces of apparatus and that he establishes the same end-expiratory resting point on both. This assumption is more likely to be true if the child is relaxed, understands the equipment, and if the spirometer used does not add a significant respiratory load.

FRC, measured as VTG, is one of the best-characterized lung volumes in infants and children, and data are available for age 12 hr and older. Weng and Levison[15] measured VTG at the end of a quiet expiration using a variable-pressure, 600-liter body plethysmograph in 42 boys and 41 girls. They did not, however, report RV and TLC calculated from this measurement.

Helium Dilution

Helium dilution FRC is not difficult to obtain in children as FRC measurement requires only tidal breathing and the spirometric maneuver can be done slowly rather than as a forced maneuver. Thus, children who will cooperate with little else can often perform well enough for an accurate assessment of FRC by helium dilution. Weng and Levison[15] performed measurements of FRC by helium dilution using a 9-liter, closed-circuit residual helium apparatus on 139 normal, healthy children. Using contemporaneously recorded spirometry, they calculated RV and TLC and the RV/TLC ratio.

Determination of FRC by gas dilution is dependent on good mixing of the trace gas (helium) in all lung spaces and may underestimate FRC, and hence, TLC, in those children with obstructive pulmonary disease. Body plethysmography measures all gas that is compressed during panting and so does not depend on unobstructed airways for its accuracy. In patients with airway obstruction, FRC with body plethysmography will be larger and more accurate than that obtained with helium dilution. What seems at first a disadvantage in the estimate of an accurate gas volume at FRC can be turned to clinical advantage by comparing the two measurements. Although in patients without airway obstruction the two measurements will be nearly identical, the difference will increase in proportion to the amount of gas trapped behind closed or severely narrowed airways. Thus, the difference between FRC measured by helium dilution (FRCHE) and FRC measured by body plethysmography (FRCBP) is the *trapped gas volume* that can be used to follow the course of patients with cystic fibrosis and asthma.

In children with muscular weakness the RV calculated by subtracting ERV from FRC will be increased (see page 235) because the patient is unable to expel gas from his lungs by forceful thoracic compression with the expiratory muscles.

The resulting RV will be high, but because the airways are not obstructed the trapped gas volume will be low and RV by helium dilution and plethysmography will be similar.

DYNAMIC MEASUREMENTS

Spirometry

If the technical quality of the tracing is adequate, one can measure lung volumes and flows from spirometry in children over age 6 with no special difficulties. However, there are clear differences between the sexes that should be taken into account when making comparisons with the reference population.

Suitable reference values are more difficult to obtain when the effect of puberty and the adolescent growth spurt are considered. Dickman and associates[16] divided their population of 482 healthy boys and 468 healthy girls into two groups by height, height being chosen as a more reliable index of puberty than age. At 60-in. standing height, FVC and flow began to increase at a different rate than in shorter children, and greater divergence was seen between the sexes. Although it is often throught that the main value of a pediatric pulmonary function laboratory is testing younger children, the data of Dickman et al. emphasize the dangers of lumping all older children together and comparing them to adult reference standards. This practice can lead to a mistaken diagnosis of abnormality in children with late-onset puberty who have perfectly normal lung function.

Peak lung function is reached at an earlier age in girls than boys,[17] but the exact age at which maximum function occurs differs from author to author. Knudson et al.[18] found maximum flows and FVC to increase with age to 20 years in women and 27 years in men. Seely et al.[17] calculated the maximum to occur at 14 years in girls and 18 years in boys. Dickman[16] found maximum FEV_1 and FVC occurring at 16 and 18 years in girls and boys, respectively. These diverse findings point out the need for further studies of adolescents who fulfill the criteria for normality and for extreme care by the clinician in comparing values obtained from individual patients with reference groups.

Peak Expiratory Flow Rate (PEFR)

PEFR is an especially useful test for obtaining information on lung function in children younger than 5 years old. Bjure and coworkers[19] have shown that five or more peak flow attempts will result in somewhat higher values than only three attempts in girls but not in boys. This is probably a factor related to effort; therefore it is best to give all children the opportunity for five peak flow attempts before deciding a maximal value has been reached. Milner and Ingram[20] were able to obtain data on 92 normal children ages 35 to 60 months of age (heights less than 95 to 115 cm) using low range (maximum flow 200 liters/min) Wright peak flowmeter. Children under age 3 were also tested, but reliable results could not be obtained either because of refusal or inability to cooperate. In seven children, each tested three or four times over 1 month, the mean coefficient of variation was 7.8 percent. Results were scattered over a wide range and there was no consistent reduction of standard deviation with increasing age in this group. A large standard deviation reduces the value of a single test in assessing the presence of airway obstruction, but does not reduce the usefulness of PEFR for serial followup of young children.

The summary data from Polgar and Promadhat[21] show that the regression lines of the data for the European and North American population run closely together, but that Chinese girls have peak flows 2 standard deviations (s.d.) lower than the summary curves at any given height above 120 cm. It is speculated that this difference may result from a cultural phenomenon related to cooperation rather than a physical cause.

Hsu and coworkers[22] have conducted a comprehensive study of peak flow measurements in children. Studying 1,805 children in the Houston public school system, these workers found racial differences in peak flow, as it related to height, at all ages (7 to 20 years) and heights (111 to 190 cm). Blacks had lower and Mexican-Americans higher flows at all heights. Hsu noted that maximum flows obtained from the peak flowmeter and those measured as FEFmax from the flow-volume display of spirometry differed in their regression against height, especially at flows above 325 liters/min (Fig. 11-4).

In Hsu's study and that of Murray and Cook,[23] the only two performed on U.S. children using a Wright peak flowmeter, separate regression equations were generated for boys and girls. These data differ from the summary data of Polgar and Promadhat, which generated a single regression line for both sexes. The summary data of Polgar and Weng,[24] generated by including data reported since 1970, include separate regression equations of peak flow versus height for boys and girls. The author suggests using separate equations for each sex.

Inspiratory Force

The measurement of inspiratory force is a valuable technique for following children with muscular weakness. TLC falls and RV increases as the inspiratory and expiratory muscles, respectively, lose strength, resulting in a reduction in VC. However, this reduction in VC takes place late in the course of the disease and a better early indication can be obtained by measuring inspiratory and expiratory force. This is achieved with an anaeroid manometer and does not require cooperation. In children too young to cooperate, we apply the manometer, connected to a tight-fitting face mask, by a tube containing a single hole. The airway is occluded by placing a finger over the hole in the tube at the end of a quiet expiration. The first few breaths against the closed system give a good measure of inspiratory force at FRC and the mask is lifted off the child's face. The

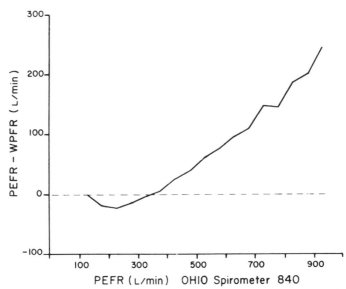

Fig. 11-4. The differences between peak flow rate obtained from a spirometer (PEFR) and a Wright peak flowmeter (WPFR). Differences become significant in children producing flows of 350 liters/min or greater. (Reproduced with permission from Hsu KHK et al: Ventilatory functions of normal children and young adults — Mexican American, white and black. II. Wright peak flow meter. J Pediatr 95:192, 1979)

entire process takes only 10 to 15 sec and children rarely become distressed by it. Inspiratory force should be measured at the same lung volume each time. Although cooperative children can be measured at RV or TLC, it is generally easier to test inspiratory force at FRC.

Racial Differences

Racial and ethnic differences are accentuated in children because they are superimposed on changes in normal values induced by growth and the physical changes brought about by the onset of puberty. For a given standing height, blacks have a longer lower body segment and consequently a shorter upper body segment than whites. This results in predicted pulmonary function values for white children that overestimate "normal" if used for black children. Stated differently, the sitting-to-standing height ratio is smaller in blacks than in Caucasians. When vital capacity of black children is compared with that of white children on the basis of sitting height, no difference is found. These racial differences appear to be genetic and not related to social or economic factors. They are greater with increasing height and age, indicating that puberty contributes to the divergence in body habitus.

Similar differences between Caucasians and Mexican-Americans have been shown by Hsu et al.[23,25] She found Mexican boys to have a slightly larger FVC and greater flows for standing height than Caucasians, a difference that was not seen in comparison of girls of the two ethnic groups. Hsu gave separate regression equation curves for Caucasians, Mexican-Americans, and blacks of each sex (see Appendix B).

Sensitivity

Which of the above tests is the "most sensitive" in judging childhood lung function? This of course depends on the clinical context. For airway obstruction, the maximal midexpiratory flow rate is a sensitive indicator of mild disease. MMEF ($FEF_{25-75\%}$) is the average flow over the middle 50 percent of the vital capacity and is in the effort-independent portion of the forced expiratory maneuver. It is sensitive to the absolute lung volume at which it is measured and so may actually increase in severely obstructed patients when RV rises, pushing the vital capacity to a higher absolute lung volume. When testing children with more severe disease, FEV_1 and peak flow are more appropriate and will not be confounded by changes in absolute lung volume.

DIAGNOSIS OF EARLY DISEASE

Volume of Isoflow

The comparison of a flow-volume curve performed while the patient breathes air with one obtained after inhaling a helium-oxygen mixture of 80 and 20 percent, respectively, is another sensitive test that can identify the presence of airway disease in the absence of gross abnormalities on spirometry.

Flows at 50-percent vital capacity ($\Delta \dot{V}max_{50\%}$) can be compared or the curves can be superimposed and the lung volume at which flows become equal can be measured. This is the volume of isoflow ($V_{iso}\dot{v}$) or point of identical flow (PIF). Normal children show density dependence. A reduction in density dependence (i.e., a higher volume of isoflow), has been seen in children who had bronchiolitis as infants and in those with mild cystic fibrosis. The specificity of the test in distinguishing small from large airways as the site of disease has recently been questioned,[26] but whatever the site, the test does seem to identify groups that are at variance with normal subjects.

Closing Volume

Closing volume by the single-breath oxygen method has been advocated as a tool for detecting mild small airway disease. This test has limited usefulness in

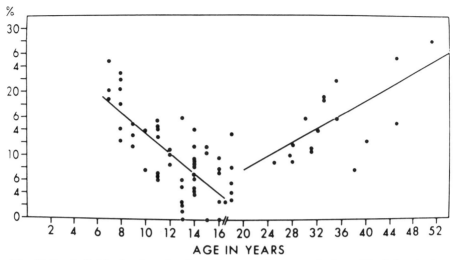

Fig. 11-5. Individual values for the volume as the start of phase IV of the single-breath oxygen (closing volume) test as a percentage of VC. Extrapolating from adult values to those predicted for children would give erroneous results. (Reproduced with permission from Mansell A, Bryan C, Levison H: Airway closure in children. J Appl Physiol 33:711, 1972)

children because by the time a child is old enough to perform it many diseases (e.g., cystic fibrosis) have become full-blown. Data for closing volume in children are presented in Figure 11-5. This not only shows the high values found in children but points out the necessity of using predicted values that are age-specific and not extrapolated from adult data. Extrapolating the closing volume of a 12-year-old child from that of a normal adult might lead one to believe that a normal 12-year-old had markedly abnormal lung function.

DIFFUSING CAPACITY

This test is used for long-term followup of patients on chemotherapy for malignancy, those with sarcoidosis, and other specialized uses, such as evaluation of fibrosing diseases.

The technical difficulties involved in testing children are related to their small lung volumes. Many automated systems with manifolds and solenoid-controlled sampling valves have large dead space volumes that make accurate sampling difficult. If such a system is employed, the dead space should be measured (by gas dilution) for both the inspiratory and expiratory circuits and used to correct the apparent lung volumes. We prefer a low dead space system incorporating a spirometer and a five-way control valve for sampling (e.g., Model 21051, W. E. Collins, Inc., Braintree, Mass.). Data from reference populations are available (see Appendix B) and intrasubject variability is shown to be less than 10 percent. Training and careful observation of the child are especially important to be certain that he is relaxed during the breathholding period of the single-breath diffusion test, as Valsalva or Mueller maneuvers, respectively, can decrease or increase apparent $D_{L_{CO}}$.[27]

$D_{L_{CO}}$ has been recommended in diagnosing drug-induced lung disease from cytotoxic agents used for treating malignancies. Bleomycin, methotrexate, and cyclophosphamide have all been shown to reduce D_L in the range of 50 percent. However, this is often accompanied by significant clinical findings (cough, dyspnea, rales), radiographic findings (diffuse infiltrates), and arterial oxygen desaturation. Often, the decrease in $D_{L_{CO}}$ cannot be measured prior to the onset of more obvious changes. This test is affected by weakness and anemia, and with bleomycin there is a high incidence of finding a decrease in $D_{L_{CO}}$ without further consequences.[28] Still, there are data that show the usefulness of careful pulmonary function testing in identifying pulmonary toxicity before clinical symptoms occur.[29]

BRONCHIAL CHALLENGE TESTING

Bronchial challenge testing is an extremely useful modality in children. Commonly used challenge agents include inhalation of histamine, methacholine, antigen (e.g., ragweed aerosol), and exercise. A large number of children have asthma, yet in many wheezing is not among the first clinical manifestations. Cloutier and Loughlin[30] and Konig[31] described groups of children with cough who had positive bronchial challenge tests to exercise and who responded to bronchodilator. We have described a group of children with recurrent pneumonia diagnosed as having asthma by methacholine challenge.[32] Children who have had lung injuries in early childhood (e.g., near-drowning, bronchiolitis, tracheoesophageal fistula, croup, and meconium aspiration) are left with long-lasting bronchial reactivity that can be diagnosed using a bronchial challenge. In 1965, Parker et al.[33] described the use of methacholine aerosol as a test for bronchial asthma in children and adults. None of the normal children responded to five inhalations of methacholine (25 mg/ml) with a decrease in FEV_1 of more than 20 percent. Eighteen of 20 asthmatic children responded with a decrease of 25 percent or more over one to five inhalations. The difference in group means in the decrease in FEV_1 from baseline was highly significant.

Standardized techniques for this test were proposed in 1975 and since then most studies using bronchial challenge have followed these procedures.[34] Though it is not necessary to follow the standardized methodology when doing a clinical assessment, the standard protocol is recommended because it is a safe and proven method and makes comparisons of tests performed on the same patient at different times more meaningful. It is important that the laboratory performing such challenges do so frequently enough that personnel become expert. Once it has been diluted to the standard concentrations, methacholine remains potent for 2 to 4 weeks under refrigeration. Drug dilutions for aerosol inhalation should be made fresh monthly to ensure accurate results. There is no need for a dosimeter.

There appear to be no problems specific to children in relating responses to challenge and clinical reactivity. Ninety to 98 percent of children with symptomatic asthma are sensitive to methacholine or histamine inhalation; however, it is assumed there is a wide separation between asthmatics and normals in their responsiveness to inhaled methacholine. Upper respiratory infections can cause a transient increase in bronchial reactivity[35] for 6 weeks or longer. Because of the frequency of upper respiratory infection in children, one may not have a long enough interval from the child's last respiratory infection to permit a definite distinction between transient, injury-induced bronchial hyperreactivity and that resulting from asthma.

In lieu of a formal challenge, some physicians perform unstandardized tests, such as having the child jump up and down or run around the office or hallway, then listening to the chest for wheezes. These tests should be avoided because they cannot be interpreted in the light of a negative test and cannot be quantified. In asthmatics, bronchodilation usually precedes bronchoconstriction as a response to exercise and this of course would be missed without a quantitative measurement of flow.

Methacholine and histamine have been shown to be equally effective in provoking a response, as have histamine and exercise. Because we find it technically easier to perform, we use methacholine in preference to exercise challenge for diagnosing of children suspected of having exercise-induced bronchospasm.

Shapiro et al.[36] have reviewed their experience with methacholine bronchial challenge in 166 children and young adults and point out its usefulness in clinical practice. Sixty-five percent of patients tested were sensitive to the agent, leading to appropriate use of bronchodilators. In the 35 percent of patients who were negative, asthma was effectively ruled out, a decision that was confirmed at reexamination 1 year later. Patients with marked sensitivity to methacholine were more likely to use medication regularly, as judged at the 1-year followup.

The usefulness of methacholine challenge in cystic fibrosis is often overlooked clinically. Mitchell demonstrated bronchial hyperreactivity to methacholine in 51 percent of 113 children tested.[37] Eighty percent of those patients with FEV_1 below 40 percent of predicted value responded to methacholine. Bronchospasm may be an important cause of episodic disease in cystic fibrosis, especially in patients who have exacerbations following viral respiratory infections. A positive response to methacholine challenge is a good indicator for a bronchodilator trial in cystic fibrosis patients, whereas the mere presence of obstructive disease on pulmonary function testing is not.

A summary of indications for methacholine challenge testing in the clinical setting is given in Table 11-4.

Table 11-4 Indications for Bronchial Challenge Testing

History of wheezing with normal pulmonary function tests
Chronic cough
Exercise tolerance
Unexplained dyspnea
Cystic fibrosis
Recurrent pneumonia
History of bronchiolitis or other early lung injury

CLINICAL USES OF PEDIATRIC PULMONARY FUNCTION TESTING

Discussion of the interpretation of pulmonary function tests is best done in the context of specific diseases once the basic testing principles as they apply to children are understood.

Asthma

Asthma is the most common chronic respiratory disease of childhood. Its diagnosis and therapy are aided by the use of lung function tests. The old saw that "All the wheezes are not asthma" is true, but it must also be recognized that "All that is asthma does not wheeze." So we must be prepared, through the use of pulmonary function testing, to ferret out children with airway hyperreactivity that may not cause wheezing.

In our laboratory we have often been presented with a child who had either chronic cough or recurrent pneumonia as an initial manifestation of asthma. Cloutier and Loughlin[30] used bronchial challenge by treadmill exercise to uncover bronchial hyperreactivity in 15 children with chronic cough and essentially normal pulmonary function tests. Methacholine bronchial challenge is also effective in diagnosing children with cough as having bronchial hyperreactivity. Any children referred for persistent or recurrent pneumonia[32] may also have bronchial hyperreactivity demonstrated on methacholine inhalation testing.

Pulmonary function testing without airway challenge can be useful in documenting the severity of chronic obstruction in children who present with a history of wheezing. First, the question of whether a child with a history compatible with, but not characteristic of, asthma actually has airway obstruction can be answered by forced exhalation spirometry. Second, in children with more typical clinical disease the degree of obstruction can be determined. This is especially useful in the child who has continued to wheeze despite a trial of therapy and who is referred to the laboratory for further evaluation. Lung function testing allows the pulmonologist to document for parents, patient, and physician the need for more aggressive treatment. Later, the efficacy of the revised treatment plan can be judged by whether or not pulmonary function has improved. Measuring lung volumes by plethysmography is useful in determining the degree of hyperinflation, which in turn may have prognostic value. Recent work by Kraemer and colleagues[38] found that the best response to albuterol inhalation is seen in children with bronchial obstruction alone, as compared to children having bronchial obstruction with hyperinflation and those with hyperinflation alone. They also expressed concern that chronic hyperinflation may lead to permanent lung changes. The ability to classify asthmatic children on the basis of degree of hyperinflation may provide the impetus for more frequent measurements of FRC by plethysmography.

An important goal of therapy in asthmatic children is to achieve not just freedom from wheezing, but normal spirometry. This is done by routinely testing children at all office visits. Failure to identify subclinical airway obstruction may lead a child to adopt a sedentary life-style to suppress symptoms, and though the history at each subsequent visit will indicate the child is free of wheezing, he may actually be severely limited by his disease.

The question frequently arises as to when to reduce or discontinue medication in children under treatment for asthma. The approach used is similar to a clinical experiment. Assuming the child has been without symptoms for several months, the physician stops the drug and observes the child until a predetermined end point is reached. The end point can be a clinical one, such as return of the wheezing or cough, but we prefer to detect the need for a return to daily therapy by noting a reduction in flow on pulmonary function testing. Our procedure is to stop the medication, then retest the child in 2 to 4 weeks whether or not there has been a reappearance of symptoms. If pulmonary function has deteriorated, we reinstate bronchodilator therapy. This approach is dependent on conducting a series of lung function tests on each child so that an appropriate baseline of responses may be established.

Home testing using a peak flowmeter is another adjunct in the management of the severe asthmatic. Interpretation of individual results is based on peak expiratory flow rates performed when the child is well and not on comparison with a reference population. Many children awaken at night with respiratory complaints that may or may not be related to an increase in airway obstruction. Peak flow measurements taken at the time of such complaints can identify asthma as the cause of this nocturnal distress. In patients who live a considerable distance from our facility, we use PEFR to guide the course of an acute episode by giving the mother instructions on what action to take for various PEFR values. For example, we would instruct her that if PEFR ranges between 200 and 300 liters/min to administer an inhaled bronchodilator; if between 100 and 200 liters/min to give the inhalation treatment and call us or bring the child to the hospital; if less than 100 liters/min to go immediately to the local hospital emergency room. Of course, the absolute values vary with the clinical circumstances but the approach is very useful (Fig. 11-6).

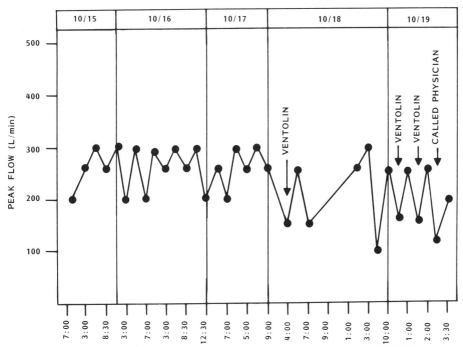

Fig. 11-6. Data from an 11-year-old asthmatic patient who used a mini-Wright peak flowmeter. (Manufactured by Armstrong Industries, Northbrook, Ill) The course of a single asthma attack is well documented, as are responses to inhaled albuterol (Ventolin).

Cystic Fibrosis

Cystic fibrosis is another disease in which pulmonary function testing plays a major role in guiding management of individual cases. Children will first develop an obstructive pattern with gas trapping. This can be measured easily on spirometry as a reduction of MMEF, or FEV_1, or both. Trapped gas will manifest as an increase in RV by body plethysmography (but not as great an increase if measured by helium dilution). Calculation of trapped gas volume, as described previously, may also be useful.

We frequently use changes in pulmonary function tests to decide on the need for hospitalization. If FVC and FEV_1 have decreased by 1 s.d., we take steps to increase the intensity of therapy. If the reduction in function is combined with weight loss or new infiltrates on chest radiographs, then admission is warranted. Improvement in pulmonary function tests is not likely to be rapid; often, patients who feel and look better after a course of intensive therapy in the hospital will not have a significant improvement in pulmonary function. Lung function usually improves by 6 to 8 weeks posthospitalization and is monitored closely after discharge (Fig. 11-7). Many patients with cystic fibrosis have a reversible obstruc-

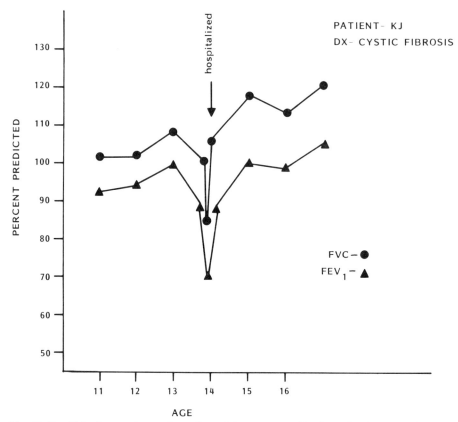

Fig. 11-7. This demonstrates the value of long-term collection of pulmonary function data in cystic fibrosis. The patient was hospitalized when function deteriorated, despite the fact that FVC was 80 percent of predicted. Recovery of pulmonary function after hospitalization is also documented.

tive component that can be detected by a rise in FEV_1 in response to an inhaled bronchodilator. Excessive bronchial reactivity can be detected by challenge testing with methacholine.

In a disease with the great inertia of cystic fibrosis, it is critical to maintain long-term records of lung function tests and make comparisons periodically with tests from at least 1 year earlier. This approach often uncovers a patient whose pulmonary function has decreased at a rate so slow that it goes unnoticed until a long-term comparison is made.

Lung Injury

There is now ample evidence that children who suffer a serious lung injury by infection (e.g., bronchiolitis or croup), by accident (e.g., near-drowning), or by aspiration (e.g., tracheoesophageal fistula) will have long-term sequellae of varying degrees of severity. Acute lung injury in near-drowning results in a severe restrictive ventilatory defect with a reduced FVC.[39,40] One reported patient experienced a reduction of DL_{CO}.[40] In two children and two adults followed serially, lung volumes returned to normal by 6 and 16 weeks postinjury, respectively. The best way to assess children with lung injury as they mature is not yet known, but studies show a pattern of residual bronchial hyperreactivity and a high isoflow volume. In such children, periodic testing of lung function by spirometry is useful for identifying any subclinical disease before it becomes symptomatic, of if no abnormalities are identified, to reassure parents their child remains healthy.

Evaluation for Surgery

Preoperative evaluation is an important use of pulmonary function testing in children as well as adults. There are no comprehensive studies in children to assist us in assessing risk on the basis of specific test results. Studies in adults that have attempted to correlate preoperative abnormalities of pulmonary function and postoperative complications have not been conclusive. Some tests are sensitive to abnormalities but are not specific and will be abnormal in many patients who come through surgery without difficulty. Despite the specific limitations of pulmonary function testing in predicting risks, lung function tests can provide an important baseline measurement for assessing the progress of patients in the postoperative period, may influence the choice of surgery, and can be used to prepare both patient and physician for the likelihood of postoperative complications.

Although it is unlikely an elective procedure would be cancelled for a child because occult disease is uncovered on preoperative pulmonary function tests, such testing may modify the surgical approach or indicate the need for presurgical therapy. For example, during routine screening of children about to undergo repair of pectus excavatum, we have identified a number of children with asthma and have delayed surgery until pulmonary function returned to normal by medication with bronchodilators. Froese[41] points out the usefulness of inspiratory capacity in trying to predict patients' ability to breathe unaided postoperatively. Even with perfectly normal pulmonary parenchyma, it is rare for a person to sustain ventilation for long periods and clear secretion with an inspiratory capacity of less than 15 ml/kg. Similarly, PEFR can give a rough estimate of whether a patient can generate flows adequate for raising secretions by coughing.

Scoliosis

Pulmonary function testing is especially useful in evaluating children with scoliosis. Idiopathic adolescent scoliosis is the most frequently encountered form of scoliosis and usually occurs in females. Respiratory abnormalities are common and progress in relationship to the degree of deformity as expressed by the angle of scoliosis, resulting in a decrease in lung volumes, small airway function, and gas exchange. TLC and its subdivisions all decrease as the angle of scoliosis increases. The use of helium-air flow-volume curves increases the sensitivity of lung function testing, permitting detection of small airway obstruction in scoliosis patients with normal spirometry.[42] The risk of surgery in most patients must be undertaken, because failure to perform it would lead to a progressive loss of lung function. Kafer[43] has demonstrated a correlation betwen increasing angle of scoliosis and decreasing arterial oxygen tension and lung volumes. The advantage of pulmonary function tests here is that they allow us to prepare the patient for surgery by improving lung function as much as possible and by planning a course of action for the postoperative period, especially at a time when pain and immobility cause further reduction in lung volumes and cough effectiveness.

Muscle Weakness

Simple measurement of pulmonary function is essential in patients with progressive muscle weakness to help the physician decide when to institute supportive measures before the patient deteriorates into frank respiratory failure. In acute diseases, such as Guillain-Barré syndrome, testing should be performed at least every 8 hr for as long as the paralysis is ascending. In cooperative children, bedside VC measurement can be made as well. This is best done using a mechanical spirometer, for example, the Breon spirometer (Model 2400, Breon Laboratories, New York, N.Y.) which gives a tracing of the volume-time curve and allows assessment of effort. Electronic models that give only numerical values but no tracing are unsatisfactory, as an assessment of effort cannot be made.

A FVC reading of less than 6 ml/kg or one less than twice the predicted tidal volume indicates respiratory failure, even if arterial Po_2 and Pco_2 have not attained values usually assigned to the diagnosis of respiratory failure. If blood gas determinations are used in the evaluation of patients with acute muscle weakness, a Pa_{O_2} of less than 70 torr breathing-room air or a Pa_{CO_2} of greater than 45 torr indicates respiratory failure. The object of these measurements is to permit intervention (intubation and mechanical ventilation) before the patient completely decompensates, thus avoiding the risk of central nervous system damage.

Inspiratory force measurements are also useful, usually in the child who is too young to cooperate with testing. Respiratory failure is indicated by an inspiratory force of less than 25 cm H_2O at FRC. The technique has been discussed previously.

Deterioration in muscle strength over months or years can be assessed by serial determinations over many months of the same parameters. Because children with slowly progressive muscle weakness may begin to accumulate secretions or develop pneumonia, vital capacity may have large swings and one must be careful to look for long-term trends when judging the progression of the underlying disease. Because peak flow and inspiratory capacity are both good measures of the ability to clear secretions, these too should be followed and charted over time. Deterioration in these functions, even if FVC has not been significantly reduced, is a sign of poor prognosis. Patients with muscle weakness may hypoventilate during sleep, resulting in early morning hypercarbia and the complaint of morning headaches. Arterial Pco_2 measurements, preferably from samples drawn from an indwelling catheter, can be helpful in recognizing sleep hypoventilation.

Testing Healthy Children

Physicians should have a low threshold for using pulmonary function tests in the diagnosis of children with signs or symptoms of pulmonary dysfunction, for example, those with a family history of asthma, a personal history of asthma, allergic rhinitis, or a disease known to cause residual lung injury. This would permit early diagnosis and treatment and avoid the problems associated with exercise intolerance, or vague but troublesome respiratory symptoms, for example, cough and easy fatigue.

In the child with no indication of pulmonary disease, either by history or physical examination, pulmonary function screening is not likely to be helpful. Boggs and coworkers[44] tested 789 healthy volunteers ages 9 to 18 and found only 5 who had abnormal lung function as judged by an $FEF_{25-75\%}$ or $FEF_{75-85\%}$ greater than 2 s.d. below the mean. None of the five had abnormal FEV_1 or FVC and so would have been missed on the usual screening exams. On reevaluation none had evidence of pulmonary abnormalities nor did they develop any during 4 years of followup.

REFERENCES

1. Mansell A, Dubrawsky C, Levison H, et al: Lung recoil in cystic fibrosis. Am Rev Resp Dis 109:190, 1974
2. Bryan AC, Mansell AL, Levison H: Development of the mechanical properties of the respiratory system. p. 445. In Hodson WA (ed): Development of the Lung. Marcel Dekker, New York, 1977
3. Leith D, Mead J: Mechanisms determining residual volume of the lungs in normal subjects. J Appl Physiol 23:221, 1967
4. Mansell A, Bryan AC, Levison H: Airway closure in children. J Appl Physiol 33:711, 1972
5. Krauss AN, Klain DB, Dahms BB, Auld PAM: Vital capacity in premature infants. Am Rev Resp Dis 108:1361, 1973
6. Duffty P, Spriet L, Bryan MH, Bryan AC: Respiratory induction plethysmography (Respitrace): An evaluation of its use in the infant. Am Rev Resp Dis 123:542, 1981
7. Taussig LM: Maximal expiratory flows at functional residual capacity: A test of lung function for young children. Am Rev Resp Dis 116:1031, 1977

8. Illiff A, Lee VA: Pulse rate, respiratory rate and body temperature of children between 2 months and 18 years of age. Child Dev 23:237, 1952
9. Waring WW: The history and physical examination. p. 77. In Kendig EL, Chernick V (eds): Disorders of the respiratory tract in children. 3rd Ed. W.B. Saunders, Philadelphia, 1977
10. Taussig LM, Chernick V, Wood R, et al: Standardization of lung function testing in children. J Pediatr 97:668, 1980
11. Lemen RJ: Pulmonary function testing in the office and clinic. p. 166. In Kendig EL, Chernick V (eds): Disorders of the respiratory tract in children. 3rd Ed. W.B. Saunders, Philadelphia, 1977
12. Brough FK, Schmidt CD, Dickman M: Effect of two instructional procedures in the performances of the spirometry test in children 5 through 7 years of age. Am Rev Resp Dis 106:604, 1972
13. American Thoracic Society: ATS statement—Snowbird workshop on standardization of spirometry. Am Rev Resp Dis 119:831, 1979
14. Lindemann H: Body plethysmograph measurements in children with an accompanying adult. Respiration 37:278, 1979
15. Weng TR, Levison H: Standards of pulmonary function in children. Am Rev Resp Dis 99:879, 1969
16. Dickman ML, Schmidt CD, Gardner RM: Spirometric standards for normal children and adolescents (ages 5 years through 18 years). Am Rev Resp Dis 104:680, 1971
17. Seely JE, Guzman CA, Becklake MR: Heart and lung function at rest and during exercise in adolescence. J Appl Physiol 36:34, 1974
18. Knudson RJ, Slatin RC, Lebowitz MD, et al: The maximal expiratory flow volume curve: Normal standards, variability, and effects of age. Am Rev Resp Dis 113:587, 1976
19. Bjure J, Dalen G, Kjellman B: Peak expiratory flow rate. Reference values for Swedish children. Acta Paediatr Scand 68:605, 1979
20. Milner AD, Ingram D: Peak expiratory flow rates in children under 5 years of age. Arch Dis Child 45:780, 1970
21. Polgar G, Promadhat V: Pulmonary Function Testing in Children: Techniques and Standards. W.B. Saunders, Philadelphia, 1971
22. Hsu KHK et al: Ventilatory functions of normal children and young adults—Mexican American, white and black. II. Wright peak flow meter. J Pediatr 95:192, 1979
23. Murray AB, Cook CD: Measurement of peak flow rates in 220 normal children from 4.5 to 18.5 years of age. J Pediatr 62:186, 1963
24. Polgar G, Weng TR: The functional development of the respiratory system: From the period of gestation to adulthood. Am Rev Resp Dis 120:625, 1979
25. Hsu KHK, et al: Ventilatory functions of normal children and young adults—Mexican American, white and black. I. Spirometry. J Pediatr 95:141, 1979
26. Mink S, Ziesmann M, Wood LDH: Mechanisms of increased maximum expiratory flow during HeO_2 breathing in dogs. J Appl Physiol 47:490, 1979
27. Giammona STJ, Daly WT: Pulmonary diffusing capacity in normal children, ages 4 to 13. Am J Dis Child 110:144, 1965
28. Lewis BM, Izbicki R: Routine pulmonary function tests during bleomycin therapy. JAMA 243:347, 1980
29. Pascual RA, Mosher MB, Sikand RS, et al: Effects of bleomycin on pulmonary function in man. Am Rev Resp Dis 108:211, 1973
30. Cloutier MM, Loughlin GM: Chronic cough in children: A manifestation of airway hyperreactivity. Pediatrics 67:6, 1981
31. Konig P: Hidden asthma in childhood. Am J Dis Child 135:1053, 1981
32. Eigen H, Laughlin JJ, Homrighausen JE: Recurrent pneumonia in children and its relationship to bronchial hyperreactivity. Pediatrics 70:698, 1982

33. Parker CD, Bilbo RE, Reed CE: Methacholine aerosol as a test for bronchial asthma. Arch Int Med 115:452, 1965
34. Chai H, Farr RS, Froehlich LA, et al: Standardization of bronchial inhalation challenge procedures. J Allergy Clin Immunol 56:323, 1975
35. Empey DW, Laitinen LA, Jacobs L, et al: Mechanisms of bronchial reactivity in normal subjects after upper respiratory tract infection. Am Rev Resp Dis 113:131, 1976
36. Shapiro GG, Furukawa CT, Pierson WE, Pierman WE: Methacholine bronchial challenge in children. J Allergy Clin Immunol 69:365, 1982
37. Mitchell I, Corey M, Woenne R, et al: Bronchial hyperreactivity in cystic fibrosis and asthma. J Pediatr 93:744, 1978
38. Kraemer R, Meister B, Schaad UB, Rossi E: Reversibility of lung function abnormalities in children with perennial asthma. J Pediatr 102:347, 1983
39. Laughlin JJ, Eigen H: Pulmonary function abnormalities in survivors of near drowning. J Pediatr 100:26, 1982
40. Jenkinson SG, George RB: Serial pulmonary function studies in survivors of near drowning. Chest 77:777, 1980
41. Froese AB: Preoperative evaluation of pulmonary function. Pediatr Clin North Am 26:645, 1979
42. Pierce JA: Superiority of helium-air flow-volume curves to routine spirometry in the preoperative pulmonary evaluation of teenage scoliotics. Conn Med 41:280, 1977
43. Kafer ER: Idiopathic scoliosis: Mechanical properties of the respiratory system of the ventilatory response to carbon dioxide. J Clin Invest 55:1153, 1975
44. Boggs PB, et al: The usefulness of spirometric screening of young children for the detection of previously unsuspected abnormal lung function. Clin Res 26:823A, 1978

12

Exercise Testing and Disability Evaluation

Gary T. Kinasewitz, M.D.

The use of exercise testing in the evaluation of the pulmonary patient is increasing. While it has long been recognized that impaired pulmonary function and gas exchange will limit an individual's ability to exercise, early testing techniques focused on steady-state exercise and timed collection of samples of expired air in Douglas bags for subsequent determination of the concentration of expired O_2 and CO_2. This was time consuming and required special analyzers generally available only in research laboratories. An exercise test in most clinical pulmonary function laboratories consisted of measuring arterial Po_2 during exercise to determine whether desaturation had occurred.

The development of rapidly responding gas analyzers and on-line data processing systems during the last decade has simplified exercise testing and made it feasible to monitor ventilation and pulmonary gas exchange continuously during exercise in the typical large clinical pulmonary function laboratory. The high prevalence of both cardiac and pulmonary disease in our society means that many people will be suffering from coexistent disorders of both the cardiovascular and respiratory systems, for example, coronary artery disease in a heavy smoker with obstructive lung disease. Furthermore, severe cardiac dysfunction can produce secondary abnormalities of pulmonary function, just as severe lung disease may eventually produce cor pulmonale.[1,2] In such a situation it is often difficult to determine clinically whether a patient's symptoms are the result of cardiac or pulmonary dysfunction. Exercise testing enables us to determine accurately the cause of the symptoms as well as the severity of the functional impairment.

The onset of physical activity elicits a predictable, albeit complex, interaction of the cardiovascular and respiratory systems to provide adequate oxygen for the increased metabolic requirements of exercising tissue. Ventilation increases to facilitate the augmented exchange of oxygen and carbon dioxide across the alveolar-capillary membrane. In concert with this increase in ventilation, cardiac output rises so oxygen delivery to peripheral tissue to satisfy its increased oxygen demand can be accomplished. Patients with a reduced work capacity and shortness of breath or fatigue at low work levels are generally limited by an impairment of either pulmonary gas exchange or systemic oxygen transport or both. The noninvasive monitoring of respiratory gas exchange during exercise allows the clinician to compare each patient's exercise response to the normal response. There is an expected series of graduated changes that increase oxygen uptake and transport in the normal individual; deviations from this expected series of changes are what characterize a given test as abnormal and indicate the etiology of the patient's effort intolerance.

This valuable information can be readily obtained by monitoring the patient during the course of a standardized exercise protocol, such as those routinely employed in the cardiac laboratory for the evaluation of chest pain. The patient exercises in the usual manner on a treadmill or cycle ergometer while breathing through the mouthpiece of a low-resistance nonrebreathing valve. In an incremental exercise test, the workload is increased at fixed time intervals by altering the resistance to pedaling the cycle or increasing the speed or grade of the treadmill. In addition to monitoring the electrocardiogram to determine heart rate and detect cardiac arrhythmias, a pneumotachograph on the expiratory side of the valve allows one to measure expiratory flow rates and, by integration of its signal, tidal volume. Minute ventilation ($\dot{V}E$) is then calculated as the product of tidal volume and respiratory rate. Samples of expired air are passed through rapidly responding O_2 and CO_2 analyzers so that the end-tidal and mixed expired concentration of these gases may be measured (Fig. 12-1), thereby enabling O_2 consumption and CO_2 production to be determined on a breath-by-breath basis.[3] It is changes in the magnitude and interrelationships of these responses during progressive exercise that delineate a patient's functional capacity.

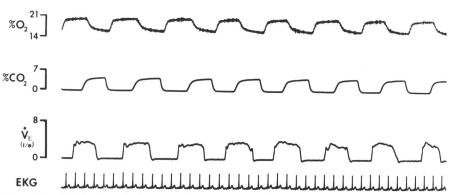

Fig. 12-1. Monitoring during exercise testing. In addition to the EKG, expiratory airflow ($\dot{V}E$) and the concentration of oxygen and carbon dioxide in the expired air must be determined in order to evaluate gas exchange during exercise.

AEROBIC AND ANAEROBIC METABOLISM
DURING EXERCISE

Every activity, whether it be in the course of one's normal daily activities or in the exercise laboratory, requires an increase in oxygen consumption over the basal metabolic rate to provide the energy necessary for performing work. Monitoring gas exchange during exercise permits the accurate determination of an individual's *maximal oxygen consumption* ($\dot{V}_{O_2}$max), thereby defining his aerobic work capacity, that is, the maximal amount of work he can perform utilizing aerobic metabolism to provide the necessary energy (Fig. 12-2). When an individual exercises, each incremental increase in workload elicits a proportionate rise in oxygen consumption.[4] Oxygen demand (energy cost) to perform the work is increased immediately, yet there is a brief but finite delay between the onset of this increased energy need and the time that peripheral blood flow to exercising muscle increases to meet this new demand.

At low levels of exercise, muscle energy stores in the form of oxygen bound to myoglobin and high-energy creatine phosphate are sufficient to supply the necessary power until the cardiopulmonary oxygen transport system has in-

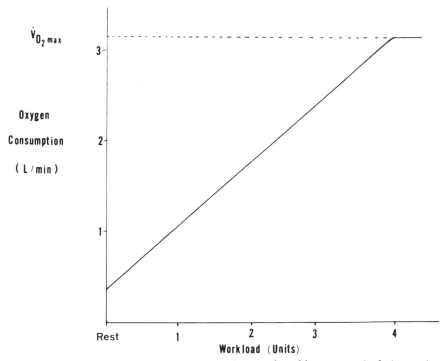

Fig. 12-2. The change in oxygen consumption produced by progressively increasing workloads (expressed in arbitrary units). The dashed line indicates the maximal oxygen uptake.

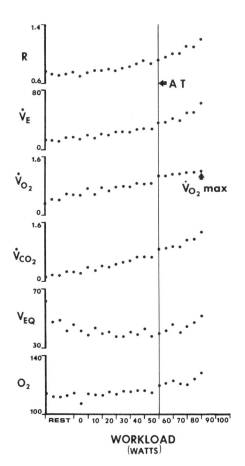

Fig. 12-3. Gas exchange data calculated from monitored airflow and expired O_2 and CO_2 signals during incremental exercise. Oxygen production ($\dot{V}_{O_2}$, liters per minute STPD) increases linearly during exercise, whereas CO_2 production ($\dot{V}_{CO_2}$ liters per minute STPD) and minute ventilation ($\dot{V}_E$, liters per minute BTPS), increase disproportionately once the anaerobic threshold (AT, indicated by the vertical line) is exceeded. R is the respiratory exchange ratio ($\dot{V}_{CO_2}/\dot{V}_{O_2}$), V_{EQ} the ventilatory equivalent for O_2 (calculated as $\dot{V}_E/\dot{V}_{O_2}$) and O_2 indicates the P_{O_2} of end-tidal expired air, which increases once the anaerobic threshold is exceeded.

creased the delivery of oxygen to peripheral tissue. At higher workloads, or if the ability to increase cardiac output is compromised, these tissue stores are inadequate to supply the entire energy demand and additional anaerobic sources of energy are utilized, with the consequent generation of lactic acid.[5] The monitoring of gas exchange during exercise permits one to identify the anaerobic threshold, that is, the workload at which the muscle stores of energy are inadequate to maintain aerobic metabolism during the delay between increased oxygen demand and cardiopulmonary adjustment to it. The lactic acid generated reacts with the body's buffer system with the consequent formation of CO_2 and lactate from bicarbonate and lactic acid. Carbon dioxide production therefore rises out of proportion to its generation from oxidative metabolism and is reflected by a rise in the respiratory exchange ratio ($\dot{V}_{CO_2}/\dot{V}_{O_2}$) (Fig. 12-3). The *anaerobic threshold* can be identified by a rise in $\dot{V}_{CO_2}$ and minute ventilation that is disproportionate to the level of oxygen consumption.[6,7]

The measurement of oxygen consumption during exercise allows one to identify $\dot{V}_{O_2}$max as the point where oxygen consumption peaks or plateaus during incremental exercise.[4,8,9] Oxygen consumption determined during exercise may be expressed in absolute terms, for example, 500 ml/min (STPD), or it may be related to that individual's resting oxygen consumption by the MET (multiple of resting O_2 consumption), an arbitrary unit approximately equivalent to 3.5 ml/kg/min. The advantage of expressing oxygen consumption in terms of METs is related to the different energy cost of various forms of activity. To lift a heavy object and carry it across a room requires a certain energy expenditure regardless of an individual's size. In contrast, when an individual walks or climbs stairs, the work performed is proportional to one's body mass and therefore is correspondingly greater in a large individual.

CARDIOVASCULAR RESPONSE TO EXERCISE

A normal individual's maximum oxygen consumption is determined by his ability to increase the peripheral delivery of oxygen to exercising muscle by increasing cardiac output and oxygen extraction.[4,8,10] While a fit subject may increase his oxygen consumption to a level that is 20 times its resting value during maximal exertion, his cardiac output generally undergoes no more than a fivefold rise from a resting level of 5 liters/min to a maximum of approximately 25 liters/min (Fig. 12-4). Simultaneously, the metabolizing muscles progressively

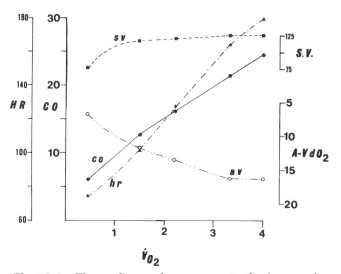

Fig. 12-4. The cardiovascular response to the increase in oxygen consumption produced by performing incremental exercise to $\dot{V}_{O_2}$max. $\dot{V}_{O_2}$, oxygen consumption (liters per minute); HR, heart rate (beats per minute); CO, cardiac output (liters per minute), SV, stroke volume (cubic centimeters); a-vD_{O_2}, arterial-venous oxygen difference (milliliters per deciliter of blood).

increase their extraction of oxygen from the arterial blood to as much as 18 ml/dl blood to provide the oxygen required for aerobic work.[11] This more efficient oxygen extraction during exercise is facilitated by the local conditions of increased muscle temperature and decreased pH, which shift the hemoglobin dissociation curve to the right and increase the unloading of oxygen at the tissue level.[8] In patients with cardiac disease, however, the capacity for O_2 extraction remains unaltered[9,11]; their maximal oxygen consumption is diminished because their maximal cardiac output, the product of stroke volume and heart rate, is depressed.

During incremental exercise, cardiac output increases proportionately to the rise in oxygen consumption. When an individual exercises in the erect position the increase in cardiac output is accomplished by increasing both heart rate and stroke volume (the volume of blood ejected during each cardiac contraction). The constriction of venous capacitance vessels, a more negative intrathoracic pressure (which increases the hydrostatic gradient for venous flow), and the pumping action of exercising muscle all facilitate an increased venous return to provide adequate ventricular filling pressures. The increase in stroke volume occurs predominantly during the early stages of exercise and its nearly complete at a level that corresponds to 40 percent of aerobic capacity.[12,13] Further incremental increases in cardiac output to perform at workloads exceeding this level are accomplished by increases in cardiac frequency until the maximal heart rate and therefore maximal cardiac output are attained. Some individuals can achieve a small increase in $\dot{V}o_2$ beyond that determined at their maximal cardiac output. This presumably reflects an internal redistribution of flow to deliver an increased percentage of cardiac output to the exercising muscle bed.[10] The efficiency of this redistribution is reflected by the Po_2 of the venous effluent from nonexercising tissue, which can fall as low as that from the exercising limbs, indicating a reapportionment of flow according to metabolic needs.[11]

The normal variation of aerobic capacity among individuals of different body habitus, age, and sex is a reflection of the differences in their oxygen transport systems.[14] A large individual has a proportionately greater heart size and stroke volume so that at any given heart rate he can generate a greater cardiac output; at the same maximal heart rate he will have a higher blood flow to his exercising muscles and therefore a greater $\dot{V}_{o_2}$max. The maximal cardiac rate one can achieve during exercise declines with age; although stroke volume and hemoglobin concentration do not alter appreciably with age, an individual's systemic oxygen transport must necessarily decline because of this decrease in maximal heart rate. Women have a smaller ratio of lean body mass to body weight and a lower hemoglobin concentration than men so that at submaximal work rates they exhibit higher heart rates and cardiac outputs than males. As would be expected, the $\dot{V}_{o_2}$max of women is generally lower than that of their male counterparts.

When two individuals perform the same amount of work aerobically, they consume the same quantity of oxygen regardless of their age, sex, or body habitus. Similarly, the cardiac patient requires the same oxygen consumption to perform a given workload aerobically as does a healthy individual. The severely compromised patient with a depressed resting stroke volume who tries to maintain his cardiac output via a compensatory tachycardia is generally easy to recognize clinically. Frequently, however, the degree of functional impairment cannot be determined at the bedside. The patient with mild cardiac dysfunction generally has a normal stroke volume at rest, but because of his limited reserve he may be able to generate little or no increase in stroke volume as his oxygen consumption increases. Another individual with a greater degree of myocardial impairment may be able to maintain an adequate resting stoke volume by virtue of an increased left ventricular filling pressure but suffer a decrease in stroke volume during the stress of exercise.[15]

In an attempt to maintain their oxygen delivery during exercise, patients with mild to moderately severe cardiac impairment compensate for a subnormal stroke volume by a greater-than-normal increase in heart rate at a given workload. The relationship of $\dot{V}o_2$ to heart rate, termed the O_2 *pulse,* is the amount of oxygen delivered in each cardiac cycle. The change in O_2 pulse, calculated as the difference between the resting and end-exercise values, is a useful indicator of the patient's stroke volume response to exercise.[9] More severely compromised patients have a greater diminution in stroke volume and therefore less of an increment in their O_2 pulse. In addition to their reduction in stroke volume, the maximal heart rate achieved during exercise is also reduced, further accentuating the disparity in systemic oxygen transport between normal and cardiac patients. Not only is the maximal oxygen uptake of the patient with cardiac disease limited because of his depressed cardiac output during exercise but, in addition, the onset of anaerobic metabolism (which reflects the capacity of the cardiovascular system to increase the delivery of oxygen to peripheral muscle) occurs earlier in these individuals.[9] In contrast, the patient with a reduced aerobic capacity because of lung disease will not manifest an early onset of anaerobiasis in the absence of heart failure.[16] Neither clinical examination nor resting hemodynamic measurements can substitute for the actual measurement of gas exchange in evaluating functional impairment of the cardiac patient.[17]

RESPIRATORY RESPONSE TO EXERCISE

Normal ventilatory responses to exercise are characterized by a series of changes designed to maximize the transfer of oxygen and carbon dioxide across the alveolar-capillary membrane of the lung. Minute ventilation rises to satisfy the increased oxygen demands of progressive exercise, a consequence of increases in both tidal volume and respiratory frequency. In contrast to cardiac output, minute ventilation shows no evidence of plateauing as $\dot{V}_{O_2}$max is attained, and it is generally agreed that ventilation does not impose a limit upon the capacity of the normal individual to exercise.[4,10,18]

The pattern in which tidal volume and respiratory rate increase to produce the high minute ventilation typical of muscular exercise has been demonstrated

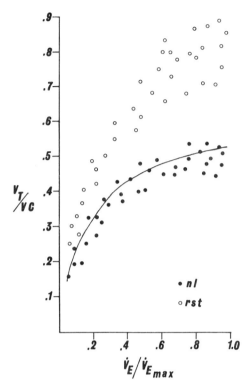

Fig. 12-5.   The changes in tidal volume that occur as ventilation increases during progressive exercise in normal individuals (nl) and patients with restrictive lung disease (rst). $\dot{V}E/\dot{V}E$max, ratio of minute ventilation at a given level of exercise to the maximal minute ventilation at end exercise; VT/VC, tidal volume (VT) expressed as a fraction of vital capacity (VC).

to be fairly characteristic in individuals free of pulmonary disease.[19] During the early stages of progressive exercise, incremental increases in minute ventilation are produced by proportionate rises in tidal volume with only modest increases in respiratory frequency. At high workloads, once tidal volume reaches 50 percent of vital capacity, the increase in minute ventilation is primarily caused by an increase in respiratory frequency. Even during maximal exercise, tidal volumes are only half of vital capacity and peak expiratory flow rates are only half of maximal values measured at rest, indicating a very large potential ventilatory reserve in the normal individual.[20]

Patients whose exercise capacity is limited because of pulmonary dysfunction will frequently encroach upon their ventilatory reserve in one of two ways (Figs. 12-5, 12-6). Those with restrictive lung disease will utilize a greater portion of their vital capacity during maximal exercise, whereas individuals with obstructive pulmonary disease may approach or even exceed their peak expiratory flow as determined at rest.[19]

Normally, at rest about one-third of each tidal breath remains in the non-gas-exchanging areas of the lung, such as the trachea and major bronchi. In addition, a portion of each breath goes to the apices of the lung that, because of the influence of gravity on pulmonary artery pressure, are poorly perfused. The consequent high ventilation-perfusion ($\dot{V}/\dot{Q}$) ratio of these alveoli results in an

Fig. 12-6. The increase in peak expiratory airflow during progressive exercise in normal individuals (dots) and patients with obstructive lung disease (circles). $\%\dot{V}_{O_2}$max, oxygen consumption expressed as a percentage of the maximal oxygen uptake. $\dot{V}ex_{pk}/\dot{V}rest_{pk}$ peak expiratory airflow at a given level of exercise expressed as a fraction of the peak expiratory flow measured during a FVC maneuver at rest.

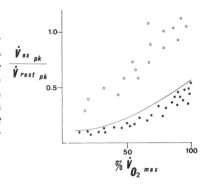

inefficient utilization of ventilation (physiological dead space). Pulmonary artery pressure rises abruptly with the onset of exercise so that ventilation-perfusion ratios throughout the lung become more uniform, and consequently, physiological dead space decreases. At the same time during the early stages of exercise, as the depth of each breath increases the relative proportion of the tidal volume retained within the anatomic dead space decreases and a greater fraction of minute ventilation is available for gas exchange. This more efficient utilization of alveolar ventilation combined with the relative decrease in anatomic dead space results in a 50 percent reduction in the V_D/V_T ratio during moderate exercise.[21]

Monitoring mixed expired CO_2 and end-tidal CO_2 as a reflection of alveolar P_{CO_2} during exercise allows one to calculate physiological dead space. In patients with lung disease and marked mismatching of ventilation and perfusion, the increased ventilation that occurs during exercise may occur in the poorly perfused regions of the lung.[22] The V_D/V_T ratio of such patients may remain constant or even rise during exercise, so that they will require an abnormally high minute ventilation to maintain their alveolar ventilation at any given level of oxygen consumption. An extreme example of this is noted in patients with obliterative disorders of the pulmonary vasculature, such as thromboembolic disease, in whom an abnormally high V_D/V_T ratio may be the major functional abnormality detected.[23]

Carbon dioxide is the main stimulus to respiration at rest; normally, ventilation is regulated to maintain arterial P_{CO_2} at approximately 40 torr.[24] During low levels of exercise, increased CO_2 production as a consequence of aerobic metabolism stimulates a proportionate rise in minute ventilation so arterial P_{CO_2} may be maintained at a normal level. Once the intensity of exercise exceeds an individual's anaerobic threshold and additional CO_2 is generated from the reaction of lactic acid with bicarbonate, there is a parallel rise in both ventilation and CO_2 production disproportionate to the increment in oxygen consumption. When the workload exceeds 75 percent of an individual's aerobic capacity, lactic acid accumulates in the blood with the development of a metabolic acidosis, which provides a further stimulus to ventilation. Minute ventilation exceeds CO_2 production at these high workloads, resulting in a fall in arterial P_{CO_2} and a respiratory alkalosis that partially compensates for the lactic acidemia.[5]

The patient with pulmonary disease and an increase in wasted ventilation from lung regions with high ventilation-perfusion ratios will require a higher-than-normal minute ventilation to maintain his arterial P_{CO_2}. This places an additional stress upon his respiratory muscles, which are already laboring under the mechanical disadvantage of an increase in airway resistance and/or a decrease in lung compliance. If, as the intensity of exercise is increased, minute ventilation approaches the patient's maximal voluntary ventilation or fails to increase, one may infer that the patient's ventilatory limit has been reached. Other patients with an equally severe pulmonary impairment maintain a relatively normal resting minute ventilation at the expense of alveolar hypoventilation. In addition to the resting hypercapnia that may be suspected on the basis of their elevated end-tidal P_{CO_2} they typically display an inappropriately low ventilatory response during exercise as a result of their depressed chemosensitivity.[25,26]

By monitoring arterial oxygen saturation via an ear oximeter or sampling arterial blood from an indwelling catheter, the clinician can document the development or worsening of hypoxemia during exercise in patients with lung disease. The healthy individual maintains relatively constant arterial P_{O_2} during progressive exercise. During the early stages of exercise, arterial P_{O_2} may even rise slightly as a result of improvement in the matching of ventilation and perfusion within the lung and the recruitment of additional pulmonary capillaries, which increases the potential surface area available for gas exchange. At high workloads, as the extraction of oxygen by exercising muscle becomes more complete and mixed venous P_{O_2} falls, the contribution of the small, physiological right-to-left shunt to arterial P_{O_2} is magnified. Despite the fact that alveolar P_{O_2} increases during the hyperventilation characteristic of the later stages of exercise, the alveolar-arterial oxygen gradient widens at high workloads and arterial P_{O_2} may fall, generally by less than 10 torr. Normally, at sea level the alveolar-arterial oxygen gradient during exercise can be accounted for on the basis of ventilation-perfusion inhomogeneity and a small physiological shunt.[27] Some patients with obstructive lung disease may actually improve their arterial oxygenation during exercise, presumably by improving their ventilation-perfusion relationships.[25] Other patients with a similar degree of obstruction will experience a marked decrease in arterial P_{O_2} as a result of their unfavorable $\dot{V}/\dot{Q}$ matching during exercise.[22] Monitoring of arterial oxygen saturation or P_{O_2} is particularly helpful in evaluating patients with interstitial pulmonary disease. Such patients may manifest only minimal derangements in their resting pulmonary function tests and blood gases, yet display dramatic falls in arterial P_{O_2} and saturation with exercise.[28]

INDICATIONS FOR EXERCISE TESTING

Exercise testing with assessment of gas exchange is capable of delineating cardiopulmonary responses to exercise in patients with disease. It can also demonstrate the absence of disease in individuals who complain of symptoms that appear to have no organic basis. Such individuals may exhibit a variety of breathing patterns and hyperventilate during low workloads; however, this can be detected by inspection of their breathing pattern and by noting the reciprocal increase in end-tidal O_2 and decrease in end-tidal CO_2 concentration of expired gas characteristic of hyperventilation. They will not be able to mask the fall in their VD/VT ratio that occurs with exertion, nor can they produce arterial hypoxemia on this basis. Their heart rate and oxygen consumption will increase linearly as the workload is increased and neither will show evidence of plateauing at the point of symptomatic limitation. Quite often they will stop exercising even before their anaerobic threshold is exceeded. Monitoring gas exchange during exercise enables the physician to identify the malingerer who may require psychiatric guidance, whereas the neurotic who imagines himself severely limited often responds to the knowledge that his cardiopulmonary function is intact with a spontaneous increase in physical activity.

Measurement of ventilation and gas exchange are important if one wishes to determine the cause of a reduced work capacity or to define more precisely an individual's ability to perform physical work. The latter is important both in deciding an individual's capacity to perform a given task and in designing an exercise program to improve his performance. If a person is stressed by a workload that exceeds his aerobic capacity, he may be able to briefly sustain the effort via anaerobic metabolism, but in a few minutes he will become exhausted and be unable to continue. The length of time an individual can perform a particular task is inversely related to that portion of his aerobic capacity required to sustain the effort.[5] An exercise that utilizes 60 percent of one individual's aerobic capacity might leave that person exhausted after 1 hr, whereas another person with a greater aerobic capacity might require only 40 percent of his $\dot{V}_{O_2}$max to perform the same task and be capable of continuing indefinitely. Studies of subjects employed in occupations that require physical labor have shown that when one is free to choose his own workrate, he will select a pace that utilizes about 40 percent of his aerobic capacity, a work level that is below his anaerobic threshold.[14] However, once this level is exceeded, intermittent rest periods must be provided to avoid exhaustion. If one wanted to improve an individual's performance, he would design an exercise program that stressed him to 60 to 70 percent of his aerobic capacity. This slight exceeding of the anaerobic threshold would promote improved efficiency in oxygen transport and, in time, the anaerobic threshold and capacity for sustained work would increase.

Dynamic assessment of exercise capacity also provides the physician with a yardstick to measure the effectiveness of his therapeutic interventions. As with any disease process, limited exertional tolerance is influenced by the patient's attitude and expectations. Objective evidence of improvement, coupled with a positive therapeutic attitude, can reinforce the need for continuing a therapeutic regimen. Alternatively, no change or a deterioration in exercise capacity may alert the physician to potential adverse effects of his therapy or to the superimposition of a second process, for example, congestive failure in the patient with lung disease, that requires further therapeutic manipulation. A comprehensive exercise study permits the physician to delineate accurately the physical work capacity of his patients, tailor a medical regimen to maximize their performance, and evaluate its effectiveness.

DISABILITY EVALUATION

Patients are often referred for pulmonary function testing by a governmental agency or attorney to evaluate their disability claims. Strictly speaking, disability cannot be measured in the pulmonary function laboratory, as it is a legal judgment that indicates the inability to perform a specific task because of an impairment, physical or otherwise. What is determined in the pulmonary function laboratory is the degree of impairment, that is, the functional abnormality that persists after treatment of the underlying condition. Degree of impairment must be interpreted in the context of other factors to determine disability. Two people with the same functional impairment may be affected differently, depending on their occupation. The loss of a lung may severely disable a construction worker but not affect the ability of an office clerk to perform his job. Decisions as to whether disability is present as a result of measured functional impairment are generally made by a committee representing the referring agency, which reviews the disability claim.

Generally, before the patient arrives at the pulmonary function laboratory he has already had a complete history and physical examination. Virtually all patients who claim disability from respiratory disease complain of dyspnea. Degree of dyspnea should be categorized according to its severity by the criteria presented in Table 12-1. The claimant should be questioned about the presence of cough, the quantity of sputum production, wheezing, and hemoptysis. A detailed occupational history with specific emphasis on exposure to hazardous fumes and dusts should be obtained and the smoking history recorded. In addition to a detailed examination of the chest, the physical examination should include specific references to the presence or absence of extrathoracic manifestations of pulmonary disease, such as cyanosis or clubbing of the fingers. The chest

Table 12-1 Grading of the Severity of Dyspnea

Grade	Symptoms
0	None with normal activity
1	Shortness of breath when hurrying or climbing stairs
2	Shortness of breath when walking on level ground with people of same age
3	Shortness of breath while walking on level ground at own pace
4	Shortness of breath while dressing or walking within the home

radiograph should be examined for abnormalities. In certain disorders, for example, coal worker's pneumoconiosis, the radiographic demonstration of characteristic abnormalities is considered sufficient evidence to document disability.[29] However, in many disorders, for example, siderosis or arc welder's pneumonitis, the correlation between radiographic abnormalities and the degree of functional impairment is poor. The chest radiograph may appear normal in some individuals impaired as a result of airway obstruction or interstitial lung disease, whereas others with radiographic evidence of diffuse pulmonary opacification may suffer little functional impairment.[30-32]

The initial screening test performed in the evaluation of an individual's functional pulmonary impairment should include the measurement of the forced expiratory volume in 1 sec (FEV_1), forced vital capacity (FVC), ratio of forced expiratory volume in 1 sec to forced vital capacity ($FEV_1/FVC\%$), and diffusing capacity (DL_{CO}). In obstructive lung disease FEV_1 and $FEV_1/FVC\%$ correlate well with the individual's work status.[30] An FEV_1 of less than 40 percent of predicted or an $FEV_1/FVC\%$ ratio of less than 40 percent indicates a severe ventilatory impairment. In restrictive lung disease FVC and DL_{CO} are good indicators of impairment and, if either of these is less than 40 percent of predicted, the patient is considered to have severe pulmonary impairment.[31,32] Arterial blood gases may be misleading because in obstructive lung disease FEV_1 correlates better with functional status than Pa_{O_2}.[33] In interstitial lung disease Pa_{O_2} may be normal at rest but fall markedly during physical activity.[28]

If the results of these initial screening tests indicate a severe impairment of pulmonary function, further studies are not warranted. Normal results on all of these tests suggest that the individual's complaints are not caused by pulmonary dysfunction, and another etiology, such as cardiovascular disease, should be sought. Exercise testing with an analysis of gas exchange should be employed to quantitate the severity of functional impairment in those individuals with mild-to-moderate abnormalities on the screening pulmonary function tests and disproportionately severe symptoms. A maximal oxygen consumption of less than 10 ml/kg/min indicates severe functional impairment, whereas the individual whose maximal oxygen uptake exceeds 20 ml/kg/min can perform jobs that entail a moderate amount of physical labor, such as carpentry, without undue stress. Relating the individual's measured maximal oxygen consumption to the O_2 cost of his particular job permits one to make an intelligent decision on whether the degree of functional impairment is sufficient to constitute a true disability.[14]

REFERENCES

1. Cosby RS, Stowell EC, Hartwig WR, Mayo M: Pulmonary function in ventricular failure including cardiac asthma. Circulation 15:492, 1957
2. Fishman AP: Chronic cor pulmonale. Am Rev Resp Dis 114:775, 1976
3. Beaver WL, Wasserman K, Whipp BJ: On-line computer analysis and breath-to-breath graphical display of exercise function tests. J Appl Physiol 34:128, 1973

4. Mitchell JE, Sproule BJ, Chapman CB: The physiological meaning of the maximal oxygen intake test. J Clin Invest 37:538, 1958
5. Wasserman K, Kessel A. van, Burton, G: Interaction of physiological mechanisms during exercise, J Appl Physiol 22:71, 1967
6. Wasserman K, McElroy MB: Detecting the threshold of anaerobic metabolism in cardiac patients during exercise. Am J Cardiol 14:844, 1964
7. Wasserman K, Whipp BJ, Kogal SN, Beaver WL: Anaerobic threshold and respiratory gas exchange during exercise. J Appl Physiol 35:236, 1973
8. Rowell LB: Human cardiovascular adjustments to exercise and thermal stress. Physiol Rev 54:75, 1974
9. Weber KT, Kinasewitz GT, Janicki JS, Fishman AP: Oxygen utilization and ventilation during exercise in patients with chronic cardiac failure. Circulation 65:1213, 1982
10. Ouellet Y, Poh SC, Becklake MR: Circulatory factors limiting maximal aerobic exercise capacity. J Appl Physiol 27:874, 1969
11. Donald KW, Bishop JM, Wade OL: A study of minute to minute changes of arterio-venous oxygen content difference, oxygen uptake and cardiac output and the rate of achievement of a steady state during exercise in rheumatic heart disease. J Clin Invest 33:1146, 1954
12. Astrand PO, Cuddy TE, Saltin B, Stenberg J: Cardiac output during submaximal and maximal work. J Appl Physiol 19:268, 1964
13. Chapman CG, Fisher JN, Sproule BJ: Behavior of stroke volume at rest and during exercise in human beings. J Clin Invest 39:1208, 1960
14. Astrand PO, Rodahl K: Textbook of Work Physiology. McGraw-Hill, New York, 1977
15. Ross J, Gault JH, Mason DT, et al: Left ventricular performance during muscular exercise in patients with and without cardiac dysfunction. Circulation 34:597, 1966
16. Daly JJ, Duff RS, Jackson E, Turino GM: Effect of exercise on arterial lactate, pyruvate and excess lactate in chronic bronchitis. Br J Dis Chest 61:193, 1967
17. Franciosa JA, Park M, Levine TB: Lack of correlation between exercise capacity and indexes of resting left ventricular performance in heart failure. Am J Cardiol 47:33, 1981
18. Saltin B, Blomqvist G, Mitchell JH, Chapman CB: Response to exercise after bedrest and after training. Circulation, 38: suppl. VII, 1, 1968
19. Hey EN, Lloyd BB, Cunningham DJC, et al: Effects of various respiratory stimuli on the depth and frequency of breathing in man. Resp Physiol 1:193, 1966
20. Wasserman K, Whipp BJ: Exercise physiology in health and disease. Am Rev Resp Dis 112:219, 1975
21. Jones NL, McHardy GJR, Naimark A, Campbell EJM: Physiological dead space and alveolar-arterial gas pressure differences during exercise. Clin Sci 31:19, 1966
22. Wagner PD, Dantzker DR, Dueck R, et al: Ventilation-perfusion inequality in chronic obstructive pulmonary disease. J Clin Invest 59:203, 1977
23. Nadel JA, Gold WM, Burgers JH: Early diagnosis of chronic pulmonary vascular obstruction. Value of pulmonary function tests. Am J Med 44:16, 1968
24. Oren A, Wasserman K, Davis JA, Whipp BJ: Effect of CO_2 set point on ventilatory response to exercise. J Appl Physiol: Resp Environ Exer Physiol 51:185, 1981
25. Jones NL: Pulmonary gas exchange during exercise in patients with chronic airway obstruction. Clin Sci 31:39, 1966
26. Ingram RH, Miller RB, Tate LA: Ventilatory response to carbon dioxide and to exercise in relation to the pathophysiologic type of chronic obstructive pulmonary disease. Am Rev Resp Dis 105:541, 1972
27. Sylvester JT, Cymerman A, Gurnter G, et al: Components of alveolar-arterial O_2 gradient during rest and exercise at sea level and high altitude. J Appl Physiol: Resp Environ Exer Physiol 50:1129, 1981
28. Fulmer JD, Roberts WC, Gal ER von, Crystal RG: Morphologic-physiologic correlates

of the severity of fibrosis and degree of cellularity in idiopathic pulmonary fibrosis. J Clin Invest 63:665, 1979

29. Morgan WKC, Lapp NL: Respiratory disease in coal miners. Am Rev Resp Dis 113:531, 1976
30. Gilbert R, Keighley J, Auchincloss JH: Disability in patients with obstructive pulmonary disease. Am Rev Resp Dis 90:383, 1964
31. Ziskind M, Jones RN, Weill H: Silicosis. Am Rev Resp Dis 113:643, 1976
32. Eppler GR, McLoud TC, Gaensler EA, et al: Normal chest roentgenogram in chronic diffuse infiltrative lung disease. N Engl J Med 298:934, 1978
33. Kass I, Dyksterhuis JE, Rubin H, Patil KD: Correlation of psychophysiologic variables with vocational rehabilitation outcome in patients with chronic obstructive pulmonary disease. Chest 67:433, 1975

13

Bedside Assessment of Acutely Ill Patients

Ronald B. George, M.D.

A major advance in pulmonary medicine during the past few years has been the extension of the pulmonary function laboratory to the patient's bedside. This is of utmost importance for acutely ill patients as it is often difficult or impossible to move them to the laboratory. It has also been useful as a cost-effective measure in office practice and for patients who have disabilities that impede their transport to a centralized laboratory. This chapter discusses the common bedside testing techniques that are most often performed by respiratory therapists and pulmonary function laboratory technicians and emphasizes less-invasive tests. A brief discussion of the more-invasive monitoring techniques used in an intensive care setting is also presented.

BEDSIDE TESTING OF VENTILATORY FUNCTION

Measurement of ventilatory function utilizing spirometry at the bedside, in the outpatient clinic, the emergency room, and even the home has been made possible by the development of reliable portable equipment. Several portable spirometers are available and the practitioner should choose one that meets established criteria, as outlined in Table 13-1.[1] The equipment should be sturdy and lightweight, should be relatively inexpensive, and should be calibrated with a standard spirometer or other measuring device at approximately monthly intervals. A major consideration is the availability of a permanent graphic record that may be evaluated in interpreting the results and may be reviewed at a later date. Electronic spirometers that yield only numerical data are not acceptable because they do not show the degree of patient effort or technical problems with the measurement. The graph should allow at least 7 sec for forced expiration because patients with airway obstruction have a "tail" at the end of the curve of continued airflow for as long as they can continue to expire. A minimum of three

Table 13-1 Guidelines for Selection of Portable Spirometers

A. General
 1. It should be practical and reliable, and should include a recording of the expiratory spirogram.
 2. Its operation should be simple enough to be readily understood by practicing physicians, nurses, technicians, and therapists.
 3. It should be durable and of modest price, and thus realistic to bedside use.
B. Specific
 1. The clinic or portable spirometer must accurately measure forced vital capacity (FVC) and forced expiratory volume in 1 sec (FEV_1). These devices should also be capable of accurately measuring forced expiratory flow rate during the middle 50% of the spirogram tracing ($FEF_{25-75\%}$).
 2. It should be capable of measuring a minimum of 7 liters expired volume and recording expiratory airflow for at least 7 sec. A longer recording time, i.e., up to 10 sec, is desirable in patients with very severe expiratory flow limitation, to measure most or all of forced vital capacity in patients with very prolonged expiratory times.
 3. It should demonstrate accuracy in clinical testing to $\pm 3\%$ of volume compared to an accepted laboratory standard, such as a water-sealed or syringe graduated-type volumetric system of 3 liters capacity or more. FEV_1 and $FEF_{25-75\%}$ accuracy against such a system should be $\pm 5\%$.
 4. The recording should be calibrated in BTPS gradations at 25°C.
 5. A "back-extrapolation" method should be allowed in analysis of the expiratory flow curve in devices that do not record the initial portion of the expiratory spirogram because of small volume thresholds or time lags.

Source: Modified from Permutt S, Chester E, Anderson A, et al: Office spirometry in clinical practice. Chest 74:298, 1978

forced expiratory tracings should be made and the largest forced vital capacity should be chosen. Variation in forced expiratory curves of more than 10 percent among the three measurements suggests the patient may be uncooperative or unable to perform optimally. If significant obstruction is present, it is important to repeat the spirogram after administration of a bronchodilator aerosol to determine reversibility.

There are several methods of interpreting the forced expiratory curve in order to determine the severity of airway obstruction. The most common methods used are forced expiratory volume in 1 sec (FEV_1), the ratio of FEV_1 to forced vital capacity ($FEV_1/FVC\%$), and maximum midexpiratory flow rate ($FEF_{25-75\%}$). Although all three measurements are useful, FEV_1 is the easiest to measure and has the least intrinsic variation because it is not influenced by changes in vital capacity.[2] The interpretation of these values is given in Chapter 10.

An acceptable substitute for the forced expiratory curve in selected patients is *peak flow*. The peak flow maneuver is very simple to perform and therefore is often used in younger children. Peak flowmeters are relatively inexpensive and portable and yield a single number that the patient may record at home and show to the physician on his regular clinic visits. A trend toward decreasing peak flow may alert the physician to failure of current therapy and may signal an impending acute asthmatic attack. An inexpensive mini-peak flowmeter has recently become available.[3]

Total lung capacity is difficult to measure outside the pulmonary function laboratory as current techniques of measurement involve gas dilution, washout techniques, or body plethysmography. A simple and fairly accurate estimate of total lung capacity may be obtained from an erect posteroanterior (EPA) chest radiograph or even a portable sitting anteroposterior (AP) radiograph, provided the standard 6-ft distance is maintained. Measuring techniques have been proposed for estimating total lung capacity from the EPA chest radiograph[4,5] and are discussed in Chapter 6; however, a simple assessment of the film will allow an estimate of whether total lung capacity is increased or decreased in the presence of a small vital capacity. The presence of a normal or large total lung capacity with a small vital capacity suggests air trapping caused by obstructive airway disease. A decrease of both vital capacity and total lung capacity suggests a true restrictive defect, whereas a marked decrease in vital capacity with an essentially normal total lung capacity suggests either lack of patient effort or weakness of the respiratory muscles.

MONITORING OF PATIENTS DURING MECHANICAL VENTILATION

Some relatively simple bedside maneuvers allow for evaluation of serial changes in respiratory mechanics, alveolar ventilation, gas exchange, and oxygen delivery in the critically ill patient. Although a moderate degree of invasiveness is required to monitor oxygen delivery, less-invasive observations, such as airway pressure measurements, analysis of expired gases, and determination of arterial gases and pH, provide information regarding respiratory mechanics, ventilation, and gas exchange while the patient is being ventilated mechanically.

Respiratory Mechanics

The relationship of changes in lung volume to changes in airway pressure is relatively easy to measure when a person is being ventilated mechanically because of the presence of a cuffed tube sealed in the upper airway. Pressure-volume curves are determined beginning at full inspiration by occluding the exhalation valve and recording the resulting airway pressure. If airway pressure is plotted during inspiration and a subsequent 1-sec inflation hold is produced by occluding the expiration valve, the resulting curve is shown in Figure 13-1. Initially, there is a peak that occurs during maximum inflation of the lungs. This is followed by a plateau, which occurs after inhalation ceases but before exhalation begins. *Peak pressure* is determined both by the elastic properties of the respiratory system and by the amount of resistance to airflow in the conducting airways. The *plateau pressure,* which is measured in the absence of airflow, is related to elastic properties but is not affected by obstruction to airflow because no flow is occurring. The difference between airway plateau and end-expiratory pressure is

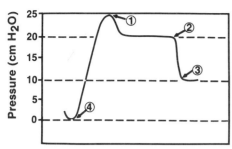

Fig. 13-1. Pressure changes that occur in the ventilator tubing during a positive-pressure inhalation and exhalation, with and without PEEP. Initially, there is a peak pressure of 25 cm H_2O maximum inflation of the lungs (1), followed by a "plateau" pressure of 20 cm H_2O during stabilization of pressures with the exhalation port occluded (2). Assuming a stable tidal volume, pressure change is less with 10 cm H_2O of PEEP (3) than without PEEP [ambient pressure (4)]. If the tidal volume is 800 ml, the effective static compliance with 10 cm PEEP is 800/10 = 80 ml/cm H_2O, while without PEEP it is 800/20 = 40 ml/cm H_2O.

related to the static compliance of the lung and chest wall. A correction factor is used to subtract the volume loss from compliance of the tubing connecting the patient to the ventilator. This measurement has been called *effective static compliance*[6]:

$$Cst_{EFF} = \frac{V_T - Psys(Cvent)}{Psys - PEEP} \qquad \text{(Eq. 13-1)}$$

where V_T is the delivered tidal volume, Cvent is the compliance of the ventilator circuit (approximately 3 ml/cm H_2O), Psys is the system plateau pressure, and PEEP is the end-expiratory pressure.

The difference between the inspiratory peak and the plateau pressures is related to the airway resistance, and is used to determine the *effective dynamic characteristics*.[6] It is calculated according to Equation 13-1, but with Psys representing peak system pressure instead of plateau pressure.

In practice, effective static compliance and effective dynamic characteristics are plotted together as curves that compare pressures to tidal volumes, which are varied over a range of about 400 to 1,400 ml. The volume change per measured peak pressure change is related to respiratory system compliance and airway resistance. The volume change per measured plateau pressure change is related to respiratory system compliance without airway resistance factors. Sample static and dynamic curves obtained with tidal volumes of 400, 600, 800, 1,000, 1,200, and 1,400 ml are shown in Figure 13-2. The test is simple to perform, requires no specialized equipment, and does not involve additional invasive procedures. It may be performed before and after new treatment modalities are initiated in order to estimate their effectiveness, and it may predict impending complications or conditions. Some of the newer mechanical ventilators are designed to measure peak and plateau airway pressures automatically.

In plotting compliance curves, careful technique is required. The inspiratory flow rate should be recorded and must not be varied during the procedure, as an increase in the flow rate will affect peak inspiratory pressure. Subsequent measurements should be taken at the same inspiratory flow rate. A Wright respirometer or the machine spirometer may be used to measure volumes,

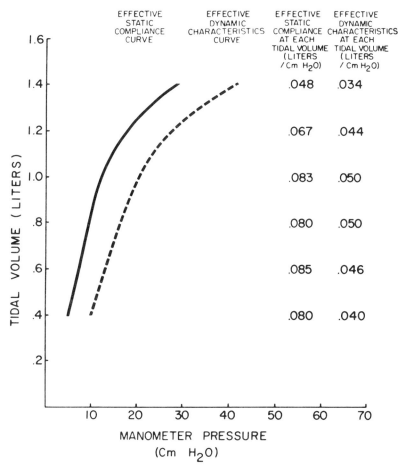

EFFECTIVE STATIC COMPLIANCE CURVE	EFFECTIVE DYNAMIC CHARACTERISTICS CURVE	EFFECTIVE STATIC COMPLIANCE AT EACH TIDAL VOLUME (LITERS /Cm H₂O)	EFFECTIVE DYNAMIC CHARACTERISTICS AT EACH TIDAL VOLUME (LITERS /Cm H₂O)
		.048	.034
		.067	.044
		.083	.050
		.080	.050
		.085	.046
		.080	.040

Fig. 13-2. Effective static compliance and dynamic characteristics curves plotted with variation of tidal volumes from 400 to 1,400 ml. The solid static compliance curve is on the left, and the dashed dynamic characteristics curve is on the right. The distance between the two curves is a measure of airway resistance. (Reproduced with permission from Bone RC: Diagnosis of causes of acute respiratory distress by pressure-volume curves. Chest 70:740, 1976)

however, the spirometer should be calibrated with a standard volume syringe or a reliable laboratory spirometer. Bedside measurements should be made with the patient completely relaxed, as chest wall compliance is measured along with lung compliance. A series of two or three deep inhalations should be given prior to performing the measurements, as the volume history of the lung affects mechanical characteristics. The volume loss resulting from compliance of the ventilator and breathing circuit should be subtracted from the tidal volume reading before recording on the graph. This is approximately 3 ml/cm H_2O system pressure increase above ambient. A nomogram for determining the correction factor has been published.[7] Average values in 14 patients obtained just prior to discontinuing mechanical ventilation were about 45 ml/cm H_2O for static compliance and 28 ml/cm H_2O for dynamic characteristics.[6] Because of the wide range of values in patients who are being ventilated mechanically, baseline measurements are not nearly as useful as serial *changes* in the curves.

Measurement of total respiratory system compliance is useful in adjusting the ventilator and in following the course of the patient's respiratory illness. A shift to the right of both the static compliance and dynamic characteristics curves has been associated with pneumothorax, atelectasis, pneumonia, pulmonary edema, and displacement of the endotracheal tube into the right main bronchus.[6] On the other hand, if the dynamic characteristic curve shifts more to the right than the static compliance curve, this suggests bronchospasm or retained secretions. Static compliance has been useful in establishing the best level of positive end-expiratory pressure (PEEP) in patients with acute respiratory failure. It has been shown that the highest level of PEEP associated with the largest effective static compliance provides optimum oxygen transport.[8] Higher levels of PEEP may produce a higher arterial Po_2, but oxygen transport is not increased because cardiac output falls.

More recently, a pulse method for measuring effective static compliance has been described.[9] This does not require an inflation hold and may be performed without disconnecting the constant-flow circuit in patients who are receiving intermittent mandatory ventilation (IMV). The pulse method is based on the principle that when a constant rate of airflow is blown into a container, the rate of change of pressure in the container is inversely related to the compliance of the container. In other words, compliance is equal to the change in volume produced per unit time (i.e., flow rate) as the result of a given change in pressure during that time. This relationship is illustrated in Equation 13-2:

$$\text{Compliance} = \frac{\dot{V}}{\Delta P/t} \qquad \text{(Eq. 13-2)}$$

This measurement requires a pneumotachometer and a pressure transducer, which are inserted in the inspiratory arm of the ventilatory circuit (Fig. 13-3). Flow and pressure are displayed against time on two separate channels of a strip chart recorder (Fig. 13-4). The ventilator is adjusted to deliver a constant rate of airflow and respiratory system compliance is calculated by dividing the flow rate (liters per second) by the slope of the pressure tracing (centimeters of H_2O per second). These measurements compared closely with the effective static compliance of nine patients undergoing mechanical ventilation with IMV for a variety of problems.[9] As with standard measurements of effective static compliance, these measurements are most useful when curves are plotted for different tidal volumes. The pulse method requires the same precautions, including complete patient relaxation and careful calibration of the instruments.

Although the pulse technique involves measurement during inflation, the values in the nine patients mentioned previously reflect static rather than

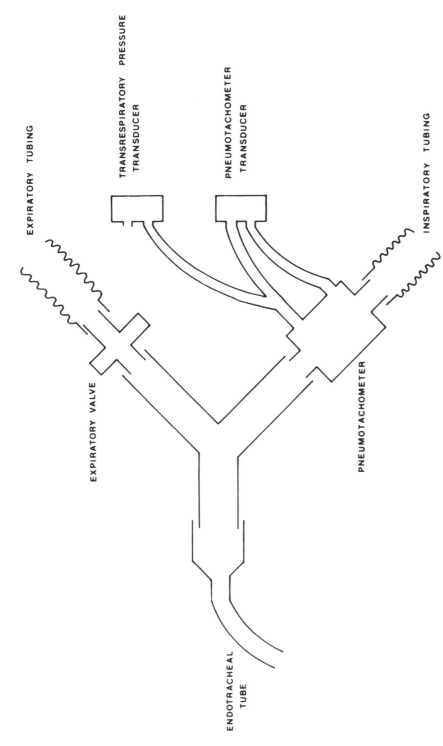

Fig. 13-3. Measurement of effective static compliance by the pulse method. Pressure and flow are measured simultaneously from the inspiratory arm of the ventilator tubing using a pneumotachometer and a pressure transducer. (Reproduced with permission from Suratt PM, Owens B: A pulse method of measuring respiratory system compliance in ventilated patients. Chest 80:34, 1981)

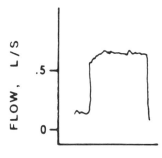 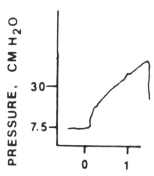

Fig. 13-4. Tracings of inspiratory flow (left) and pressure per unit time (bottom curve) recorded simultaneously in a relaxed patient without obstruction to airflow. Effective static compliance is calculated as the rate of lung inflation (flow), divided by the change in pressure per unit time (the slope of the right tracing). (Reproduced with permission from Suratt PM, Owens B: A pulse method of measuring respiratory system compliance in ventilated patients. Chest 80:34, 1981)

dynamic compliance, even in those patients with airway obstruction.[9] The authors proposed that the time constants in the lungs of their patients were not diverse enough to affect compliance measurements over a brief period of time. In patients with very low lung compliance, powerful ventilators, such as the Siemens Servo 900 series (Model S-17195, Siemens-Elema, Solna, Sweden) must be used to provide constant flows. Because the expiratory valve is inside that ventilator, measured compliance reflects the compliance of both patient and expiratory tubing. This necessitates subtracting the tubing compliance as discussed.

Minute and Alveolar Ventilation

Minute ventilation is easy to measure during mechanical assistance and, in fact, with some ventilators, like the Siemens Servo, the clinician sets the desired minute volume and the ventilator dynamically adjusts tidal volume and rate according to the patient's respiratory mechanics. Because physiological dead space is usually high, minute ventilation must often be increased during mechanical ventilation to achieve adequate gas exchange. The volume of minute ventilation required to achieve this exchange (i.e., the work of breathing) is one of the measurements used in determining whether patients can be weaned effectively, as is discussed later in this chapter.

Alveolar ventilation is more difficult to estimate than minute ventilation because physiological dead space varies tremendously in the acutely ill. Estimation of alveolar ventilation involves collection of expired gas over a period of time and comparison of the CO_2 partial pressure in the expired gas sample with arterial Pco_2, measured simultaneously. This relationship is described in the Bohr equation (see Chapters 3 and 8). In normal subjects the dead space is approximately 150 ml, or one-third of a normal tidal volume. Since approximately one-third of tidal breathing is used to ventilate dead space, expired CO_2 should be approximately two-thirds of arterial Pco_2.

In the Bohr equation, arterial Pco_2 is used as an estimate of alveolar Pco_2. Recently, expired CO_2 monitors have become available that provide instantaneous measurement of the CO_2 content of the gas at the airway opening.[10] During expiration the CO_2 concentration of expired air, measured at the mouth, increases rapidly as the anatomic dead space is cleared, then achieves a relatively steady plateau phase that represents the mean alveolar concentration of CO_2 in the lungs. A slight upward slope of the normal alveolar CO_2 plateau (about 0.6 torr/sec) results from normal fluctuation in alveolar Pco_2 during each respiratory cycle. In the person with a normal distribution of ventilation and perfusion, Pco_2 measured at the end of expiration (end-tidal Pco_2) is a reasonably accurate measurement of arterial Pco_2. However, most patients undergoing mechanical ventilation have markedly distorted ventilation-perfusion relationships as well as abnormal gas exchange. In these patients the difference between end-tidal Pco_2 and arterial Pco_2 has been used as an estimate of inhomogeneity of ventilation and perfusion. Thus, a patient who has interruption of blood flow to a large area of ventilated lung will have a relatively low end-tidal Pco_2, whereas a patient who has more homogenous perfusion and ventilation will demonstrate a close relationship between the two factors.[11,12]

In practice, there is wide variation among end-tidal versus arterial Pco_2 relationships during mechanical ventilation. The expired CO_2 plateau may have a fairly sharp rise, and there may be a terminal increase in expired CO_2 as poorly ventilated portions of the lung empty, so that during maximal expiration end-tidal Pco_2 may approach arterial Pco_2, even in the face of marked $\dot{V}/\dot{Q}$ mismatching. Furthermore, because $\dot{V}/\dot{Q}$ mismatching is so common in patients who are being ventilated, the presence of a wide end-tidal versus arterial Pco_2 gradient is very nonspecific and occurs in most of the diseases that necessitate mechanical ventilation. The potential variability of the arterial versus end-tidal Pco_2 gradient is from -6 to $+20$ torr, so that monitoring of end-tidal Pco_2 is useful mainly as an indication of a *change* in a particular patient's condition.

In a deteriorating patient, an *increase* in end-tidal Pco_2 may reflect a decrease in minute ventilation with elevation of alveolar CO_2 or a decrease in cardiac output, which increases mixed venous Pco_2. A *fall* in end-tidal Pco_2 may reflect a sudden increase in alveolar dead space as may occur with a large pulmonary embolus,[13] or an increase in minute ventilation, resulting in a drop in alveolar CO_2.

Thus, whereas a change in end-tidal CO_2 and its relationship to arterial P_{CO_2} in a given patient may signal a change in his clinical status, it does not identify the cause of this change or even tell with certainty whether that change is for the better or the worse. End-tidal P_{CO_2} provides no information regarding the adequacy of oxygen transport; arterial blood gas levels are more sensitive to changes in cardiac output and $\dot{V}/\dot{Q}$ matching. Once the physiological background for changes in expired P_{CO_2} are fully understood, expired P_{CO_2} may be used in conjunction with arterial blood gas and pH measurements for assessing the overall status.[13]

Gas Exchange

Mechanical ventilation is usually indicated because of the inadequacy of gas exchange, that is, the patient is not oxygenating his blood adequately and/or he is not removing CO_2 in sufficient quantities to maintain a normal pH. Thus, the easiest way to assess the adequacy of gas exchange in a patient undergoing mechanical ventilation is the measurement of arterial blood gases and pH. Inspired fractional concentration of oxygen ($F_{I_{O_2}}$) is generally adjusted so that arterial P_{O_2} is maintained between 60 and 100 mmHg, and arterial pH is maintained at or slightly below 7.4 by adjusting minute ventilation. In acutely ill patients arterial blood gas measurements must be taken repeatedly because of rapidly changing conditions. This is facilitated by placement of an arterial cannula, usually in the radial artery. Pressure in the cannula must be maintained above mean arterial blood pressure, and a small constant infusion is used to prevent clotting in the tube. This permits continuous monitoring of systemic blood pressure as well as an atraumatic means of sampling arterial blood gases as frequently as necessary.

The relationship of alveolar to arterial oxygen is determined by the effectiveness of gas transfer in the lungs. If we compare alveolar oxygen tensions to arterial oxygen tensions, the effectiveness with which mechanical ventilation is achieving its desired goal may be determined. Serial changes in the alveolar-arterial oxygen gradient $P(A-a)_{O_2}$ may indicate whether the patient's gas exchange is improving or deteriorating. Though Pa_{O_2} is easy to measure, PA_{O_2} is a problem. Fortunately, alveolar P_{O_2} may be estimated with sufficient reliability for clinical purposes by using a simplified version of the alveolar gas equation. This is shown in Equation 13-3, where $P_{I_{O_2}}$ equals the barometric pressure minus water vapor (713 torr at sea level), multiplied by the fraction of inspired oxygen as determined by ventilator settings, which can be checked with a portable oxygen analyzer.

$$P_{A_{O_2}} = P_{I_{O_2}} - P_{A_{CO_2}} \left[\frac{F_{I_{O_2}} + (1 - F_{I_{O_2}})}{R} \right]$$

$$\approx P_{I_{O_2}} - \frac{Pa_{CO_2}}{R} \qquad \text{(Eq. 13-3)}$$

Pa_{CO_2} is used to estimate alveolar CO_2 and R is the respiratory exchange ratio (the ratio of carbon dioxide production to oxygen consumption), which can be estimated as 0.8. The alveolar-arterial oxygen gradient, $P(A-a)_{O_2}$, is calculated by subtracting measured arterial oxygen tension from calculated alveolar oxygen tension. The normal value on room air for young people is up to 10 torr, whereas the normal range increases to about 20 torr in people over age 65.

It is important that serial $P(A-a)_{O_2}$ values are determined while breathing with the same F_{IO_2}, as $P(A-a)_{O_2}$ increases as F_{IO_2} increases. This may be impossible in patients who are being ventilated mechanically. Therefore a substitute measurement, the arterial-to-alveolar oxygen tension ratio (a/A ratio) may be substituted, as it does not vary as much with varying F_{IO_2}.[14] A normal a/A ratio is 0.8 or greater, and a decrease in the a/A ratio on serial measurements implies a deterioration of gas exchange.

Noninvasive Monitoring of Oxygen Transfer

In patients with marked defects in oxygen transfer, frequent blood gas determinations are necessary because of rapidly changing conditions. Thus, attempts have been made to measure arterial hemoglobin saturation and oxygen tension noninvasively. A significant advance in the noninvasive monitoring of arterial hemoglobin saturation is the *ear oximeter*.[15] This device, when attached to the ear, has a heated element that dilates the capillaries in the ear lobe (to "arterialize" the capillary blood) and calculates hemoglobin saturation colorimetrically. Because a reference color measurement is included, skin pigment does not affect the calculations. The ear oximeter measures arterial O_2 saturation within 95 percent confidence limits of ± 4 percent when hemoglobin saturation is more than 65 percent, but may be inaccurate at lower levels. Elevated bilirubin levels and the use of cardiogreen dye for estimating cardiac output will distort the readings. The oximeter is sensitive to carboxyhemoglobin and will overestimate arterial saturation if carboxyhemoglobin levels are high.[15]

Significant strides have been made in recent years in the development of transcutaneous blood gas electrodes. Both oxygen and carbon dioxide electrodes are available and can be built into a common electrode body with a single membrane and a single electrolyte.[16] In general, skin P_{CO_2} measurements are more accurate than skin P_{O_2} measurements. This is unfortunate because in severe defects in gas exchange it is arterial oxygenation that we would most like to determine. However, skin P_{O_2} measurements are most accurate in the lower range of arterial P_{O_2}, and diffusion from capillary blood to the electrode is improved by warming the electrode and keeping the skin moist.

Skin electrodes are most useful in monitoring oxygen tensions in infants as diffusion of oxygen across the skin is related to age and skin thickness. It is important that the electrode be calibrated carefully, that temperature be maintained at close to 44°C, and that the electrode be placed on the lateral side of the abdomen, chest, or buttocks or on the inside of the upper thigh where capillary pressure is high. To avoid burning the skin, temperature of the electrode should be checked frequently and it should be moved every 4 hr. Clinically useful hints for the measurement of transcutaneous blood gases are provided in Ref. 16. Generally, Ps_{O_2} is reasonably accurate when Pa_{O_2} is below 60 torr, provided the hemodynamic status is not compromised.

Oxygen Transport

The actual delivery of oxygen to the tissues is determined not only by Pa_{O_2}, but by the amount of hemoglobin available, the saturation of that hemoglobin, and cardiac output. Thus, determination of systemic oxygen transport requires calculation of whole blood oxygen content (see Chapter 4).

Cardiac output is usually measured by inserting a Swan-Ganz triple-lumen, balloon-directed catheter into the pulmonary artery.[17] This catheter contains a proximal lumen 30 cm from the catheter tip and a thermistor located near the tip. For thermodilution cardiac output studies, a 10-ml bolus of cold 5 percent dextrose or normal saline is injected through the proximal lumen and the thermistor senses a temperature change that is based on the dilution of the cold liquid by the blood. Temperature change is inversely related to the volume of blood flow, allowing a reliable estimate of cardiac output. The Swan-Ganz catheter also permits determination of mixed venous Po_2 ($P\bar{v}_{O_2}$) and oxygen saturation ($S\bar{v}_{O_2}$) as well as pulmonary artery pressure and pulmonary artery wedge pressure (a reflection of left atrial pressure). The level of $P\bar{v}_{O_2}$ is a reflection of the relationship between oxygen delivery and tissue utilization, and with inadequate perfusion of the tissues $P\bar{v}_{O_2}$, which is normally about 40 torr, progressively decreases. At levels of $P\bar{v}_{O_2}$ below about 32 torr anaerobic metabolism results in increasing metabolic acidosis. Pulmonary artery catheters are available that can continuously monitor mixed venous oxygen saturation through the use of fiberoptics,[18] thereby providing early detection of changes in cardiovascular function or tissue oxygen utilization.

Major complications resulting from pulmonary artery catheter insertion include local bleeding, pneumothorax, ventricular arrhythmias, sepsis, rupture of a pulmonary artery caused by overinflation of the balloon, and pulmonary infarction from prolonged arterial occlusion. The catheter must be placed below the level of the heart or falsely high pressures may be obtained during mechanical ventilation, especially when PEEP is used. In patients with adult respiratory distress syndrome (ARDS) a decrease in delivery of oxygen to the tissues may lead to decreased uptake of oxygen, so that changes in mixed venous Po_2 may not always bear a consistent relationship to cardiac output or oxygen delivery.[19] Thus, $P\bar{v}_{O_2}$ should not be relied on alone in determining the adequacy of tissue oxygenation in patients undergoing mechanical ventilation for ARDS. A detailed introduction to pulmonary artery catheterization is available in a monograph by Sprung.[20]

WEANING FROM MECHANICAL VENTILATION

Various methods of measuring the strength of the respiratory muscles may be used to predict whether a patient can be safely weaned from the respirator.[21,22] Proposed criteria indicating that the patient may be weaned satisfactorily include some simple ones and some more sophisticated ones, as outlined in Ref. 22.

Because none of these measurements is reliable by itself, a combination of measurements is employed; in the individual patient no completely reliable criteria exist for predicting successful weaning. However, if the four minimum criteria in Table 13-2 are met, weaning should be considered. Additional criteria for successful weaning that are relatively simple to determine at bedside include a resting minute ventilation of less than 10 liters/min and a maximum voluntary ventilation (MVV) at least double the resting minute ventilation.

Factors that interfere with weaning include respiratory muscle weakness or exhaustion,[23] poor nutrition,[24] and the excess elimination of bicarbonate during mechanical ventilation in patients with chronic CO_2 retention. They become acidotic when their usual levels of Pa_{CO_2} are reached during spontaneous ventilation.

These criteria are useful in attempting to wean patients with either a T-tube or intermittent manditory ventilation. In a study that compared tidal volume, respiratory rate, vital capacity, peak negative pressure (PNP), functional residual capacity, pulse rate, blood pressure, and arterial blood gas and pH levels, Downs et al. found the criteria that correlated best with the patients' ability to breathe spontaneously were vital capacity and PNP.[25]

The techniques and equipment for the determination of weaning criteria (Table 13-2) at bedside are simple and readily available. The Wright respirometer may be used to measure tidal volume, vital capacity, minute ventilation, and MVV. Several pressure manometers designed to measure both inspiratory and expiratory pressures while the airway is occluded are marketed. In general, PNP is related to muscle *strength* whereas MVV is related to muscle *endurance*. Because strength and endurance affect spontaneous ventilation, both measurements are useful. Peak *negative* pressure is related to inspiratory muscle function, which governs quiet breathing, whereas peak expiratory *positive* pressure is related to

Table 13-2 Criteria for Weaning from Mechanical Ventilation

Minimal
Clinical status stable or improving
Pa_{O_2} of 55 torr or greater with an F_{IO_2} of 0.6 or less and PEEP of 5 cm H_2O or less
Peak negative pressure (PNP) following maximum expiration of 20 cm H_2O or greater
Vital capacity 10 ml/kg or greater
Additional
Resulting minute ventilation less than 10 liters/min
Maximum voluntary ventilation at least twice the resting minute ventilation

Source: Adapted from Light RW: Acute Respiratory Failure. p. 601. In George RB, Light RW, Matthay RA (eds): Chest Medicine. Churchill Livingstone, New York, 1983

the ability of the patient to cough successfully. Thus, both inspiratory and expiratory peak pressures provide useful information.

In addition to the selection of patients for weaning from mechanical ventilation, these simple bedside tests are also useful in following patients with neuro-muscular diseases, such as ascending polyneuritis (Guillain-Barré syndrome) or polymyositis, to obtain a quantitative evaluation of their progress. They are also useful for following patients who are being treated conservatively on an intensive care unit for acute respiratory failure in an attempt to avoid the necessity of mechanical ventilation. Deterioration of these parameters suggest exhaustion of the muscles of breathing and may predict a failure of conservative management.[23] Similarly, serial bedside measurements in patients who are being weaned may predict failure of the weaning process from muscular tiring.

REFERENCES

1. Permutt S, Chester E, Anderson A, et al: Office spirometry in clinical practice. Chest 74:298, 1978
2. Light RW, Conrad SA, George RB: The one best test for evaluating the effects of bronchodilator therapy. Chest 72:512, 1977
3. Perks WH, Tanis IP, Thompson DA, Prowse K: An evaluation of the mini-Wright peak flow meter. Thorax 34:79, 1979
4. Harris TR, Pratt PC, Kilburn KH: Total lung capacity measured by roentgenogram. Am J Med 50:756, 1971
5. Barnhard HJ, Pierce JA, Joyce JW, et al: Roentgenographic determinations of total lung capacity. Am J Med 28:51, 1960
6. Bone RC: Diagnosis of causes for acute respiratory distress by pressure-volume curves. Chest 70:740, 1976
7. Saklad M, Paliotta J: A nomogram for the correction of needed gases during artificial ventilation. Anesthesiology 29:150, 1968
8. Suter PM, Fairley B, Isenberg MD: Optimum end-expiratory airway pressure in patients with acute pulmonary failure. N Engl J Med 292:284, 1975
9. Suratt PM, Owens B: A pulse method of measuring respiratory system compliance in ventilated patients. Chest 80:34, 1981
10. Prakash O, Meij S: Use of mass spectrometry and infrared CO_2 analyzer for bedside measurement of cardiopulmonary function during anesthesia and intensive care. Crit Care Med 5:180, 1977
11. Robin ED, Julian DG, Travis DM, et al: A physiologic approach to the diagnosis of acute pulmonary embolism. N Engl J Med 260:586, 1959
12. Hatte L, Rosketh R: The arterial to end-expiratory carbon dioxide tension gradient in acute pulmonary embolism and other cardiopulmonary diseases. Chest 66:352, 1974
13. Kinasewitz GT: Use of end-tidal capnography during mechanical ventilation. Resp Care 27:169–171, 1982
14. Gilbert R, Keighley JF: The arterial/alveolar oxygen tension ratio. An index of gas exchange applicable to varying inspired oxygen concentrations. Am Rev Resp Dis 109:142, 1974
15. Douglas NJ, Bash HM, Wraith PK, et al: Accuracy, sensitivity to carboxyhemoglobin, and speed of response of the Hewlett-Packard 47201A ear oximeter. Am Rev Resp Dis 119:311, 1979
16. Severinghaus JW: Transcutaneous blood gas analysis. Resp Care 27:152, 1982

17. Swan HJC, Ganz W, Forrester J, et al: Catheterization of the heart in man with use of a flow-directed balloon-tipped catheter. N Engl J Med 283:447, 1970
18. Baele PL, McMichan JC, Marsh MD, et al: Continuous monitoring of mixed venous oxygen saturation in critically ill patients. Anesthesiology 55:A113, 1981
19. Danek SJ, Lynch JP, Weg JG, Dantzger DR: The dependence of oxygen uptake on oxygen delivery in the adult respiratory distress syndrome. Am Rev Resp Dis 122:387, 1980
20. Sprung CL: The Pulmonary Artery Catheter: Methodology and Clinical Applications. Univ. Park Press, Baltimore, Md, 1983
21. Sahn SA, Lakshminarayan MB: Bedside criteria for discontinuation of mechanical ventilation. Chest 63:1002, 1973
22. Sahn SA, Lakshminarayan MB, Petty TL: Weaning from mechanical ventilation. JAMA 235:2208, 1976
23. Macklem PT: Respiratory muscles: The vital pump. Chest 78:753, 1980
24. Arora NS, Rochester DF: Respiratory muscle strength and maximal voluntary ventilation in undernourished patients. Am Rev Resp Dis 126:5, 1982
25. Downs JB, Klein EF Jr., Desautels D, et al: Intermittent mandatory ventilation: A new approach to weaning patients from mechanical ventilators. Chest 64:331, 1973

14

Sleep-Related Breathing Disorders and Their Monitoring

Andrew L. Chesson, Jr., M.D.

Today's specialists in the field of respiratory diseases have recently awakened to the connection between sleep disorders and respiratory dysfunction. During the last two decades the field of sleep studies has expanded rapidly. With this expansion has come the observation that sleep-related respiratory dysfunction is more common than formerly realized and, in fact, some disorders once considered cardiac or pulmonary in nature may be induced by sleep-related respiratory dysfunction.

To facilitate an understanding of the procedures used to study these disorders, a review of central respiratory control mechanisms, the physiology of sleep and respiration, and the modifying effect of sleep on respiratory control is presented. This chapter also discusses general concepts concerning sleep disorders and their classification, and current methodology used in polysomnography.

Sleep is a common process familiar to all but fully understood by none. Many of the most basic facts, such as the purpose of sleep, and the fundamental pathophysiological processes by which sleep affects other organ systems, are yet to be revealed.

Sleep is not a single state, or a series of distinct steps, but is rather a continuum of stages through which one gradually passes and to which one may return many times a night in a gradual or abrupt manner, depending on both internal and external influences. For convenience, sleep may be classified into stages on the basis of changes in the electroencephalogram (EEG) that occur during the sleep state. The EEG recording is usually augmented by EOG (electrooculogram or recording of eye movements) and EMG (electromyogram or recording of muscle activity). Although division of sleep into stages is helpful in trying to classify and understand physiological observations, the significance of these subdivisions, formed by arbitrary definitions, should not be overemphasized.

CLASSIFICATION OF SLEEP STAGES

Sleep classification was first approached systematically following the description of rapid eye movement (REM) sleep by Aserinsky and Kleitman.[1] Dement and Kleitman,[2] on the basis of a large number of all-night recordings of undisturbed sleep, defined five electroencephalographic stages of sleep; stages 1 through 4 during which rapid eye movements (REMs) are absent and a fifth stage that was accompanied by REMs. Rechtschaffen and Kales[3] modified the Dement-Kleitman system and their data form much of the conventional system for classifying sleep stages. Table 14-1 summarizes the electroencephalographic, eye movement, chin electromyographic, and other physiological features that accompany wakefulness and the various stages of sleep. Figure 14-1 provides examples of these stages as recorded in a normal sleeping adult and should be used for reference during the ensuing discussion of sleep stages.

A number of laboratories have helped define the characteristics of a typical night's sleep in a young adult subject.[2,4-6] Following the awake state the subject usually "descends" serially from stage 1 to stages 2, 3, and 4, in that order. The EEG reflects these changes by a progressive decrease in frequency and increase in the amplitude of EEG waveforms. The sleeping individual becomes progressively less sensitive to external stimuli and has less active control over motor function in the deeper stages of sleep.

After approximately 70 min of predominantly stages 3 and 4 non-REM (NREM) sleep, the first REM period occurs. The termination of the REM period is often followed by a brief awakening and then a return to a stage 1 pattern of sleep that soon gives away to stage 2, and so on. This REM-NREM sleep cycle averages 70 to 90 min in length and is generally repeated four to six times during a night. In later cycles, stage 4 is likely to be omitted and the REM segments are usually longer. About 20 to 25 percent of total sleep time in young adults is spent in REM, 5 percent in stage 1, 50 percent in stage 2, and 20 percent in stages 3 and 4 combined.[7] Specific criteria for standardized scoring of sleep stages are described by Rechtschaffen and Kales.[3]

For an individual sleeping in familiar surroundings, the pattern of sleep from night to night remains relatively constant. In an unaccustomed setting there may be a change in the patient's typical sleep pattern,[8] called the "first-night effect." This factor may be of significance in interpreting a single night's sleep in a laboratory setting and has to be considered in both studies of sleep physiology and interpreting possible sleep pathology.

Classification of REM sleep is more elusive than the NREM stages. The designation "rapid eye movement sleep" might suggest that REM is a lighter stage of sleep, whereas the accompanying reduced sensitivity to external stimuli

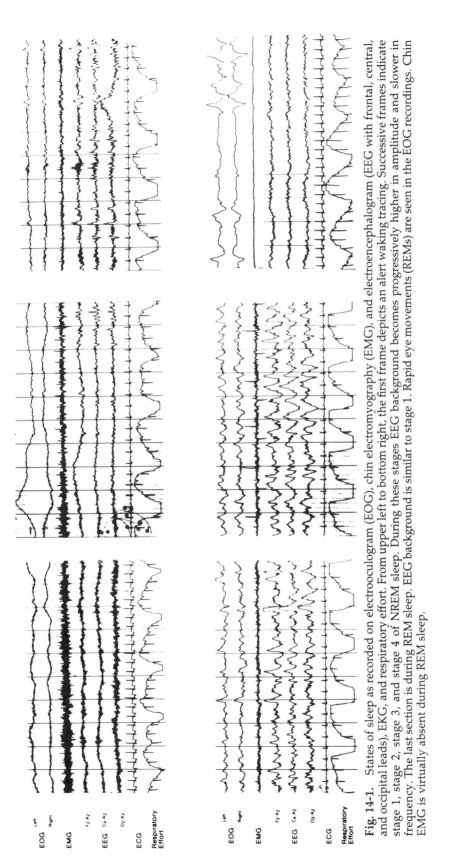

Fig. 14-1. States of sleep as recorded on electrooculogram (EOG), chin electromyography (EMG), and electroencephalogram (EEG with frontal, central, and occipital leads), EKG, and respiratory effort. From upper left to bottom right, the first frame depicts an alert waking tracing. Successive frames indicate stage 1, stage 2, stage 3, and stage 4 of NREM sleep. During these stages EEG background becomes progressively higher in amplitude and slower in frequency. The last section is during REM sleep. EEG background is similar to stage 1. Rapid eye movements (REMs) are seen in the EOG recordings. Chin EMG is virtually absent during REM sleep.

Table 14-1 Characteristics of Wakefulness and the Stages of Sleep

Sleep Stages	Clinical Correlation	EEG	EMG[a]	EOG[a]	% Time in Each Stage	Breathing Pattern
Relaxed wakefulness	Awake, relaxed	Sinusoidal alpha activity (8–12 Hz), with some lower voltage activity of mixed frequency	Muscle tone high	Eyelid blinks and intermittent eye movements		Steady, regular, slow
1	Dozing state— transition from wakefulness	Loss of alpha with transition to low voltage, mixed frequency background	EMG activity low voltage	Slow, side-to-side rolling eye movements	5%	Shifts to include some cyclic waxing and waning with episodes of apnea of ≤ 15 sec
2	Sleepy, but easily arousable, including spontaneous arousals	Background activity low voltage, mixed frequency; appearance of 12–14 Hz sleep spindles and K complexes	EMG activity low voltage	Less rolling or brief episodes related to arousal	50%	
3	Moderately deep sleep, few gross body movements	High voltage, slow waves of 1–2 Hz; 20–50% of recording contains this activity	EMG activity low voltage	Stage of minimal eye movement	20% Stages 3 and 4 combined	Breathing becomes regular without apneic pauses

| 4 | Deep sleep, difficult to arouse, few gross body movements | High voltage, slow waves 1–2 Hz; more than 50% of background consists of this slow wave activity | EMG activity low voltage | Stage of minimal eye movement | | |
| REM | Most dreams, most gross body movements, episodic penile erections; may be increased irregularity of respiration and heart rate | Similar to stage 1 with low voltage, mixed frequency background | Marked reduction in EMG activity with occasional gross body | Conjugate, rapid horizontal and vertical bursts of large-amplitude rapid eye movements (REMs) | 20–25% | Irregular patterns that include 15–20 sec apneic episodes |

aEEG, electroencephalogram; EMG, submental electromyogram; EOG, electrooculogram and progressive muscular flacidity would suggest REM to be a deeper stage. In addition, there are two probably physiologically different components within the REM stage — *tonic* events that are continuously present, such as EMG suppression and low voltage, mixed-frequency EEG background, and *phasic* events associated with bursts of rapid eye movements.

To reduce this confusion, Remmers et al.[9] suggest the use of broader "active" and "quiet" sleep categories. "Quiet" sleep with synchronized high-voltage, slow-wave EEG recordings suggests a relatively neuronally inactive central nervous system. "Active" sleep with a desynchronized low-voltage, mixed-frequency EEG suggests a period of intense neuronal activity in the brain. During the "active" sleep of the REM period, the ability of sensory input to excite the central nervous system is markedly reduced and the translation of central motor activity in the brain into muscular activity is severely compromised. Skeletal motor tone, as monitored by submental EMG activity, is extremely low. The REM stage of sleep is associated with dreaming as well as numerous autonomic changes, including changes in circulation,[1,7,10] temperature regulation,[11] penile erections,[12,13] and cerebral blood flow.[14]

REGULATION OF RESPIRATION

The central and peripheral nervous system structures involved in the control of respiration and their interactions were described in Chapter 1. However, a review of these concepts will provide a basis for better understanding the implications of central nervous system-associated respiratory dysfunction.

Physiology of Respiratory Control

As the respiratory muscles have no intrinsic automaticity of their own, the rhythmic nature of respiration, whether one is awake or asleep, comes from centers in the region of the brain stem near the pontine-medullary junction. The major centers located in this region are the medullary and pneumotaxic centers (see Fig. 1-2). The medullary center, located beneath the floor of the fourth ventricle, is the neuronal group responsible for initiation and maintenance of spontaneous respiratory patterns and is self-sustaining, even when afferent stimuli have been interrupted.[15] Within the medullary center there are two distinct electrically excitable cell populations that induce sustained inspiration or forced expiration. The anatomic overlap of the two areas suggests that the two nuclei may be interconnected locally with feedback inhibition for coordinated responses.[16]

The other brain stem respiratory control region, the pneumotaxic center, is located in the lower portion of the pons. It lacks inherent rhythmic pacing, but has been postulated to act as a patterning area for producing cyclic respiration.[17] The medullary center thus seems to provide the respiratory stimulus to breathe, whereas rhythm is integrated in the more rostral pneumotaxic center. Both areas are affected by their central and peripheral connections. The dorsal and ventral respiratory groups in the substance of the medulla, in addition to providing respiratory automaticity, receive sensory input regarding lung inflation as well as laryngeal and pharyngeal states.[18] This provides an arrangement for coordinating breathing with upper airway behavior. Breathing patterns are also influenced by cortical modulation, which allows complex voluntary respiratory acts, such as talking, singing, exercising, and so on, to be under planned cortical control.

Chemical control of breathing depends on changes in central and peripheral Po_2, Pco_2, and pH in the arterial blood. Chemoreceptors on the ventral medullary surface (central chemoreceptors) and at the level of the bifurcation of the common carotid (peripheral chemoreceptors) are stimulated by O_2, CO_2, and pH changes. Alterations usually evoke a compensatory change in respiration that tends to restore these parameters toward normal. The combination of hypoxia and even a mild degree of hypercapnea form a particularly powerful synergistic respiratory stimulus,[18] which produces an increase in minute ventilation.

Normal Respiratory Responses During Sleep

During the normal transition from wakefulness to sleep, ventilatory patterns change. Experimentally, in the early stages of sleep, minute ventilation ($\dot{V}$) declines,[19,20] Pa_{CO_2} rises,[21,22] and Pa_{O_2} drops slightly.[23] During deeper NREM sleep, ventilatory responses to CO_2 appear reduced compared to the waking state, whereas O_2 drive appears unaltered. Effects of pulmonary, upper airway, and chest wall receptor stimulation all appear to be similar to those observed during wakefulness.[24] During sleep stages 1 and 2, periodic (Cheyne-Stokes) respiration is frequently encountered in normal individuals; this cyclic pattern is not a characteristic of stages 3 and 4.[24,25] The mechanism is unclear but may reflect the fluctuating activity of the cortical respiratory drive system in lighter stages of sleep.

Changes in respiration during REM sleep are rather nonhomogenous. Pa_{O_2} may be high, low, or unchanged.[23] Pa_{CO_2} also appears to be variable in different studies. The confusion in some of this data may reflect the variable responses during phasic and tonic aspects of REM sleep. During the phasic portion (associated with bursts of eye movement) breathing is more irregular, with a rapid rhythm and a variable tidal volume. With bursts of increased muscular activity, alveolar ventilation may even be greater with ventilatory volume increases of 10 to 15 percent.[24] The hypercarbic ventilatory drive is decreased in REM sleep compared to NREM but the hypoxic drive may be intact, although there is limited data in humans. Proprioceptive and pulmonary components of respiratory control appear to have reduced effect during REM sleep.[20,26] The afferent input in the upper airway may, however, have an enhanced effect on respiration in the dog, and stimulation elicits periods of apnea,[27] suggesting a lowered threshold for apneic episodes during REM sleep in people.

Abnormal Respiratory Responses During Sleep

Normal subjects have been shown to have nocturnal apneic episodes and periodic breathing, with males much more likely to be affected than females.[25,28] The presence of a rather wide variation in "normal" apneic episodes raises a question regarding the number of episodes needed to establish an "abnormal" state. For the purpose of sleep apnea studies, an apnea has been defined as cessation of airflow at the nose and mouth lasting for at least 10 sec[29] or for three respiratory periods.[9] Sleep apnea syndrome is diagnosed if, during 7 hours of nocturnal sleep, at least 30 apneic episodes are observed, occurring in both REM and NREM sleep. Some of these episodes must appear in a repetitive sequence in NREM sleep.[29] Apneic episodes at sleep onset or with an accompanying burst of eye movement during REM periods may not be pathological.[30] There are also formulas, such as the apnea index, which some authors feel better define how many apneic episodes are necessary for a polysomnographic study to be considered abnormal.[31] The apnea index equals the total number of apneic episodes during sleep divided by the sleep time in minutes, then multiplied by 60. The number derived with the apneic index takes into account variation in total sleep time and could be considered the density of apneic episodes during a night's sleep. It allows partial quantification of the severity of an apneic syndrome.[32]

Monitoring arterial oxygen desaturation helps gauge the significance of apneic or hypopneic episodes. The fact that, during sleep, an asymptomatic subject can occasionally show oxygen desaturation as low as 68 to 72 percent[28,33] suggests caution must be exercised in interpreting tests from a single study on an individual patient.

SLEEP APNEA

Types of Apnea

For clinical purposes, apnea associated with sleep may be divided into three categories: (1) central or nonobstructive apnea, (2) obstructive or occlusive apnea, and (3) mixed apnea. Characteristics of these three types are noted in Table 14-2. Central apnea may be defined as lack of all respiratory effort for a period exceeding 10 sec or three respiratory periods.[29,33,34] This type of apnea implies loss of the rhythmic central respiratory drive and is identified by the simultaneous cessation of airflow (measured at the nose and the mouth) and respiratory effort (measured by chest wall excursions or their generated intrathoracic pressure). The frequency of pure central apnea is unclear. Recent literature suggests this category may have been overestimated because the techniques used to monitor chest wall excursions may have been suboptimal in some studies. Much of the dispute centers around whether esophageal manometry (which reflects pleural pressure changes) provides higher sensitivity in detecting respiratory efforts than methods used in other studies.[9]

Table 14-2 Types of Sleep Apneas

Type	Features
Obstructive (occlusive)	Absence of airflow despite continued respiratory effort
Nonobstructive (central, diaphragmatic)	Absence of airflow and absence of respiratory effort
Mixed	Initial absence of airflow and absence of respiratory effort, progressing to active respiratory effort without resumption of airflow

Occlusive or obstructive apnea results from upper airway occlusion. This seems to be the most common cause of periodic breathing during sleep and is probably the most frequently seen sleep-related ventilatory disturbance.[35,36] Obstruction, as used in this sense, indicates complete occlusion of the airway, which would imply that if the occlusion is at a single location, it must lie at the level of trachea or above. Most evidence suggests that the occlusive process starts in the oropharynx, usually at the level of the soft palate, and results in inspiratory obstruction to airflow.[37] During monitoring, obstructive apnea is characterized by lack of airflow from the nose and mouth despite the presence of continued evidence of respiratory effort, as indicated by chest wall and abdominal movements or esophageal pressure changes.

Mixed apnea is characterized initially by cessation of both airflow and respiratory movements. When respiratory efforts return, however, they are unsuccessful in establishing airflow for an additional period of time.[29] Some individuals may demonstrate a combination of both central and obstructive episodes during a night's recording.

Because of the intermittent nature of the apneic episodes, O_2 and CO_2 recordings will show periodic fluctuations. During the obstructive phase alveolar Po_2 falls and Pco_2 rises. These tend to correct during the ventilatory phases. Alveolar gas changes, caused by lack of ventilation, are reflected in the peripheral arterial blood. If tracings are closely correlated there is a 10 to 15 sec delay between cessation of airflow and oxygen desaturation in the blood. After breathing resumes there is a similar delay between the return of respiratory movement and subsequent increase in arterial oxygen saturation. These changes correlate with the lung-to-periphery circulation time.

Clinical Presentation

The four major headings for the classification of disorders of sleep and arousal are given in Table 14-3.[38] The sleep apnea syndrome can be classified with the DIMS or DOES groups, depending on the predominant clinical symptoms.

The sleep apnea syndrome is primarily a disease of males, with the reported

Table 14-3 Diagnostic Classification of Sleep and Arousal Disorders

1. Disorders of initiating and maintaining sleep, DIMS (the insomnias)
2. Disorders of excessive somnolence, DOES
3. Disorders of the sleep-wake schedule
4. Dysfunctions associated with sleep, sleep states, or partial arousals (parasomnias)

male-to-female ratio varying from 10 : 1 to 60 : 1. Most patients are 30 to 50 years of age and overweight, although many are not obese[29] and some are within their normal weight range.[39] Patients with nonobstructive sleep apnea are more likely to be of normal weight or underweight and tend to be older than those of obstructive sleep apnea.[31] The common clinical features of the sleep apnea syndrome are listed in Table 14-4.

Snoring is almost always present in those with obstructive apnea and may be loud, sonorous, and of long duration, with onset before age 21 in most patients. Those with central apnea tend to have light and intermittent snoring.[32] Sleeping difficulty is also a common complaint. Excessive daytime somnolence is present in over 80 percent of patients with obstructive sleep apnea and may be severe.[32,39] Others, especially those with central apnea, may go to sleep easily but complain of difficulty staying asleep, with frequent awakening, sometimes associated with gasping for breath or a choking sensation. Complaints of personality changes or intellectual deterioration may be elicited with careful questioning of spouses or close family members. Anxiety and depression occur commonly, and job or marital difficulties related to excessive somnolence are an additional problem. Inattentiveness, reduced concentration, and hallucinatory states are less frequently reported.[39-41] Morning headaches of a frontal or diffuse nature are common, although the etiology is not clear.[39] Impotence and nocturnal enuresis may also be present.[32,39,41] Disorders associated with sleep apnea syndromes are shown in Table 14-5.

**Table 14-4 Clinical Features of Sleep Apnea
Syndrome**

Snoring, especially sonorous with intermittent pauses
Excessive daytime sleepiness
Abnormal motor activity during sleep
Personality or intellectual changes
Hypertension
Morning headaches
Sexual impotence
Cardiorespiratory failure
   Congestive heart failure
   Dependent edema
   Shortness of breath on exertion
   Polycythemia
   Pulmonary hypertension
Nocturnal enuresis

Table 14-5 Disorders Associated with Sleep Apnea Syndromes

Disorders	References
Disrupted integrity of brain stem-cervical pathways	
Bulbar poliomyelolitis	26, 42
Bilateral cervical cordotomy	26, 43
Brainstem infarction	26, 44 – 46
Arnold-Chiari malformation	47
Ondine's curse (idiopathic alveolar hypoventilation)	26
Disruption of oropharyngeal airway structures	
Enlargements of tonsils and adenoids	47, 48
Micrognathia	49, 50
Acromegaly	9, 26, 47
Myxedema	9, 47
Neck infiltration secondary to Hodgkin's disease or lymphoma	26
Associated with neurological disorders	
Myotonic dystrophy	5, 26, 33
Muscular dystrophies	47
Parkinson's disease and Shy-Drager syndrome	26, 33, 51, 52
Associated with other disorders of "idiopathic" nature	
Obstructive lung disease	33, 53
Kyphoscoliosis	54

SLEEP APNEA MONITORING (POLYSOMNOGRAPHY)

To adequately evaluate a patient for a possible sleep-related respiratory disturbance, several parameters should be studied while the patient sleeps. Polysomnography is the process of monitoring physiological phenomena associated with sleep, and a laboratory should be able to perform the techniques outlined in Table 14-6. An attempt is made to monitor these parameters in as natural a sleep setting as possible. The laboratory should be comfortable and quiet. The technician and equipment need to be isolated from the patient, but visualization of the patient during recording is helpful. This can be accomplished by one-way windows or via video monitoring. The laboratory should be located where emergency care can be provided rapidly if severe respiratory insufficiency

Table 14-6 Parameters for Recording During Polysomnography

1. Electroencephalography (EEG monitoring)
2. Electrooculogram (EOG or eye movement monitoring)
3. Evaluation of airflow at the nose and mouth
4. Monitoring of oxygenation
5. Recording respiratory muscle excursions
6. Heart rate monitoring (EKG)
7. Electromyography (EMG or monitoring muscle activity)
8. Limb lead monitoring (monitoring leg or arm movements)

occurs. Though this monitoring is hardly the same as sleeping at home, generally patients with hypersomnia will be able to fall asleep under study conditions. One night of adaptation to the laboratory and equipment may be necessary before a representative night's sleep can be obtained.

A number of different methods are available for evaluating many of the parameters listed and new devices or improvements are steadily being developed to make these studies more accurate and comfortable for the patient. Because familiarity with a variety of methods allows selection of the most useful technique for an individual laboratory and patient, a general overview of the types of equipment available is presented.

EEG Monitoring

EEG monitoring can be performed in a simple or an extensive manner. A single-vertex channel or the use of a few leads involving the vertex, frontal, and occipital areas confirms the presence of sleep. It also allows identification of the particular stage of sleep during which an abnormality may occur, makes it possible to identify the amount of time a patient spends in each sleep stage, and enhances the polysomnographer's ability to follow the transition from one stage of sleep to another. The use of more extensive monitoring with numerous leads may be indicated in situations where seizures may be suspected or if an electroencephalographer is doing detailed EEG-related sleep analysis.

EOG Monitoring

An electrooculogram is performed to characterize eye movement. Observations regarding rate, direction, and speed of eye movements, including the presence or absence of rapid eye movements, help in sleep staging and delineating REM sleep.

Measurement of Airflow

Airflow at the nose and mouth must also be monitored. There are a number of ways of detecting airflow but care must be taken to monitor both the nose and mouth. Thermocouple leads consist of two dissimilar metals that generate a voltage when warmer, exhaled air causes a temperature change compared with cooler, inhaled air. The voltage generated by the thermocouple is proportional to the temperature change, which corresponds to the rate and depth of respiration. High-gain amplification is required. Other methods for recording airflow include thermistors,[55] which are temperature-sensitive flow-sensing devices that can be placed in front of the nose and mouth, a carbon dioxide analyzer that can be used to detect expiratory flow high in carbon dioxide,[56] and laryngeal sound recordings.[57,58] The laryngeal sound is produced as air flows across the glottis. Apnea can be identified by cessation of laryngeal sounds during continuous monitoring. This type of recording usually takes the form of a specialized microphone coupled to a stethoscope head and taped to the neck. Sounds are filtered to reduced cardiac and carotid artifacts, and the sound-intensity voltage produces corresponding pin deflections.

An alternative method, which also has the advantage of quantifying the amount of air moved by the patient, is a pneumotachygraph.[59] This device is placed on a face mask and worn by the patient during sleep. The disadvantage is that the presence of the mask may increase discomfort and interfere with sleep. For routine monitoring, a thermocouple or thermistor is less expensive than other techniques and more comfortable than using a mask. Sound recording equipment and carbon dioxide analyzers are expensive. The latter also requires either a mask or placement of a sampling probe in the posterior nasopharynx. Frequent filter changes resulting from clogging by secretions may also necessitate intermittent disruptions in recording data.

Arterial Oxygen Saturation and Po_2 Monitoring

Arterial oxygenation can be measured most easily in a noninvasive manner using an ear oximeter.[60] An earpiece transmits wavelengths of light through the pinna of the ear. From the wavelengths transmitted, oxyhemoglobin saturation is calculated by an internal computer and the percentage of saturation is displayed. Although not as precise as direct arterial blood gas measurements, especially in the lower ranges, this technique indicates the severity of oxygen desaturation and has the advantages of allowing continuous measurements, being easier to monitor, and being less invasive than frequent blood gas analysis. Depending on the oximeter model, disadvantages may include reduced accuracy in blacks because of darker ear pigmentation, reduced accuracy in patients with jaundice or poor cardiac output, and heat buildup during prolonged monitoring that may require changing the earpiece from side to side. Recently introduced models have greatly reduced these problems.

Other techniques for blood gas monitoring include single-sample percutaneous arterial puncture, an indwelling arterial catheter, and transcutaneous blood gas electrodes.[61] These techniques are discussed in more detail in Chapter 13. Single-sample punctures and indwelling arterial catheters are painful and share the risk of hematoma formation, bleeding, and arterial occlusion. Both are also likely to disrupt sleep during collection procedures. Transcutaneous blood gas electrodes can measure both Pco_2 and Po_2, but measurements of Po_2 are less accurate at $Pa_{O_2} > 60$ torr and in older patients with thicker skin. Careful electrode calibration is required. Electrode temperature must be checked frequently and moving them to prevent skin burns is mandatory. The ear oximeter is used in most laboratories because it allows continuous monitoring with reasonable reliability when arterial oxygen saturation is between 50 and 100 percent.

Measurement of Respiratory Effort

Respiratory efforts can be monitored either by assessing chest wall and abdominal excursions or by measuring the pressure differential created by the force of these movements. Several types of motion detection devices can be used to measure respiratory excursions. Strain gauge devices[55] that fit around the rib cage or abdomen measure circumferential changes during respiration. Other devices include respiratory impedance plethysmographs,[57,62] which fit over the patient as a vest; detectors that measure impedance changes in the chest cavity as the lungs fill or collapse; EEG cardiopneumographs; and magnetometers on the anterior and posterior aspects of the rib cage and abdomen to measure thoracoabdominal motion.[57,63,64] The latter devices utilize magnetic fields, generated at one body surface and measured at another, to detect changes in body wall position.

Strain gauge devices are perhaps the simplest to use, but are position-dependent and tend to move on obese patients. EEG cardiopneumographs cause minimal discomfort and are relatively inexpensive, but placement of leads for clear recording may be difficult and artifacts are frequent in obese patients. New or improved respiratory motion detecting devices are appearing on the market regularly and it seems that a "best method" that is useful for a wide range of laboratory applications, relatively inexpensive, and does not interfere with the patient's comfort and sleep has not yet been found.

As an alternative to monitoring thoracoabdominal movement directly, the pressure changes generated by the respiratory movements can be measured by esophageal manometry.[57] A small balloon is placed in the lower third of the esophagus where pressure is equivalent to pleural pressure. This allows quantitation of ventilatory effort rather than merely detecting its presence. The disadvantages of this system are its invasiveness, the special equipment required, and the time necessary for balloon placement. Strain gauges and magnetometers have been calibrated to reflect *volume* changes, whereas the other techniques primarily detect the *presence* of respiratory movements.

A type of respiratory inductive plethysmography system (Respitrace, Ambulatory Monitoring, Inc., Ardsley, N.Y.) has also developed a system for combining quantification and detection of respiration. Two coils of wire sewn into stretch bands encircle the abdomen and rib cage. With expansion and contraction of the chest and abdomen, changes in frequency of electrical signals produce changes in voltage output. If proper initial recumbent calibration of respiratory volume is performed, an assessment of tidal volume can be made. The major disadvantage of this system is the high cost.

EMG Monitoring

Monitoring the EMG via a surface electrode under the chin[65] allows an assessment of muscular tone in the tongue and oral musculature. This contributes to assessment of sleep staging by indicating loss of muscular tone during REM sleep. It also provides information about reduced muscle tone that may coincide with upper airway obstruction in obstructive apnea. Sampling of selected muscles using needle electrodes can also be done if special conditions warrant a more invasive approach.[37] EMG recording is also helpful in evaluation of limb movements, identification of nocturnal myoclonus, and confirmation of bruxism. Most commonly, surface electrodes are placed on the tibialis anterior to assess leg movement.

EKG Monitoring

Electrocardiographic monitoring can be performed by using standard EKG leads attached to the arm or chest[66] to provide documentation of heart rate and rhythm. This makes it possible to detect any arrhythmias that occur during or after apneic periods. Because many patients have both cardiac and respiratory disorders, the problem of whether an arrhythmia may be a primary problem or secondary to sleep-related hypoxia may be resolved via this technique.

ANALYSIS OF DATA

The simultaneous recording of these parameters allows the polysomnographer to assess the presence of apneic episodes. If they occur, the number can be recorded and the significance with regard to the presence of cardiac arrhythmias and the accompanying degree of oxygen desaturation can be assessed. During apneic episodes, the timed relationship between changes in airflow and changes in chest wall or abdominal movements can determine whether the apnea is central, obstructive, or mixed in nature. EEG recordings, along with EMG and EOG data, allow assessment of the sleep architecture and the sleep stages involved in any abnormalities. Figure 14-2 is a recording from a patient with central apnea. Simultaneous cessation of airflow and respiratory effort occurs. The apneic episode depicted is accompanied by a mild to moderate reduction in oxygen saturation. Arousal movements can be seen on the EMG monitor and EOG irregularity can also be noted. Repeated episodes with recurrent arousals may prevent restful sleep and result in excessive daytime sleepiness.

The tracings pictured in Figure 14-3 were recorded during episodes of obstructive apnea. Cessation of airflow occurs despite the persistence of respiratory effort. Paradoxical abdominal and thoracic movements occur during efforts against the obstructed airway and efficient respiratory movement returns only when airway patency is restored. The lowest oxygen saturation, as measured by the ear oximeter, occurs after resumption of airflow. This lag reflects lung-to-periphery circulation time, with Sa_{O_2} continuing to fall until the effects of restored airflow are apparent at the ear 10 to 15 sec after air exchange resumes.

Figure 14-4 depicts an episode of mixed apnea. Airflow and thoracoab-

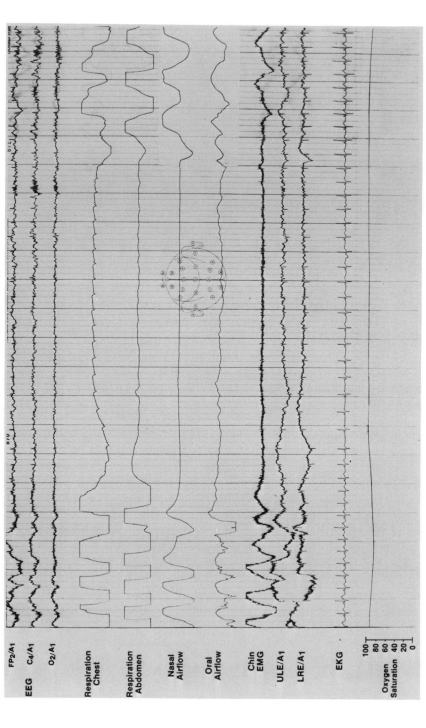

Fig. 14-2. In central apnea, simultaneous cessation of airflow and respiratory effort occurs. Arrow represents maximal desaturation. Arousal can be noted by EMG changes, and EOG rhythm disturbances can be seen.

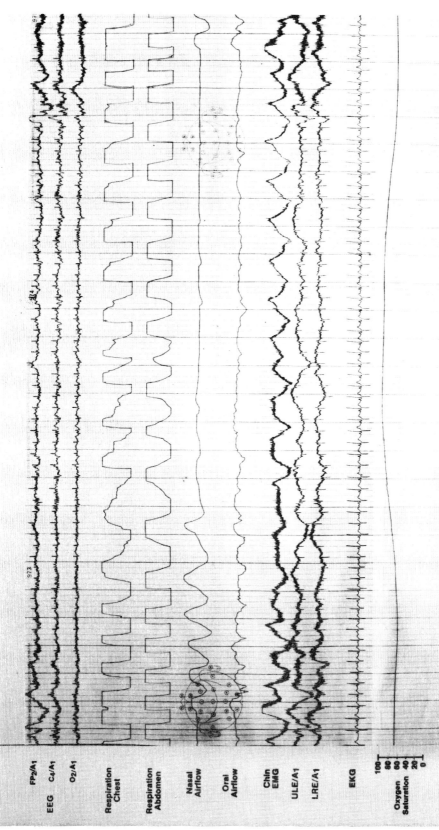

Fig. 14-3. In obstructive apnea, cessation of airflow occurs despite the persistence of respiratory effort. Paradoxical abdominal and thoracic movements are recorded during the apneic periods. Oximetry indicates maximum oxygen desaturation occurs after resumption of airflow, which reflects the lung-to-periphery circulation delay.

EEG { FP2/A1 C4/A1 O2/A1

Respiration Chest

Respiration Abdomen

Nasal Airflow

Oral Airflow

Chin EMG

ULE/A1

LRE/A1

EKG

Oxygen Saturation

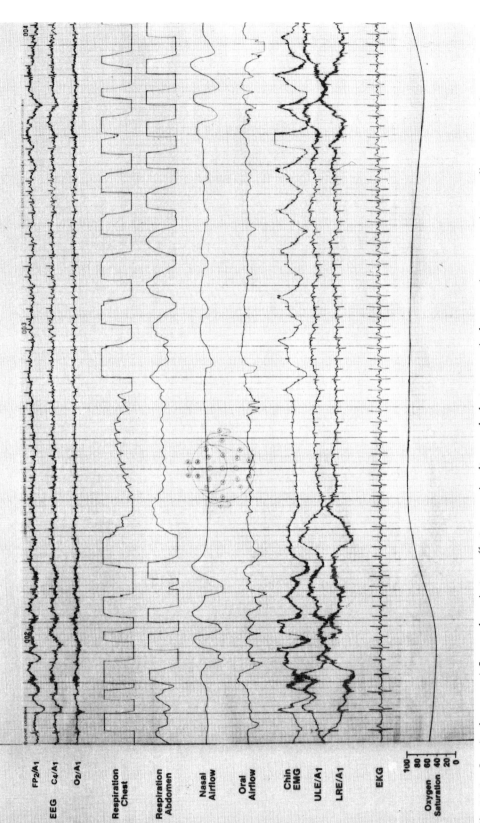

Fig. 14-4. In mixed apnea, airflow and respiratory efforts cease simultaneously, but progressively more vigorous respiratory effort occurs before airflow is reinstated. Arousal, reflected by increased EMG activity, is associated with return of effective respiratory effort.

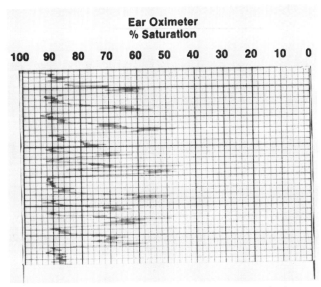

Fig. 14-5. Ear oximeter recording in a patient with obstructive and mixed apneic episodes. This continuous 25-min period shows multiple episodes of oxygen desaturation to values below 60 percent.

dominal effort cease simultaneously, but respiratory effort resumes five breaths prior to the return of airflow. Chin and extremity movements occur during arousal following the apneic episodes.

Special monitoring can also be performed in selected situations. Figure 14-5 shows an ear oximeter recording of a patient with both obstructive and mixed apneic episodes who had multiple episodes of rather marked oxygen desaturation. This 25-min epic, taken during sleep, shows multiple episodes with oxygen saturation values of less than 60 percent. Figure 14-6 depicts airflow movements in the same patient using a carbon dioxide analyzer measuring gas samples from the upper oropharynx. Note the repeated episodes of apnea in this 30-min segment, one of which exceeded 80 sec. Blood gas sampling confirmed very low saturation levels.

THERAPY

Although a number of therapeutic measures have been tried in patients with sleep apnea syndromes, success has been limited. The procedure of choice in an individual patient depends on both the type of sleep apnea and severity of symptoms.

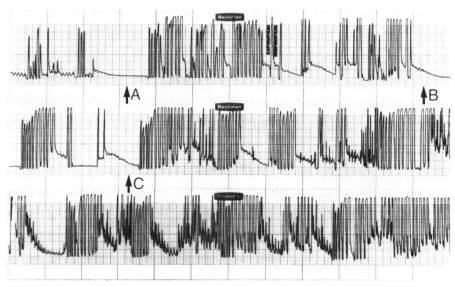

Fig. 14-6. This CO_2 analyzer recording of a sampling from the upper oropharynx identifies inspiratory and expiratory airflow by its CO_2 content. A continuous 30-min segment reveals repeated episodes of inspiratory obstruction of airflow. The longer episodes, marked A, B, and C in the earlier portions, reflect more complete obstruction than the hypopneic episodes in the later segments. Episode B exceeds 80 sec in duration.

Tracheostomy

This procedure, which allows air to bypass supralaryngeal obstructions, is the most effective treatment for "idiopathic" obstructive sleep apnea. It should be considered in patients with significant drops in oxygen saturation, disabling hypersomnia, severe cardiac arrhythmias associated with hypoxia, and secondary cardiopulmonary changes.[21,31,67,68] Dramatic symptomatic improvement may begin within a few days, although nocturnal sleep abnormalities, systemic and pulmonary hypertension, and cardiovascular abnormalities may take longer to disappear.[69,70] This procedure is not without potentially significant sequelae, however, and should not be considered without adequate documentation. Permanent tracheostomy requires psychological and social adjustment; recurrent tracheobronchitis, stomal infections, stomal granulomas, and bleeding are among reported complications.[18] For daytime use a fenestrated cannula can be used to permit normal speech and the site concealed with clothing or jewelry. Other mechanical attempts at maintaining a patent oropharynx by nightly insertion of airways, nasopharyngeal tubes,[71] tongue retractors,[72] nasal CPAP,[73] and so on, have been used only in small trials or have been poorly tolerated by patients on a long-term basis.

Surgical Correction of Obstruction

Surgical correction of a specific obstruction to airflow should be performed, if possible. Enlarged tonsils and adenoids may be resected and orofacial abnormalities require appropriate reconstruction; polypectomy may be of help if nasal polyps are present. A uvulopalatopharyngoplasty may be considered if redundant mucosa is noted in the pharyngeal and pharyngopalatal arch and if the uvula is large and narrows the airway lumen.[74,75] Special studies, such as fluoroscopic examination of the upper airway during sleep, may indicate the site of obstruction in selected cases.[76]

Weight Reduction

Most patients with obstructive sleep apnea are obese. Weight loss may improve symptoms in some patients but not in others.[29] Weight loss may be difficult in these patients and some may be able to lose weight only after tracheostomy to correct excessive daytime sleepiness. Weight loss is particularly desirable in motivated patients with minimal disability.

Pharmacological Therapy

Sedative-hypnotic drugs and alcohol worsen obstructive sleep apnea and should be avoided. Progesterone, doxapram, theophylline, and protriptyline[9,24,26,32,47,74,77-79] have been reported to benefit a limited number of patients with central and occasionally obstructive sleep apnea, perhaps on a basis of central respiratory stimulation. Acetazolamide has been reported to improve both apneic episodes and symptoms in central sleep apnea.[80] Strychnine-induced activation of oropharyngeal muscle tone has also been reported to be beneficial in obstructive sleep apnea.[18]

Oxygen

Nocturnal oxygen therapy has been useful in some patients with sleep apnea to relieve hypoxemia; however, some patients have an associated increase in CO_2 retention and longer apneic episodes.[55] Nocturnal oxygen may be more effective in patients with associated chronic obstructive pulmonary disease.[81] Trials should be monitored cautiously to detect any detrimental side effects.

Rocking Beds and Negative-Pressure Ventilators

Rocking beds have been used in central sleep apnea on a long-term basis.[82,83] Man et al.[84] reported a 14-year-old girl with central apnea managed with a negative-pressure (tank) ventilator during the night and Chaudhary and Spier reported a negative-pressure chest shell (cuirass) used for more than 1 year with good results.

Diaphragm Pacing

Electrode placement around the phrenic nerve permits long-term diaphragm pacing. This technique is useful in the central type of sleep apnea. It may accentuate obstructive apnea in mixed apnea syndromes or unmask or produce obstructive apnea in others. The resulting obstructive apnea may be the result of lack of coordination between the diaphragm and oropharynx if the diaphragm contracts when the oropharynx is closed. In patients with mixed apnea, diaphragm pacing or negative-pressure ventilators may be combined with tracheostomy.[85] A summary of therapeutic approaches, classified according to the type of apneic syndrome in which they are most useful, is given in Table 14-7.

Table 14-7 Treatment of Sleep Apnea Syndrome

Type of Apnea	Therapeutic Considerations
Obstructive apnea	Surgical correction of specific structural causes
	Weight reduction
	Tracheostomy
	Nasopharyngeal tube
	Uvelopalatopharyngoplasty
	Progesterone
	Strychnine
	Oxygen therapy
Central apnea	Progesterone
	Theophylline
	Doxapram
	Protriptyline
	Acetazolamide
	Oxygen therapy
	Rocking bed
	Negative pressure ventilation
	Diaphragm pacing
	Chronic nighttime ventilation
Mixed apnea	One or combination of above treatments, depending on the prominent component
	Negative pressure ventilation or diaphragmatic pacing only accompanying tracheostomy

REFERENCES

1. Aserinsky E, Kleitman N: Two types of ocular motility occurring in sleep. J Appl Physiol 8:1, 1955
2. Dement WC, Kleitman N: Cyclic variations in EEG during sleep and their relation to eye movements, body motility, and dreaming. Electroenceph Clin Neurophysiol 9:673, 1957
3. Rechtschaffen A, Kales A (eds): A manual of standardized terminiology, techniques and scoring system for sleep stages of human subjects. National Institutes of Health, publication 204, U.S. Government Printing Office, Washington, D.C., 1968.
4. Kales A, Jacobson A, Kales JD, et al: All-night EEG sleep measurements in young adults. Psychon Sci 7(2):67, 1967
5. Williams RL, Agnew HW Jr, Webb WB: Sleep patterns in young adults: An EEG study. Electroenceph Clin Neurophysiol 17:376, 1964
6. Williams RL, Agnew HM Jr, Webb WB: Sleep patterns of the young adult female: An EEG study. Electroenceph Clin Neurophysiol 20:264, 1966
7. Berger RJ: The sleep and dream cycle. p. 17. In Kales A (ed): Sleep, Physiology and Pathology: A Symposium. J.B. Lippincott, Philadelphia, 1969
8. Agnew HW Jr, Webb WB, Williams RL: The first night effect: An EEG study of sleep. Psychophysiology 2:263, 1966
9. Remmers JE, Anch AM, de Groot WJ: Respiratory disturbances during sleep. Clin Chest Med 1:1, 1980
10. Snyder F, Hobson JA, Morrison DF, Goldfrank F: Changes in respiratory, heart rate and systolic blood pressure in sleep. J Appl Physiol 19:417, 1964
11. Henane R, Brigriet A, Roussel B, Bittel J: Variations in evaporation and body temperature during sleep in man. J Appl Physiol: Resp Environ Exer Physiol 42:50, 1977
12. Fisher C, Gross J, Zuch J: Cycle of penile erection synchronous with dreaming (REM) sleep. Arch Gen Psychiatr 12:29, 1965
13. Karacan I, Goodenaugh DR, Shapiro A, Starker S: Erection cycle during sleep in relation to dream anxiety. Arch Gen Psychiatr 15:183, 1966
14. Townsend RE, Prinz PN, Obrist WD: Human cerebral blood flow during sleep waking. J Appl Physiol 35:620, 1973
15. Lumsden T: The regulation of respiration. J Physiol 58:81, 1923–1924
16. Goetz CG: Respiratory neuroanatomy. p. 1. In Weiner WJ (ed): Respiratory Dysfunction in Neurologic Disease. Futura Publishing, Mont Kisco, NY, 1980
17. Pitts RF: Organization of the respiratory center. Physiol Rev 26:609, 1946
18. Gee JBL, Remmers JE: Sleep apnea syndromes: Mechanisms and therapy. Compr Ther 7:52, 1981
19. Bulow K: Respiration and wakefulness in man. Acta Physiol Scand, suppl., 59:209, 1963
20. Phillipson EA: Respiratory adaptations in sleep. Ann Rev Physiol 40:133, 1978
21. Wurtz RH, O'Flaherty JJ: Physiological correlates of steady potential shifts during sleep and wakefulness. I. Sensitivity of the steady potential to alterations in carbon dioxide. Electroenceph Clin Neurophysiol 22:30, 1967
22. Birchfield R, Sieker HO, Heyman A, Durham NC: Alterations in respiratory function during natural sleep. J Lab Clin Med 54:216, 1959
23. Guazzi M, Freis ED: Sino-aortic reflexes and arterial pH, Po_2, and Pco_2 in wakefulness and sleep. Am J Physiol 217:1623, 1969
24. Nausieda PA, Weber S: Sleep-related respiratory disorders. p. 285. In Weiner WJ (ed): Respiratory Dysfunction in Neurologic Disease. Futura Publishing, Mont Kisco, NY, 1980

25. Web P: Periodic breathing during sleep. J Appl Physiol 37:899, 1974
26. Miranda FG: Clinical significance and dangers associated with sleep apnea syndrome, part I: Symposium on sleep apnea. Fourteenth Annual Meeting of the American Medical Electroencephalographic Association, May 20–22, Nashville, Tenn., 1980
27. Sullivan CE, Murphy E, Kozar LF, Phillipson EA: Waking and ventilatory responses to laryngeal stimulation in sleeping dogs. J Appl Physiol: Resp Environ Exer Physiol 45:681, 1978
28. Block AJ, Boysen PG, Wynne JW, Hunt LA: Sleep apnea, hypopnea and oxygen desaturation in normal subjects. N Engl J Med 300:513, 1979
29. Guilleminault C, Tilkian A, Dement WC: The sleep apnea syndromes. Ann Rev Med 27:465, 1976
30. Aserinsky E: Periodic respiratory pattern occurring in conjunction with eye movements during sleep. Science 150:763, 1965
31. Guilleminault C, Cummiskey J, Dement WC: Sleep apnea syndrome: Recent advances. Adv Intern Med 25:347, 1980
32. Chaudhary BA, Speir WA Jr: Sleep apnea syndromes. South Med J 75:39, 1982
33. Block AJ: Respiratory disorders during sleep, part II. Heart Lung 10:90, 1981
34. Sanders MH: Apnea associated with sleep. Clin Notes Resp Dis 19:3, 1980
35. Thach BT, Stark AR: Spontaneous neck flexion and airway obstruction during apneic spells in preterm infants. J Pediatr 94:275, 1979
36. Lugaresi E, Coccagna G, Mantovani M: In Weitzman E (ed): Hypersomnia with Periodic Apneas. Vol. 4. SP Medical and Scientific Books, New York, 1978
37. Remmers JE, deGroot WJ, Sauerland E, Anch AM: Pathogenesis of upper airway occlusion during sleep. J Appl Physiol: Resp Environ Exer Physiol 44:931, 1978
38. Dement WC, Guilleminault C: Diagnostic classification of sleep disorders. Sleep 2:1, 1979
39. Guilleminault C, Eldridge FL, Tilkian A, Simmons FB, et al: Sleep apnea syndrome due to upper airway obstruction. Arch Intern Med 137:296, 1977
40. Guilleminault C, Billiard M, Montplaisir JR, Dement WC: Altered states of consciousness in disorders of daytime sleepiness. J Neurol Sci 26:377, 1975
41. Fairman RP, Mathers JAL Jr, Isrow LA, et al: Sleep apnea syndrome: Clinical features and treatment. Va Med 107:490, 1980
42. Plum F, Swanson AG: Abnormalities in central regulation of respiration in acute and convalescent poliomyelitis. Arch Neurol Psychiatr 80:267, 1958
43. Krieger AJ, Rosomoff HL: Sleep-induced apnea: Part I—A respiratory and autonomic dysfunction syndrome following bilateral percutaneous cervical cordotomy. J Neurosurg 39:168, 1974
44. Deverezux MW, Keane JR, Davis RL: Automatic respiratory failure associated with infarction of the medulla. Arch Neurol 31:338, 1974
45. North JB, Jennett S: Abnormal breathing patterns associated with acute brain damage. Arch Neurol 31:338, 1974
46. Levin BF, Margolis G: Acute failure of automatic respirations secondary to a unilateral brainstem infarct. Ann Neurol 1:583, 1977
47. McCoy KS, Koopmann CF, Taussig LM: Sleep-related breathing disorders. Am J Otolaryngol 2:228, 1981
48. Noonan J: Reversible cor pulmonale due to hypertrophied tonsils and adenoids: Studies in two cases. Circulation, suppl., 32:164, 1965
49. Coccagna G, Di Donato G, Veruchi P, et al: Hypersomnia with periodic apneas in acquired micrognathia. A bird-like face syndrome. Arch Neurol 33:769, 1976
50. Weitzman ED, Pollack CD, Borowiecki B: Hypersomnia and sleep apnea due to micrognathia. Arch Neurol 35:392, 1978
51. Lehrman KI, Guilleminault C, Schroeder JS, et al: Sleep apnea in a patient with Shy-Drager syndrome. Arch Intern Med 138:206, 1978
52. Weiner WJ, Klawans HL: Respiratory dysfunction in movement disorders. p. 15. In

Weiner WJ (ed): Respiratory Dysfunction in Neurologic Disease. Futura Publishing, Mont Kisco, NY, 1980

53. Tammeling GJ, Devries G, Sluiter HJ, Ginicno F: Lung mechanics during sleep in patients with obstructive lung diseases. Prog Resp Res 6:271, 1971
54. Bergofsky EH, Turino GM, Fishman AP: Cardiorespiratory failure in kyphoscoliosis. Medicine 38:263, 1959
55. Guilleminault C, Dement WC (eds): Sleep Apnea Syndromes. Alan R. Liss, New York, 1978
56. Gillies AJD, Larkin J, Guy HJB: Nocturnal sleep apnoea: Method of diagnosis. NZ Med J 93:297, 1981
57. Krumpe PE, Cummiskey JM: Use of laryngeal sound recordings to monitor apnea. Am Rev Resp Dis 122:797, 1980
58. Cummiskey J, Williams TC, Krumpe PE, Guilleminault C: The detection and quantification of sleep apnea by tracheal sound recordings. Am Rev Resp Dis 126:221, 1982
59. Muspratt S: A simple pneumotachograph for qualitative monitoring of respiration and detection of apnea. Am Rev Resp Dis 124:650, 1981
60. Douglas NJ, Bash HM, Wraith PK, et al: Accuracy, sensitivity to carboxyhemoglobin and speed of response of the Hewlett-Packard 47201A ear oximeter. Am Rev Resp Dis 119:311, 1979
61. Severinghaus JW: Transcutaneous blood gas analysis. Resp Care 27:152, 1982
62. Nyboer J: Electrical Impedance Plethysmography. C.C. Thomas, Chicago, Ill, 1970
63. Sharp JT, Druz WS, Foster JR, et al: Use of the respiratory magnetometer in diagnosis and classification of sleep apnea. Chest 77:350, 1980
64. Mead J, Peterson N, Grimby G, Mead J: Pulmonary ventilation measured from body surface movements. Science 156:1383, 1967
65. Berendes J, Kipp J, Hansotia PL: Technique of polysomnography. Am J EEG Technol 22:63, 1982
66. Block AJ: Respiratory disorders during sleep, part I. Heart Lung 9:1011, 1980
67. Tilkian AG, Guilleminault C, Schroeder JS, et al: Sleep-induced apnea syndrome. Prevalence of cardiac arrhythmias and their reversal after tracheostomy. Am J Med 63:348, 1977
68. Simmons FB, Guilleminault C, Dement WC, et al: Surgical management of airway obstructions during sleep. Laryngoscope 87:326, 1977
69. Sackner M, Landa J, Forrest T, Greeneltch D: Periodic sleep apnea: Chronic sleep deprivation related to intermittent upper airway obstruction and central nervous system disturbance. Chest 67:164, 1975
70. Lugaresi F, Coccagna G, Mantovani M, Brignani F: Effects of tracheostomy in two cases of hypersomnia with periodic breathing. J Neurol Neurosurg Psychiatr 36:15, 1973
71. Afzelius LE, Elmqvist DE, Hougaard K, et al: Sleep apnea syndrome—An alternative treatment to tracheostomy. Laryngoscope 91:285, 1981
72. Cartwright RD, Samelson CF: The effects of a nonsurgical treatment for obstructive sleep apnea. The tongue-retaining device. JAMA 248:705, 1982
73. Wagner DR, Pollak CP, Weitzman ED: Nocturnal nasal-airway pressure for sleep apnea. N Engl J Med 308:461, 1983
74. Walsh JK, Ulett GA, Schweitzer PK, O'Regan JP: Snoring, sleepiness and the obstructive sleep apnea syndrome. Mo Med 79:21, 1982
75. Fukita S, Zorick F, Conway W, Roth T: Surgical correction of anatomic abnormalities in obstructive sleep apnea syndrome: Uvulopalato-pharyngoplasty. Otolaryngol Head Neck Surg 89:923, 1981
76. Fodor J, Malott J, Colley D: Somnofluoroscopy in the evaluation of sleep apnea. Radiol Technol 53:105, 1981
77. Strohl KP, Brown R, Hensley MJ: Progesterone therapy for obstructive sleep apnea. Am Rev Resp Dis 173:119A, 1979

78. Orr WC, Imes NK, Martin RJ: Progesterone therapy in obese patients with sleep apnea. Arch Intern Med 139:109, 1979
79. Schmidt HS, Clark RW, Hyman PR: Protriptyline: An effective agent in the treatment of narcolepsy-cataplexy syndrome and hypersomnia. Am J Psychiatr 134:182, 1977
80. White DP, Zwillich CW, Pickett C, Hudgel DW: Acetazolamide therapy for central sleep apnea. Am Rev Resp Dis 123:177, 1981
81. Kerley R, Wynne J, Block A, et al: The effect of low flow oxygen on sleep-disordered breathing and oxygen desaturation. Chest 78:682, 1980
82. Moskowitz MA, Fisher JN, Simpser MD, Strieder DJ: Periodic apnea, exercise hypoventilation, and hypothalamic dysfunction. Ann Intern Med 84:171, 1976
83. Hyland RH, Jones NL, Powles ACP: Primary alveolar hypertension treated with electrophrenic respiration. Am Rev Resp Dis 117:165, 1978
84. Man GCW, Jones RI, MacDonald GF, King GE: Primary alveolar hypoventilation managed by negative pressure ventilation. Chest 76:219, 1979
85. Glenn WL, Gee JB, Cole DR, et al: Combined central alveolar hypoventilation and upper airway obstruction. Treatment by tracheostomy and diaphragm pacing. Am J Med 64:50, 1978

15

Organization and Management of the Pulmonary Function Laboratory

Steven A. Conrad, M.D.

DEFINING REQUIREMENTS OF THE LABORATORY

Predicting the testing requirements of a pulmonary function laboratory for a particular institution is dependent on many factors, and no absolute recommendations can be made. In practice, a balance must be struck between the desires of pulmonary function laboratory staff, the needs in terms of what is required by the practicing physicians, and the financial return in terms of which tests are done frequently enough to warrant their inclusion. For purposes of recommendations, facilities are divided into four categories representing increasing levels of sophistication.

Office Setting

The physician's office should be capable of testing basic mechanics of ventilation (Table 15-1). This would include obtaining a spirometer and providing space for performing the tests, evaluating the response to bronchodilator aerosol, as well as keeping a desk and file cabinets for interpreting the results and maintaining records. A portable spirometer is also suitable for the emergency or outpatient department of a hospital and bedside testing (see Chapter 13). Equipment investment and maintenance requirements are minimal. Office spirometry should receive the same priority from the practicing physician as the routine use of electrocardiography in the diagnosis of cardiac disorders.

Table 15-1 Recommended Minimal Requirements for
Physician Office Setting[a]

Tests	Suggested Equipment/Method
Lung Mechanics	
Forced vital capacity	Portable wedge or bellows
Forced expired volumes	spirometer, or electronic
Forced expiratory flows	spirometer with graphic
	recording capability

[a] See Table 13-1 for portable spirometry recommendations.

Community Hospital

The small community hospital should be capable of performing assessment of lung volumes, mechanics, and gas diffusion to be of maximal benefit in evaluating and following common pulmonary diseases (Table 15-2). This capability may not meet the special requirements of physicians with subspecialty training in pulmonary diseases, but would provide all that is required by most internists and family practitioners.

Medical Center

The large medical center may treat a number of patients referred from a wide geographic area with uncommon or undiagnosed diseases for treatment by physicians with subspecialty training in pulmonary diseases. The requirements of a laboratory in this type of setting should be capable of most of the tests

Table 15-2 Recommended Minimal Requirements for Community Hospital or Clinic

Tests	Suggested Equipment/Method
Lung Volumes	
Functional residual capacity	Helium dilution
Vital capacity and subdivisions	Water- or dry-seal spirometer
Lung Mechanics	
Forced vital capacity	
Forced expired volumes	Water- or dry-seal spirometer with
Forced expiratory flows	graphic recorder
Flow-volume loops	
Maximal voluntary ventilation	
Bronchodilator responsiveness	Inhaled bronchodilator
Gas Diffusion	
Single-breath diffusion	CO single breath
Distribution	
Distribution of ventilation	Helium mixing time
Distribution of $\dot{V}/\dot{Q}$	Arterial blood gases

Table 15-3 Recommended Minimal Requirements for Major Medical Center

Tests	Suggested Equipment/Method
Lung Volumes	
Functional residual capacity	Nitrogen washout
	Body plethysmography
Vital capacity and subdivisions	Water- or dry-seal spirometer
Lung Mechanics	
Forced vital capacity	
Forced expired volumes	Water- or dry-seal spirometer
Forced expiratory flows	with graphic recorder
Flow-volume loops	
Maximal voluntary ventilation	
Airway resistance	Body plethysmograph
Pulmonary compliance	Esophageal balloon/transducers
Bronchodilator responsiveness	Inhaled bronchodilator
Bronchial reactivity	Methacholine challenge
Closing volume	Single-breath N_2 elimination
Gas dependent flow-volume loops	Helium-oxygen spirometry
Gas Diffusion	
Diffusing capacity	CO single-breath diffusion
Membrane/intracapillary diffusion	
Distribution	
Distribution of ventilation	Multibreath nitrogen washout
	Radionuclide ventilation scanning
	Single-breath N_2 elimination
Distribution of perfusion	Radionuclide perfusion scanning
Distribution of $\dot{V}/\dot{Q}$	Arterial blood gases
Exercise Testing	
Exercise testing	Instrumentation for exercise, and on-line expired gas and arterial blood gas analysis

discussed in Chapters 6 through 9. There are also requirements for testing outside the pulmonary function laboratory, such as nuclear medicine. Suggested capabilities are given in Table 15-3.

Research Laboratory

A research laboratory may involve both clinical trials of new modalities of treatment using standard pulmonary function tests, as well as research into new tests or new methods of analysis of pulmonary function. In general, then, such a laboratory would require the capabilities described for the major medical center. In addition, a computer system is usually employed for storage and retrieval of large volumes of data. Computer systems are also used for real-time data collection on new methods of analysis.

PERSONNEL QUALIFICATIONS

At present there are no uniform regulations for personnel employed in pulmonary function laboratories. Qualifications are set by each hospital for each laboratory. The personnel employed in the pulmonary function laboratory consist of a *medical director* and one or more *pulmonary technologists.* The medical director is a physician in charge of the laboratory. Pulmonary technologists are divided, depending on the size of the laboratory, into three levels of expertise and laboratory responsibility consisting of a chief pulmonary function technologist, supervisory staff, and the technical staff.[1]

Medical Director

Every laboratory, regardless of its size, must have a physician appointed as medical director to be in charge of the laboratory space, equipment, and personnel.[2] He must have a medical degree or equivalent, and be licensed to practice medicine in the state where the laboratory is located. The director should have training in clinical pulmonary physiology, and be certified or eligible for certification in the appropriate specialty or subspecialty. As part of his training, the medical director should be knowledgable about the procedures and instrumentation used in the pulmonary function laboratory. It is also helpful if he has had training in biomedical instrumentation, statistics and quality control, and computer applications.

Responsibilities of the medical director vary, depending on the hospital. However, he should appoint, supervise, and evaluate the technical staff. At the time of his appointment he should prepare or review the procedure manual, the charges for various tests, the laboratory budget, and organization of records and periodical reports. He should direct continuing education programs, when necessary, for the technical staff as well as interested hospital staff. A primary responsibility is interpretation of all test results. The director should keep abreast of new equipment and developments in the field, and update laboratory equipment as needed. He should ensure safety in the performance of tests. The director is accountable to the hospital administration and staff for the performance of the laboratory.

Pulmonary Technologist

The pulmonary technologist must possess the ability to provide professional services relating to the diagnostic evaluation of normal and abnormal pulmonary function under the supervision of a physician.[3] There are two avenues of preparation: (1) formal educational programs in pulmonary function technology and (2) on-the-job training in hospitals. Formal educational program curricula should encompass three areas of instruction. *General education courses*, such as math and physics, form the foundation. *Core science courses* to ensure fundamental knowledge in pulmonary function technology, such as cardiopulmonary physiology and medical instrumentation, are the next level of instruction. Finally, *technical specialty courses* are included to provide advance study in specific areas.

Specific minimal standards for personnel have been proposed for the large laboratory and are summarized according to the position level[1]:

Technical Staff   A high school education at minimum is required to initiate training in pulmonary function technology, either by formal education or on-the-job training. One or more years of college in biological science and math is preferred. Depending on the complexity of the test performed, a minimum of 6 to 12 months of laboratory training is recommended. To provide troubleshooting expertise in any problems or discrepancies, a minimum of 1 1/2 to 2 years is recommended, again depending on the complexity of the test.

Supervisory Staff   Technologists acting in a supervisory capacity should have a minimal educational background consisting of a formal training program in respiratory therapy or cardiopulmonary technology, or 2 years of college in biological science and math. A bachelor of science degree or higher in biological science or respiratory therapy is recommended. He (or she) should have a minimum of 2 years experience in routine testing and up to 4 years in more complex testing, such as exercise testing. Certification or registration by the National Board for Respiratory Care (NBRC) or National Society for Cardiopulmonary Technology (NSCPT) is recommended.

Chief Pulmonary Function Technologist   The chief technologist is selected from the supervisory staff, and it is strongly recommended that he or she have 2 to 3 years in this capacity. His minimal educational background is the same as that of the supervisory staff, but it is strongly recommended that he have a bachelor of science or higher degree (M.S., Ph.D.), or substantial experience in pulmonary function technology. His laboratory training and experience should be a minimum of 4 to 6 years, depending on the complexity of the tests involved. The acquisition of a credential is also strongly recommended.

These recommendations apply to the small as well as large laboratory, even though the number of personnel may be limited. All personnel must work under the supervision of the medical director.

PHYSICAL FACILITY REQUIREMENTS

Physical layout of pulmonary function testing facilities is important for maximizing the benefits of testing and the comfort of both technician and the patient. No specific requirements exist; some general recommendations are presented here.

Four functional areas are required (Table 15-4). The *testing* area contains the actual testing instrumentation. It should be separately enclosed from the other areas so that the technician can work with the patient in a quiet, undisturbed environment, and provide the necessary vocal stimulation without disturbing the rest of the laboratory. An *administrative* area houses report filing systems, desk space for report preparation, and offices for administrative personnel. This must be separate from the testing area if used by people other than the technician performing the tests, as patient cooperation is dependent on concentration without distraction. An equipment *storage and processing* area is used for cleaning and disinfection of reusable equipment, and storage of disposable equipment, test gases, and processed reusable equipment, such as breathing circuits. Keeping it out of sight reduces patient distraction and the "laboratory atmosphere" that is somewhat alien to the patient. It requires a sink, storage area for disinfectants, and a drying area. Finally, a patient *waiting area* is useful for patients waiting to be tested as well as those who have just been administered a bronchodilator and need to be retested.

Smaller laboratories may not have the separate physical space corresponding to the four functional areas listed. Two or more areas, such as the storage and administrative areas, are typically combined into a single area. Alternatively, the storage and administrative areas may be those of the respiratory therapy department, to reduce overall physical space requirements.

EQUIPMENT SELECTION AND STANDARDS

Although much attention is paid to the types of tests performed and their significance, the quality and reliability of the *instrumentation* used receive little attention and are often taken for granted. To assure accuracy and reproducibility in pulmonary function test results, the equipment selected for use must be of high quality, meet certain minimal standards, and be regularly maintained and calibrated. This section provides some guidelines for the selection of equipment for use in a clinical pulmonary function laboratory. Reference is made to the type of equipment and not particular manufacturer's brands.

Spirometers

In the clinical laboratory, volume-displacement spirometers are chosen over pneumotachometer-based systems because of their inherent accuracy, minimal maintenance, relative lack of interference from environmental factors, and because they can be used in gas dilution, distribution, and diffusion studies. Dry-seal spirometers are becoming more popular than water-seal types because of their increased convenience, lower maintenance requirements, lower inertia, and easy adaptability to electronic processing. In bedside spirometry, the wedge or bellows spirometers are inexpensive and easy to maintain. Pneumotachometer-based electronic spirometers are smaller and more easily transported, but are more complicated and do not offer any advantage in accuracy.

Table 15-4 Functional Areas of the Pulmonary Function Laboratory

Area	Function	Space (ft^2)^a
Testing	Performance of testing	200-400
Administrative	File storage and report generation; director's and staff offices	50-250
Storage and processing	Inventory of diposable and cleaned reusable equipment Disinfection of reusable equipment	25-75
Waiting	Patient waiting before and between tests	75-150

^{a} Depending on the amount of equipment, number of technicians, and number of patients tested daily.

Regardless of the type chosen, the spirometer should meet certain standards of performance. The minimal acceptable standards for spirometry recommended by the American Thoracic Society[4] are summarized in Table 15-5. Standards for portable spirometers in particular are discussed in Chapter 13 in the section on bedside spirometry. Recommendations for spirometers used in pediatrics have been presented in the pediatric literature and are summarized in Chapter 11.

Table 15-5 Recommended Minimal Spirometry Standards^a

Volume		
Range	All tests	0-7 liters
Accuracy	FVC, VC	±3% or 50 ml, whichever is greater
	FEV$_t$	±3%
	MVV	±5%
Flow		
Range	All tests	0-12 liters/sec
Accuracy	FEF$_{25-75\%}$	±5% or 0.1 liters/sec (greater)
	FEF$_x$	±5% or 0.2 liters/sec (greater)
Timing		
Range	VC	30 sec
	FVC, FEF$_{x-y}$, FEF$_x$	10 sec
	MVV	12 to 15 sec
Accuracy	FEV$_1$	1.0 sec
Start Point		
Method	FEV$_1$	Back extrapolation
Resistance		
Maximum	FEV$_t$, FEF$_{x-y}$, FEF$_x$	Less than 1.5 cm H$_2$O/sec/liter
	MVV	±10 cm H$_2$O @ 2 liters TV @ 2 Hz
Recorder		
Minimum	Time	10 sec
	Speed	2 cm/sec
	Volume sensitivity	1 cm/liter BTPS
	Flow sensitivity	4 mm/liter/sec BTPS

^{a} For standards for portable spirometers, see Table 13-1. For pediatric testing, see Chapter 11.

Source: Adapted from ATS statement—Snowbird workshop on standardization of spirometry. Am Rev Resp Dis 119:831, 1979

Body Plethysmography

The "body box" is a low-acoustic compliance box with associated instrumentation for which no specific standards have been adopted. The box volume ranges from 550 to 700 liters. The pneumotachometer should be linear to 2 liters/sec. The box pressure transducer must be sensitive as small pressure changes must be detected; it should be linear with full scale from -2.5 to 2.5 cm H_2O. Mouth pressure is greater than box pressure, and its transducer must be linear with a full scale of -50 to $+50$ cm H_2O.

Gas Analyzers

Gas dilution methods for FRC measurement and the single-breath diffusion method require measurement of gas concentrations. The CO analyzer should be linear to a full scale of 0.3 percent. Helium analyzers should be linear to a full scale of 15 percent. If the open-circuit nitrogen washout or single-breath nitrogen elimination method is used, the anlayzer should be linear to 80 percent. Closed-circuit nitrogen analyzers involve a lower concentration of gas, and should have a linear full-scale response of 10 percent.

QUALITY ASSURANCE

The assurance of accurate and consistent results in the pulmonary function laboratory depends on careful attention to details in technician training, patient instruction, test performance, equipment calibration, and interpretation of the results. These have been addressed in this and other chapters in Sections II and III. Some additional suggestions are discussed here.

Procedure Manual

To obtain reproducible results of tests, a protocol must be defined for each test's performance. This is best done by developing a *procedure manual* that describes in a step-by-step fashion how the test is perform_d, with details on the use of the particular equipment in the laboratory. Most of the information can be obtained from the manufacturers' literature, but should be segregated into a separate manual and supplemented as needed for readability. It should be read by all of the technical staff and made readily available at all times for any procedural questions that may arise during the course of testing. It would be of great benefit to new technicians who have experience in testing, but not necessarily for the equipment in use, and those who may not perform tests frequently. A suggested format for a pulmonary function laboratory procedure manual is listed in Table 15-6.

Table 15-6 Suggested Outline for a Pulmonary Function Laboratory Procedure Manual

Date
  Original
  Revisions
Name of Test
Patient Preparation
  Pretest instructions
  Test procedure instruction
Equipment Preparation
  Equipment configuration/assembly
  Pretest Checking
Test Procedure
Data Processing
  Data recording
  Calculations
  Data reporting
Equipment Maintenance Schedule

Equipment Calibration and Maintenance

Errors introduced into pulmonary function testing by improperly calibrated equipment is a major concern because it will often go undetected. Measures must be undertaken to assure that these errors are not permitted to develop. Aside from the selection of quality equipment at the outset, the major means of reducing instrumentation error is the regular and frequent maintenance and calibration of the equipment. Frequency of calibration checks depends on several factors, including type of equipment, number of patients tested, and environmental conditions. No uniform procedures for calibration have been adapted. Formal recommendations for quality control of spirometer systems have been published,[5] but none exist for other types of pulmonary function equipment. A suggested schedule for quality control is given in Table 15-7. Such a schedule can be modified to suit the needs of a particular laboratory.

The equipment needed to check the accuracy of pulmonary function testing equipment is minimal. A *calibrated syringe* for checking static spirometer volumes is available from manufacturers of pulmonary function testing equipment, and consists of a 3-liter calibrated hand-driven piston syringe that can deliver an accurate volume. Checking timed volumes requires an *FVC simulator,* a commercially available instrument that releases a preset volume of gas in a calibrated exponential fashion to simulate the forced expiratory spirogram. It is particularly useful for checking timed volumes and flows.[5] *Test gases,* guaranteed by the supplier to fall within a certain tolerance, are available to check the full-scale accuracy of gas and analyzers. An *isothermal lung simulator* is a device for checking the accuracy of volume measurement in a body plethysmograph. It contains a material to avoid adiabatic behavior of a simple lung. An isothermal simulator can be constructed according to the directions given in Ref. 6.

Table 15-7 Suggested Equipment Maintenance and Calibration Schedule

Control	Frequency	Equipment/Method
Spirometry		
Breathing circuit leaks	Daily	Inspection
Water level	Daily	Inspection
Mechanical linkage	Daily	Inspection
Volume accuracy	Weekly	Calibrated syringe
Timed volume accuracy	Weekly	FVC simulator
Kymograph speed	Weekly	Stopwatch
Gas Analyzers		
Point calibration	Daily	Test gas
Response time	Monthly	Test gas
Plethysmograph		
Mechanical function	Daily	Inspection
Volume accuracy	Weekly	Isothermal lung
Blood Gas		
Point calibration	2–4 hr	Calibrated gases
Accuracy	12 hr	Simulation solution
Mechanical function	Daily	Inspection

The results of calibration checks and the need for adjustment should be recorded in a logbook as a flowsheet. Graphing of the results is recommended to detect early trends or isolate problems.

SELECTION OF A LABORATORY COMPUTER SYSTEM

Because of the cost and training required to install a computer system in the pulmonary function laboratory, the decision of what system to purchase should be carefully evaluated before any commitments are made. The purpose of this section is to provide some broad guidelines to follow in making this decision.

A computer system can be used in the pulmonary function laboratory in two ways. A *general-purpose* computer system can be used for calculation of results, calculation of predicted values, and report generation using data manually entered into the system. This application provides limited advantages. A more common, albeit more expensive, approach is to use a *dedicated* computer system that can electronically interface with the equipment to obtain raw data directly from the equipment. This approach improves productivity while minimizing technician error in acquiring and transferring data.

The adaptation of a general-purpose computer for use in the pulmonary function laboratory requires considerable investment and expertise. Most laboratories do not have these resources; therefore, the purchase of a dedicated computer system custom-designed for the existing equipment is recommended. The investment in a dedicated system is greater, but it is easier to use and has fewer maintenance problems.

Hardware Considerations

There are several considerations that influence the purchase of computer system hardware.

Service Availability The availability of reliable on-site service and repair is one of the most important considerations of all. Equipment that malfunctions frequently or requires long periods for repair can reduce the effectiveness of the laboratory.

Data Acquisition The computer system should be capable of automatically acquiring the necessary data directly from the equipment without technician involvement during the performance of the test itself.

Resolution The precision of data acquired by the computer system is determined by the specifications of the analog-to-digital converter (ADC) that interfaces with the equipment. The resolution of the variable being measured, for example, volume, is equal to the full scale of the equipment divided by the number of levels that the ADC can resolve. An 8-liter spirometer with a 256-level converter has a volume resolution of about 32 ml, and a potential error of over 1 percent, whereas a 4,096-level ADC can resolve about 2 ml with a level of error that is insignificant. In general, the resolution of the converter should be better than the inherent error of the spirometer itself.

Memory Size Each pulmonary function test requires its own independent software program. Therefore the computer only requires a memory capacity large enough for one test at any given time. The internal memory capacity should thus be large enough to run that test without interruption. The software for other tests not in use can be stored in magnetic storage. Size of the memory depends on the particular software in use. Typical computer systems require 16 kilobytes (16K) for this purpose.

Magnetic Storage The popular "floppy disk" or diskette provides ample storage capacity with sufficient speed to be of general-purpose use. Larger nonremovable "hard disks" are increasingly popular, but their cost is higher, they cannot be interchanged, and they offer no advantage for the typical laboratory. Research or high-volume clinical laboratories may find justification for their use. The cassette-tape format should be avoided as its access time is slow and can hinder testing.

Software Considerations

The software distributed with a custom system is designed to acquire raw data, process it to derive standard indexes of pulmonary function, and store and report the results. The software chosen depends in part on the type of hardware, the type of functions performed, and the data storage required. Software may be distributed in "source" or "executable" format. The latter can be run but not modified by the laboratory. The former can be modified in the laboratory to fix problems with the software or make changes to meet new requirements. If the expertise is available, the former method may be desirable but will entail a much larger initial cost. If the executable format is used, changes must be made by the software supplier and costs can be considerable. Regardless of the format obtained, the software supplier should agree to fix without cost any software problems that do not meet the advertised specifications.

Though a number of computer languages are available, the two most commonly chosen are *assembly language* and *BASIC.* Of these two, assembly is tedious to use, but is fast, allowing rapid acquisition of data. It is very difficult to make changes in programs written in assembly. BASIC is a higher-level language that permits changes or additions to be made relatively easily. Some software systems combine assembly and BASIC or other high-level language to achieve both speed and flexibility.

RECORDING AND REPORTING OF DATA

The presentation of pulmonary function tests results to the interpreting physician must be organized, clear, and complete. The interpreter should not have to search for the data he requires on a sheet of paper crowded with an abundance of numbers and abbreviations.

A functioning organization provides a report that is easily readable and effective in conveying the necessary information. Table 15-8 gives an example report. The report should be accompanied by any tracings generated, especially spirograms and flow-volume loops. Special tests, such as pulmonary compliance and tests of small airway function, are not depicted unless they are routinely performed.

INFECTION CONTROL

The overall risk of transmitting communicable diseases via pulmonary function testing is essentially nonexistent, and only minimal precautions need be taken.[7] Only the mouthpiece of the breathing circuit is changed between patients, unless the patient is known to have a communicable disease. At the end of the day, the breathing circuit and manifold can be disassembled for cleaning and disinfection by gas or chemical means, depending on the composition of the equipment. Gas sterilization is safe for almost all equipment, but chemical sterilization when applicable is faster and can be performed in the laboratory area. Disinfected equipment should be stored in sealed plastic bags in preparation for use. Water-seal spirometers should be disassembled and disinfected weekly or bimonthly.

If a subject is known to have a communicable disease, he should be tested at the end of the day. If a water-seal spirometer or other easily disassembled piece of equipment is in use, the technician need only disinfect the equipment using gas or chemicals. If the equipment cannot be disassembled for cleaning, such as a

Table 15-8 Typical Clinical Pulmonary Function Report

Name:	Age:	
ID:	Sex:	Ht:
Date:	Clinical Diagnosis:	Wt:

Lung Volumes	Actual		Predicted	% Predicted	
VC					
	Gas	Pleth.		Gas	Pleth.
FRC	___	___	___	___	___
RV	___	___	___	___	___
TLC	___	___	___	___	___
RV/TLC	___	___	___	___	___
Lung Mechanics					
FVC	___		___	___	
FEV_1	___		___	___	
FEV_1/FVC	___		___	___	
FEV_3	___		___	___	
FEV_3/FVC	___		___	___	
$FEF_{25-75\%}$	___		___	___	
$FEF_{75-85\%}$	___		___	___	
MVV	___		___	___	
Raw	___		___	___	
SGaw	___		___	___	
Distribution					
7 min N_2 washout	___		___		
ΔN_2/liter	___		___		
Diffusion					
DL_{CO}	___		___	___	
DL_{CO}/VA	___		___	___	
Bronchodilator Study					

	Pre-broncho-dilator	Post-bronchodilator	% Change
FEV_1	___	___	___
FVC	___	___	___
$FEF_{25-75\%}$	___	___	___
Interpretation			

Physician _____

dry-seal spirometer, then a large surface area, low-resistance bacterial filter should be placed in the line. At the end of the testing session, the filter and breathing circuits can be cleaned and gas sterilized.

A potential route for infection is the administration of aerosolized bronchodilators for testing bronchial reversibility or agents for bronchial provocation. Two sources of infected particles are the medication delivered and the equipment used to deliver it. The handheld metered-dose inhaler (MDI) in use by most laboratories is essentially free of medication-transmitted infection. They are used with interchangeable mouthpieces that can be disinfected. Patients who cannot use the MDI, such as small children, or those undergoing methacholine challenge, require administration of medication with nebulizers. The risk of infection can be minimized by using unit-dose medication vials when available, or by strict adherence to aseptic technique if only multiple-dose vials are used. Disposable handheld nebulizers offer no risk of infection as they are sterilized before packaging. If reusable nebulization equipment is used, the equipment must be properly processed before reuse. The breathing circuit and nebulizer must be cleaned with soap and water to remove deposits that might interfere with the action of the disinfectant. Equipment subjected to chemical disinfection or sterilization, such as by glutaraldehyde, must be in full contact with the solution for the time recommended by the manufacturer. Equipment susceptible to damage by chemicals should be gas-sterilized. All equipment so treated must be thoroughly dried before sterilization. All disinfected and sterilized equipment should be dried and packaged to prevent recontamination. The principles of sterilization and disinfection of respiratory therapy equipment are presented in more detail in Ref. 7.

REFERENCES

1. ATS Ad Hoc Committee on Proficiency Standards for Clinical Pulmonary Function Laboratories: Pulmonary function laboratories—Personnel standards. ATS News 1:8, 1982
2. George RB, Chenez FW Jr., Kanner RE, et al: The ATS Respiratory Care Committee position on the director of the pulmonary function laboratory. ATS News 4:6, 1978
3. George RB: Occupational description: Pulmonary technologist. In preparation.
4. Gardner RM (chairman): Snowbird workshop on standardization of spirometry. ATS statement. Am Rev Resp Dis 119:831, 1979
5. Shigeoka JW: Calibration and quality control of spirometer systems. Resp Care 28:747, 1983
6. Kanner RE, Morris AH (eds): Clinical Pulmonary Function Testing—A Manual of Uniform Laboratory Procedures for the Intermountain Area. Intermountain Thoracic Society, Salt Lake City, Utah, 1975
7. Elder HA, Sauer RL: Infectious disease aspects of respiratory therapy. p. 400. In Burton GG, Gee, GN, Hodgkin JE (eds): Respiratory Care: A Guide to Clinical Practice. J.B. Lippincott, Philadelphia, 1977

APPENDICES

Appendix A:

Terms, Symbols, and Abbreviations*

Ronald B. George, M.D.

The terms, symbols, and abbreviations used here are based upon the most recent recommendations of the American College of Chest Physicians-American Thoracic Society Joint Committee on Pulmonary Nomenclature.[1,2] This committee, under the joint chairmanship of David Cugell and Harold Menkes, has worked for several years on this difficult task, with input from associated organizations such as the American Physiological Society.[3]

In general, a respiratory physiology term is constructed from one primary symbol followed by one or more qualifying symbols to denote a specific anatomic location, function, or physical condition. The combined symbols noted here demonstrate some of the more commonly used representations; other examples are given in the text.

RESPIRATORY PHYSIOLOGY TERMS AND SYMBOLS

A. General

P	Pressures in general
$\bar{X}$	Dash above any symbol indicates a mean value
$\dot{X}$	Dot above any symbol indicates a time derivative
$\ddot{X}$	Two dots above any symbol indicate the second derivative with respect to time

* Modified from George, RB, Light, RW, Matthay, RA: Chest Medicine. Churchill Livingstone, New York, 1983

%X	Percent sign preceding a symbol indicates percentage of the predicted normal value
X/Y%	Percent sign following a symbol indicates a ratio function with the ratio expressed as a percentage. Both components of the ratio must be designated; e.g., $FEV_1/FVC\% = 100 \times FEV_1/FVC$.
f	Frequency of any event in time, e.g., respiratory frequency — the number of breathing cycles per unit of time.
t	Time
anat	Anatomic
max	Maximum
min	Minimum

B. Gas Phase Symbols

1. Primary Symbols
V	Volume of gas
$\dot{V}$	Flow of gas
F	Fractional concentration in dry gas phase

2. Qualifying Symbols
I	Inspired
E	Expired
A	Alveolar
T	Tidal
ET	End tidal
D	Dead space
B	Barometric
STPD	Standard temperature and pressure, dry. These are the conditions of a volume of gas at 0°C and 760 mmHg without water vapor.
BTPS	Body temperature (37°C) and barometric pressure (760 mmHg at sea level), saturated with water vapor.
ATPD	Ambient temperature and pressure, dry
ATPS	Ambient temperature and pressure, saturated with water vapor.

C. Blood Phase Symbols

1. Primary Symbols

Q   Volume of blood

$\dot{Q}$ Flow of blood

C   Concentration in blood phase

S   Saturation in blood phase

2. Qualifying Symbols

b   Blood in general

a   Arterial

v   Venous

$\bar{v}$ Mixed venous

c   Capillary (exact location to be specified in text when term is used)

c′   End-capillary

D. Pulmonary Function

1. Lung Volumes (expressed as BTPS)

RV   Residual volume: volume of air remaining in the lungs after maximum exhalation.

ERV   Expiratory reserve volume: maximum volume of air which may be exhaled from the end tidal volume.

TV   Tidal volume: volume of gas which is inspired or expired during one respiratory cycle. Used to report lung volume derived from spirometry.

V_T Tidal volume: used in reporting studies of distribution of ventilation, e.g. V_D/V_T is the physiologic dead space fraction.

IRV   Inspiratory reserve volume: maximum volume that can be inspired from end tidal inspiratory level.

V_L Volume of the lung, including the conducting airways.

V_{TG} Thoracic gas volume: volume of all gas within the thorax, including any extrapulmonary gas, and all gas within the lungs and intrathoracic airways.

IC   Inspiratory capacity: volume that can be inspired from the end tidal expiratory volume.

IVC	Inspiratory vital capacity: maximum volume measured on inspiration from RV.
VC	Vital capacity: volume measured on complete expiration after the deepest inspiration but without respect to the effort involved.
FRC	Functional residual capacity: volume of gas remaining in the lungs and airways at the end of a resting tidal expiration.
TLC	Total lung capacity: volume of gas in the lung and airways after as much gas as possible has been inhaled.
RV/TLC%	Residual volume to total lung capacity ratio, expressed as a percent
V_A	Alveolar volume
V_D	Physiologic dead space: Calculated volume which accounts for the difference between the pressures of CO_2 in mixed expired gas and arterial blood. Physiologic dead space reflects the sum of anatomic dead space and alveolar dead space.
$V_{D_{anat}}$	Volume of the anatomic dead space
V_{D_A}	Volume of the alveolar dead space

2. Forced Respiratory Maneuvers (Expressed as BTPS)

FVC	Forced vital capacity: the volume of gas expired from TLC, with expiration performed as rapidly and completely as possible.
FIVC	Forced inspiratory vital capacity: Maximum volume of air inspired from RV, with inspiration performed as rapidly and completely as possible.
FEV_t	The volume of gas which is exhaled in a given time interval t during the execution of a forced vital capacity.
$FEV_t/FVC\%$	Ratio of forced expiratory volume in a given time t to forced vital capacity, expressed as a percentage.
PEF	Peak expiratory flow (liters/min or liters/sec)
$\dot{V}max_{xx\%}$	Maximum expiratory flow (instantaneous) qualified by the volume at which measured, expressed as percent of the FVC which has been exhaled. (*Example:* $\dot{V}max_{75\%}$ is the maximum expiratory flow after 75% of the FVC has been exhaled and 25% remains to be exhaled.)
FEF_{x-y}	Forced expiratory flow between two designated volume points in the FVC spirogram. These points may be designated as absolute volumes starting from the full inspiratory point or the percent of FVC exhaled may be designated. (*Examples:* $FEF_{0.2-1.2}$ is the forced

expiratory flow between 200 ml and 1,200 ml of the FVC spirogram, formerly called *maximum expiratory flow:* $FEF_{25-75\%}$ is the
forced expiratory flow during the middle half of the FVC spirogram, formerly called *maximum midexpiratory flow.*)

MVV   Maximum voluntary ventilation: maximum volume of air which
can be breathed per minute by a subject breathing quickly and as
deeply as possible. The time of measurement of this lung function
test is usually 12 to 30 seconds, but the test result is given in liters
(BTPS)/min.

FET_x Forced expiratory time required to exhale a specified FVC (*Exam-*
ples: $FET_{95\%}$ is the time required to deliver the first 95% of the
FVC; $FET_{25-75\%}$ is the time required to deliver the middle half of
the FVC.)

3. Measurements of Ventilation

$\dot{V}_E$ Expired volume per minute (BTPS)

$\dot{V}_I$ Inspired volume per minute (BTPS)

$\dot{V}_{CO_2}$ Carbon dioxide production per minute (STPD)

$\dot{V}_{O_2}$ Oxygen consumption per minute (STPD)

R   Respiratory exchange ratio. Quotient of the volume of CO_2 produced divided by the volume of O_2 taken up.

$\dot{V}_A$ Alveolar ventilation: physiological process by which alveolar gas
is completely removed and replaced with fresh gas. The volume
of alveolar gas actually expelled completely is equal to the tidal
volume minus the volume of the dead space.

$\dot{V}_D$ Ventilation per minute of the physiologic dead space (BTPS).

$\dot{V}_{D_{anat}}$ Ventilation per minute of the anatomic dead space, that portion of
the conducting airway in which no significant gas exchange
occurs (BTPS).

$\dot{V}_{D_A}$ Ventilation of the alveolar dead space (BTPS), defined by the
equation: $\dot{V}_{D_A} = \dot{V}_D - \dot{V}_{D_{anat}}$

4. Mechanics of Breathing*

(a) Pressure terms

Paw   Pressure at any point along the airways (cmH_2O)

Pao   Pressure at the airway opening, e.g., mouth, nose, tracheal cannula

---

* All pressures are expressed relative to ambient pressure unless otherwise specified.

Ppl   Pleural pressure: the pressure between the visceral and parietal pleura

Pa   Alveolar pressure

Pl   Transpulmonary pressure: Pl = Pao − Ppl, measurement conditions to be defined

Pst(l)   Static recoil pressure of the lung: Pst(l) = Pl, measured under static conditions

Pbs   Pressure at the body surface

Pes   Esophageal pressure used to estimate Ppl

Pw   Transthoracic pressure: pressure difference between parietal pleural surface and body surface. Pw = Ppl − Pbs (Transthoracic means "across the chest wall".)

Ptm   Transmural pressure pertaining to an airway or blood vessel

Prs   Transrespiratory pressure: pressure across the respiratory system Prs = Pao − Pbs = Pl + Pw.

(b) Flow-pressure relationships

R   Flow resistance: the ratio of the flow-resistive components of pressure to simultaneous flow (cmH_2O/liter/sec)

Raw   Airway resistance calculated from pressure difference between airway opening (Pao) and alveoli (Pa) divided by the air flow.

Rl   Total pulmonary resistance includes the frictional resistance of the lungs and air passages. It equals the sum of airway resistance and lung tissue resistance. It is measured by relating flow-dependent transpulmonary pressure to air flow at the mouth.

Rrs   Total respiratory resistance includes the sum of airway resistance, lung tissue resistance, and chest wall resistance. It is measured by relating flow-dependent transrespiratory pressure to air flow at the mouth.

Rus   Resistance of the airways on the upstream (alveolar) side of the point in the airways where intraluminal pressure equals Ppl (equal pressure point), measured during maximum expiratory flow.

Rds   Resistance of the airways on the downstream (mouth) side of the point in the airways where intraluminal pressure equals Ppl, measured during maximum expiratory flow.

Rs	Resistance of the airways upstream from the collapsible segment of the airway. This is used by Pride and Permutt in their analysis of the mechanics of air flow during forced expiration.
Gaw	Airway conductance, reciprocal of Raw
Gaw/VL	Specific conductance, expressed per liter of lung volume at which Gaw is measured

(c) Volume-pressure relationships

C	Compliance: The slope of a static volume-pressure curve at a point, or the linear approximation of a nearly straight portion of such a curve (liter/cmH$_2$O or ml/cmH$_2$O).
Cdyn	Dynamic compliance: the ratio of the tidal volume to the change in intrapleural pressure between the points of zero flow.
Cst	Static compliance: value for compliance determined on the basis of measurements made during periods of cessation of air flow.
C/VL	Specific compliance: compliance divided by the lung volume at which it is determined, usually FRC.
E	Elastance: the reciprocal of compliance (cmH$_2$O/liter or cmH$_2$O/ml).
Pst	Static components of pressure.
W	Work of breathing: the energy required for breathing movements.

5. Diffusing Capacity

DL	Diffusing capacity of the lung: amount of gas (O$_2$, CO, CO$_2$) commonly expressed as milliliters of gas (STPD) diffusing between alveolar gas and pulmonary capillary blood per minute per mmHg mean gas pressure difference. Total resistance to diffusion for oxygen ($1/D_{L_{O_2}}$) and carbon monoxide ($1/D_{L_{CO}}$) includes resistance to diffusion of the gas across the alveolar-capillary membrane, through plasma in the capillary, and across the red cell membrane ($1/D_M$) and resistance to diffusion within the red cell arising from the chemical reaction between the gas and hemoglobin ($1/\theta V_c$), according to the formula

$$\frac{1}{D_L} = \frac{1}{D_M} + \frac{1}{\theta V_c}$$

DM	The diffusing capacity of the pulmonary membrane
θ	The rate of gas uptake by normal whole blood at standard partial pressure. Usual units are ml STPD per ml blood per minute per mmHg.

Vc   Average volume of blood in the capillary bed

Qc   Alternate notation for Vc. This term is consistent with primary symbol recommendations, but Vc is well established in the literature.

D_L/V_A Diffusing capacity per unit of alveolar volume

6. Respiratory Gas Pressures and Content

Pa_x Arterial pressure of gas x (mmHg)

PA_x Alveolar pressure of gas x (mmHg)

PET_x End tidal pressure of gas x (mmHg)

Sa_{O_2} Arterial oxygen saturation (%)

PA-Pa   Alveolar-arterial gas pressure difference: the difference in partial pressure of a gas (e.g., O_2 or N_2) in the alveolar gas spaces and that in the systemic arterial blood, measured in mmHg. (For oxygen as an example, PA_{O_2}-Pa_{O_2})

P(A-a)   Alternate notation for PA-Pa.

Ca-Cv   Arterial-venous content difference (for oxygen as an example, $Ca_{O_2} - Cv_{O_2}$)

C(a-v)   Alternate notation for Ca-Cv.

7. Pulmonary Shunts

$\dot{Q}s$ Shunt of blood flow: vascular connections between circulatory pathways allow venous blood to be diverted into vessels containing arterialized blood (right-to-left shunt, venous admixture) or vice versa (left-to-right shunt). Flow from left to right through a shunt should be marked with a negative sign.

E. Pulmonary Dysfunction

1. Altered Breathing

Hyper-   Alveolar ventilation is excessive relative to the simultaneous
ventilation   metabolic rate. As a result, the alveolar P_{CO_2} is reduced.

Hypo-   Alveolar ventilation is small relative to the simultaneous meta-
ventilation   bolic rate, so that alveolar P_{CO_2} rises.

2. Altered Blood Gases

Hypoxia   Any state in which the oxygen in the lung, blood, and/or tissues is abnormally low compared with that of a normal resting person breathing air.

Hypoxemia   A state in which the oxygen pressure and/or concentration in arterial blood is lower than its normal value.

Hypocapnia   Any state in which the systemic arterial carbon dioxide pressure is significantly below 40 mmHg as in hyperventilation.

Hypercapnia   Any state in which the systemic arterial carbon dioxide pressure is significantly above 40 mmHg. May occur when alveolar ventilation is inadequate for a given metabolic rate (hypoventilation) or during CO_2 inhalation.

3. Altered Acid-Base Balance

Acidemia   Any state of systemic arterial plasma in which the pH is significantly less than the normal value, 7.41 ± 0.02

Alkalemia   Any state of systemic arterial plasma in which the pH is significantly greater than the normal value, 7.41 ± 0.02.

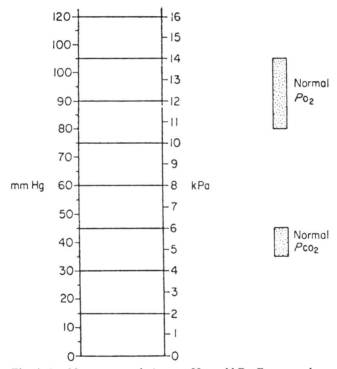

Fig. A-1. Nomogram relating mmHg and kPa. Even numbers of kPa relate exactly to convenient values of mmHg at intervals of 15 mmHg, and some of these values may be worth remembering. (Reprinted with permission from Brewis, RAL: *Lecture Notes on Respiratory Diseases.* 3rd Printing, Blackwell Scientific Publications, Oxford, 1975.)

SI UNITS

The International System of Units (Système International, SI) was proposed by the International Bureau of Weights and Measures in 1970 as an alternative to the system currently in use. A National Bureau of Standards booklet which describes this system is available from the U.S. Government Printing Office, Washington, D.C. 20402.[4] This proposed system has certain drawbacks, and traditional units are used throughout this textbook. A nomogram (Fig. A-1) has been included in this Appendix for conversion to SI units.[5]

Table A-1 Comparison of Traditional and SI Units with Factors for Conversion to SI Units

Terms	Traditional Units (a)	SI Units (b)	Conversion Factor (k)[1]
A. Gas phase:			
Gas flow	L/unit time[2]	L/unit time	1
Pressure or tension	cmH_2O	kPa	0.098
	torr (or mmHg)	kPa	0.133
B. Pulmonary function:			
Compliance	L/cmH_2O	L/kPa	10.2
Resistance	$cmH_2O/L/sec$	kPa/L/sec	0.098
Conductance	$L/sec/cmH_2O$	L/sec/kPa	10.2
Specific conductance	$L/sec/cmH_2O/V_{tg}$	$L/sec/kPa/V_{tg}$	10.2
Gas uptake	ml/min	mmol/min	0.045
Gas content in blood	ml/dl	mmol/L	0.045
Gas transfer factor			
(diffusing capacity)	ml/min/torr	mmol/min/kPa	0.336
Ventilatory response to			
CO_2	L/min/torr	L/min/kPa	7.52
C. Other:			
Energy expenditures	calories	joules	4.18
Power output	kpm/min	watts	0.164

[1] $a \times k = b$. For example, $20\ cmH_2O \times 0.098 = 1.96\ kPa$.
[2] Strictly the time should be in seconds, but minutes may be used if more convenient.

REFERENCES

1. Report of the American Thoracic Society-American College of Chest Physicians ad hoc Subcommittee on Pulmonary Nomenclature. Am Thorac Soc News 3(4):5, 1977.
2. Report from the American Thoracic Society Pulmonary Nomenclature Subcommittee on Respiratory Physiology. Am Thorac Soc News 4, No. 2:12, 1978.
3. Glossary on respiration and gas exchange. J Appl Physiol 34:549, 1973.
4. Page CH, Vigoureaux P., Eds.: *The International System of Units (SI)*. U.S. Dept. Commerce, Nat. Bur. Standards Spec. Publ. No. 330, 1974.
5. Brewis RAL: *Lecture Notes on Respiratory Diseases*, 3rd printing. Blackwell Scientific Publications, Oxford, 1975.

Appendix B:

Normal Values and Variability in Pulmonary Function Testing

Steven A. Conrad, M.D.

One of the goals of pulmonary function testing is to determine whether an individual is "normal." The term normal has many meanings; in pulmonary function testing it is used to indicate whether or not measured indices obtained from certain laboratory subjects have values expected for an individual with the subject's characteristics. This appendix first discusses some general principles of the prediction of normal values and then presents a series of tables of regression equations for most of the tests described in the book. References to the sources of the equations follow the tables and are annotated to provide brief information on the methods used in developing the equations.

DERIVATION OF REGRESSION EQUATIONS

To obtain the expected values for a group of normals, a large number of individuals who appear to be free of disease are studied and their test results are recorded. To apply this data, a regression equation is derived using statistical methods and the dependence of a given test result on certain characteristic variables, such as age, height, weight, and sex, is determined. These variables are often called characteristic variables. If a test result is found to vary independently of a characteristic variable, then that variable is excluded from the equation.

If the test result appears to vary *linearly* with all of the independent variables, then the equation is derived by multiple linear regression. These equations are similar in form to:

$$y = x_1 A + x_2 H + x_3 \qquad \text{(Eq. B-1)}$$

335

where x_1, x_2, and x_3 are equation coefficients, and A and H are selected subject measurements, of age and height in this case. These are the simplest equations to derive and apply. If the test result appears to vary *nonlinearly* with the characteristic variables, then another form of regression may be sought to better fit the data. Commonly used forms include exponential equations, such as:

$$y = x_1 e^{(x_2 H)}$$
(Eq. B-2)

or power equations, such as:

$$y = x_1 H^{x_2}$$
(Eq. B-3)

with patient height (H) used here as an example of an independent variable. The goal is to find an equation that best "fits" the data by minimizing the error obtained when the equation is applied. The statistical methods used in this process are beyond the scope of this book; the reader is referred for them to a general textbook on multivariate statistics.

Numerous problems can exist in the development of regression equations. Selection of a sample of normal individuals varied enough to represent the general population is a difficult task. For example, a random sample of normal subjects in Sweden would have different values from a random sample of normals in China. The sample must be large enough to ensure that the range of variation in normals is included. Selection of which variables to include in the regression equation can be problematic. Though each study of normal individuals attempts to minimize error from these problems, none is free from inaccuracy.

Use of Regression Equations

The application of a regression equation to a particular individual yields a single number which represents the expected value of a person with his or her characteristics. Obviously a group of normal individuals with the same characteristics will not have this expected value; there will be some variation among the values. Traditionally, those interpreting pulmonary function test results have assumed that normals vary by a certain fixed percentage from the expected value, most commonly ranging from 15 to 20 percent. Therefore, a vital capacity less than 20 percent below the expected value was reported as abnormal.

The actual variation from the expected value may be quite different from the 15 to 20 percent range. An approach which is theoretically more statistically sound is to determine a range within which the vast majority of normal individuals fall. Limits of this range, or *normal limits,* that include 95 percent of normals, can be constructed from knowledge about the variance of the test result in the population studied.

For a constant predicted value, assuming a normal distribution, the normal range is calculated by the formula:

$$y \pm 1.96\ SD \qquad \text{(Eq. B-4)}$$

where y is the expected value and SD is the *standard deviation.* For linear or multiple linear regression equations, the SD is replaced by the *standard error of the estimate* (SEE):

$$y \pm 1.96\ SEE \qquad \text{(Eq. B-5)}$$

where SEE is the standard error about the regression line of the estimate derived from the sample of normal individuals. This number is obtained from the regression analysis and its use is analogous to that of the SD.

When the results of a pulmonary function test are known to vary in only one direction in disease, such as a decrease in the vital capacity in restrictive disease, then a lower bound can be derived, above which 95 percent of normals lie. This lower bound is computed by:

$$y - 1.65\ SEE \qquad \text{(Eq. B-6)}$$

where y is the expected value derived from the regression equation. Notice that by concentrating the 5 percent of potentially misclassified normal individuals below a lower bound, a limit is obtained that is less removed from the expected value.

The computation of normal limits in nonlinear equations is less straight forward. Hsu et al,[11] who used this type of equation and report variance in percent SD, gives the following formula for the 95 percent lower limit:

$$y(1 - SD)^2 \qquad \text{(Eq. B-7)}$$

Use of the Tables

The following tables represent those studies of normal individuals that are most commonly cited. The list is by no means exhaustive but includes frequently used equations, most of which have been derived in the last twenty years. Each table contains equations for a separate test and is divided into adult and pediatric sections. The first equation in each section is the recommended one and appears to be most commonly used. Other selected equations are included in reverse chronological order and are referenced with brief annotations to aid the reader in choosing the most appropriate equations for his own laboratory.

The equations are reproduced from the original publications, with only minor changes implemented to insure uniformity. Coefficients have been rounded to four digits of precision and scaled if necessary to provide uniformity in units of measurement. Resistance values have been converted to conductance.

The following are the units used in the equations:

Measurement	Units
Volume	liters
Flow	liters/sec
Peak expiratory flow rate	liters/min
Ventilation	liters/min
Pressure	cmH_2O
Compliance	liters/cmH_2O
Conductance	liters/sec/cmH_2O
Diffusion	ml/min/torr
Ratios	percent

Abbreviations for characteristic variables in the tables are:

Abbreviation	Units
H(in)	Height in inches
H(cm)	Height in centimeters
W(lb)	Weight in pounds
W(kg)	Weight in kilograms
A	Age in years
S	Body surface area (m^2)

Formulas for the calculation of BSA for adult are:

$$\text{BSA (m}^2) = W(\text{kg})^{.425} \times H(\text{cm})^{.725} \times 7.184 \times 10^{-3}$$
$$\text{BSA (m}^2) = W(\text{lb})^{.425} \times H(\text{in})^{.725} \times 1.009 \times 10^{-2}$$

Formula for the calculation of BSA for pediatric and adult is:

$$\text{BSA (m}^2) = W(\text{g})^{(.7285 - .0188 \log W(g))} \times H(\text{cm})^{.3} \times 3.207 \times 10^{-4}$$

The standard error of the estimates are included in the tables when provided. If a prediction equation is a constant, such as 86 percent for the FEV_1/FVC percent, the SD is given instead. Some authors have reported SD or SEE as a percent of the mean value and others as a maximum or minimum value. The author's original choice is used, since the results are easily interchangeable.

Table B-1 Vital Capacity (VC) Prediction Equations

Author	Date	Sex	Ages	Regression Equation	SEE
Adults					
Knudson et al[1]	1976	M	25–90	$0.065H$(cm) $- 0.029A - 5.459$	0.601
		F	20–90	$0.037H$(cm) $- 0.022A - 1.774$	0.519
Morris et al[2]	1971	M	20–84	$0.148H$(in) $- 0.025A - 4.241$	0.74
		F	20–84	$0.115H$(in) $- 0.024A - 2.852$	0.52
Lapp et al[3]	1974	M/B[a]	35 $\pm$ 12	$0.100H$(in) $- 0.021A - 1.84$	0.32
Schmidt et al[4]	1973	M	20–94	$0.119H$(in) $- 0.022A - 2.815$	0.461
		F	20–94	$0.093H$(in) $- 0.022A - 1.924$	0.358
Bass[5]	1973	M	21–71+	$0.159H$(in) $- 0.023A - 5.720$	0.60
		F	21–71+	$0.069H$(in) $- 0.019A - 0.510$	0.38
Cherniack & Raber[6]	1972	M	15–79	$0.1210H$(in) $- 0.0136A - 3.1837$	—
		F	15–79	$0.0783H$(in) $- 0.0154A - 1.0491$	—

Continued

Table B-1 *(continued)*

Author	Date	Sex	Ages	Regression Equation	SEE
Abramowitz et al[7]	1965	M/W[a]	19–64	$0.072H(cm) - 0.016A - 7.29$	0.46
		M/B	21–51	$0.051H(cm) - 0.018A - 3.82$	0.46
		F/W	19–66	$0.0539H(cm) - 0.011A - 4.93$	0.41
		F/B	19–52	$0.0457H(cm) - 0.007A - 3.94$	0.37
Ferris et al[8]	1965	M	25–74	$0.046H(cm) - 0.027A - 2.79$	0.66
		F	25–74	$0.030H(cm) - 0.023A - 0.94$	0.47
Berglund et al[9]	1963	M	7–70	$0.0481H(cm) - 0.020A - 2.812$	0.50
		F	7–70	$0.0404H(cm) - 0.022A - 2.350$	0.40
Children and Adolescents					
Weng & Levison[10]	1969	M,F	4–18	$0.146\ e^{0.0199H(cm)}$	6.2%
Hsu et al[11]	1979	M/MA[a]	7–20	$1.06 \times 10^{-6}H(cm)^{2.97}$	13%
		M/W	7–20	$3.58 \times 10^{-7}H(cm)^{3.18}$	13%
		M/B	7–20	$1.07 \times 10^{-6}H(cm)^{2.93}$	17%
		F/MA	7–20	$1.25 \times 10^{-6}H(cm)^{2.92}$	14%
		F/W	7–18	$2.57 \times 10^{-6}H(cm)^{2.78}$	14%
		F/B	7–20	$8.34 \times 10^{-7}H(cm)^{2.98}$	15%
Knudson et al[1]	1976	M	8–24	$0.050H(cm) + 0.078A - 5.508$	0.544
		F	8–19	$0.033H(cm) + 0.092A - 3.469$	0.500
Polgar & Promadhat[12]	1971	M	—[b]	$4.4 \times 10^{-6}H(cm)^{2.67}$	—[b]
		F	—[b]	$3.3 \times 10^{-6}H(cm)^{2.72}$	—[b]
Dickman et al[13]	1971	M	5–11	$0.094H(in) - 3.042$	0.176
		M	12–18	$0.164H(in) + 0.174A - 9.425$	0.354
		F	5–11	$0.077H(in) - 2.371$	0.171
		F	12–18	$0.117H(in) + 0.102A - 5.869$	0.297
DeMuth et al[14]	1965	M	4–18	$2.157 \times 10^{-6}H(cm)^{2.81}$	—
		F	4–18	$1.858 \times 10^{-6}H(cm)^{2.82}$	—
Cherniak[15]	1962	M	3–16	$0.04053H(cm) + 0.05134A - 3.655$	—
		F	3–16	$0.02786H(cm) + 0.09096A - 2.554$	—

[a] B = black, MA = Mexican American, W = white.
[b] Composite data from several studies.

Table B-2 Functional Residual Capacity (FRC) Prediction Equations

Author	Date	Sex	Ages	Regression Equation	SEE
Adults					
Boren et al[16]	1966	M	20–66	$0.032H(cm) - 2.94$	0.63
Grimby & Soderholm[17]	1963	F	18–72	$0.0513H(cm) - 0.028W(kg) - 4.50$	0.41
		M	20–65	$0.0530H(cm) - 0.037W(kg) + 0.015A - 3.89$	0.56
Goldman & Becklake[18]	1959	M	42 ± 14	$0.0814H(cm) - 1.792S - 7.11$	17%
		F	42 ± 14	$0.53H(cm) - 0.017W(kg) - 4.74$	17%
Needham et al[19]	1959	M	20–70	$0.180H(in) - 0.018W(lb) + 0.010A - 6.56$	0.59
		F	20–70	$0.018W(lb) + 5.000S - 0.530$	0.45
Children and Adolescents					
Weng & Levison[10]	1969	M,F	4–18	$0.067e^{0.0211H(cm)}$	9.4%
Polgar & Promadhat[12]	1971	M	—[b]	$7.46 \times 10^{-7}H(cm)^{2.917}$	—[b]
		F	—[b]	$1.37 \times 10^{-6}H(cm)^{2.795}$	—[b]
DeMuth et al[14]	1965	M	4–18	$7.312 \times 10^{-7}H(cm)^{2.93}$	—
		F	4–18	$4.781 \times 10^{-6}H(cm)^{2.54}$	—
Needham et al[19]	1954	M	11–19	$0.140H^a(cm) + 0.080A - 3.60$	0.34
		F	11–19	$0.085H^a(cm) - 3.430$	0.26

[a] Sitting height.
[b] Composite data from several studies.

Table B-3 Residual Volume (RV) Prediction Equations

Author	Date	Sex	Ages	Regression Equation	SEE
Adults					
Boren et al[16]	1966	M	20–66	$0.019H(cm) + 0.0115A - 2.24$	0.53
Grimby & Soderholm[17]	1963	F	18–72	$0.0268H(cm) + 0.007A - 3.42$	0.32
		M	20–65	$0.0198H(cm) - 0.015W(kg)$	
				$+ 0.022A - 1.54$	0.36
Lapp et al[3]	1974	M/B[a]	35 ± 12	$0.07H(in) + 0.05A - 4.73$	0.59
Goldman & Becklake[18]	1959	M	42 ± 14	$0.027H(cm) + 0.017A - 3.447$	19%
		F	42 ± 14	$0.032H(cm) + 0.009A - 3.900$	24%
Needham et al[19]	1954	M	20–70	$0.100H(in) - 0.010W(lb)$	
				$+ 0.024A - 4.150$	0.41
		F	20–70	$0.009A + 1.200$	0.36
Children and Adolescents					
Weng & Levison[10]	1969	M,F	4–18	$0.033e^{0.0210H(cm)}$	11.2%
Polgar & Promadhat[12]	1971	M,F	—[b]	$4.41 \times 10^{-6}H(cm)^{2.410}$	—[b]
Needham et al[19]	1954	M	11–19	$0.110H^c(cm) - 2.460$	0.30
		F	11–19	$0.045H^c(cm) - 1.790$	0.21

[a] B = black.
[b] Composite data from several studies.
[c] Sitting height.

Table B-4 Total Lung Capacity (TLC) Prediction Equations

Author	Date	Sex	Ages	Regression Equation	SEE
Adults					
Boren et al[16]	1966	M	20–66	$0.078H(cm) - 7.30$	0.87
Grimby & Soderholm[7]	1963	F	18–72	$0.0671H(cm) + 0.015A - 5.77$	0.48
		M	20–65	$0.0692H(cm) - 0.017W(kg) - 4.30$	0.67
Lapp et al[3]	1974	M/B[a]	35 ± 12	$0.17H(in) + 0.03A - 6.57$	0.78
Goldman & Becklake[18]	1959	M	42 ± 14	$0.094H(cm) - 0.015A - 9.167$	14%
		F	42 ± 14	$0.079H(cm) - 0.008A - 7.49$	10%
Needham et al[19]	1954	M	20–70	$0.160H(in) - 0.010A$	
				$+ 1.500S - 4.210$	0.68
		F	20–70	$0.110H(in) - 0.010A - 2.180$	0.54
Children and Adolescents					
Weng & Levison[10]	1969	M,F	4–18	$0.160e^{0.0210H(cm)}$	6.4%
Polgar & Promadhat[12]	1971	M	—[b]	$5.56 \times 10^{-6}H(cm)^{2.669}$	—[b]
		F	—[b]	$4.09 \times 10^{-6}H(cm)^{2.730}$	—[b]
Needham et al[19]	1954	M	11–19	$0.200H^c(cm) + 0.100A - 6.480$	0.46
		F	11–19	$0.090H^c(cm) + 2.000S - 3.900$	0.36

[a] B = black.
[b] Composite data from several studies.
[c] Sitting height.

Table B-5 Residual Volume/Total Lung Capacity Ratio (RV/TLC%) Prediction Equations

Author	Date	Sex	Ages	Regression Equation	SEE
Adults					
Boren et al[16]	1966	M	20–66	$0.195A + 17.5$	6.25
Grimby & Soderholm[17]	1963	F	18–72	$0.27H(cm) + 0.28A - 28$	4.3
		M	20–65	$0.33A - 0.14W(kg) + 23.4$	5.5
Goldman & Becklake[18]	1959	M	42 ± 14	$0.343A + 16.7$	15%
		F	42 ± 14	$0.265A + 21.7$	18%
Needham et al	1954	M	20–70	$0.60H(in) - 0.12W(lb)$	
				$+ 0.45A - 7.1$	4.4
		F	20–70	$0.34A - 0.07W(lb) + 31.3$	5.4

Continued

Table B-5 *(continued)*

Author	Date	Sex	Ages	Regression Equation	SEE
Children and Adolescents					
Weng & Levison[10]	1969	M,F	4–18	$0.13A + 20.93$	3.46%
Polgar & Promadhat[12]	1971	M	—[b]	$77.9H(cm)^{-0.259a}$	—[b]
		F	—[b]	$107.8H(cm)^{-0.320a}$	—[b]
Needham et al[19]	1954	M	11–19	24.9	4.7
		F	11–19	25.7	4.7

[a] Derived from prediction equations for RV and TLC.
[b] Composite data from several studies.

Table B-6 Forced Expired Volume in One-Half Second ($FEV_{0.5}$) Prediction Equations

Author	Date	Sex	Ages	Regression Equation	SEE
Adults					
Knudson et al[1]	1976	M	25–90	$0.037H(cm) - 0.017A - 2.746$	0.474
		F	20–90	$0.019H(cm) - 0.014A - 0.406$	0.388
Kory et al[20]	1961	M	20–65	$0.0196H(cm) - 0.024A + 0.24$	0.51
Children and Adolescents					
Knudson et al[1]	1976	M	8–24	$0.030H(cm) + 0.043A - 3.054$	0.425
		F	8–19	$0.019H(cm) + 0.061A - 1.738$	0.364

Table B-7 Forced Expired Volume in 1 Second (FEV_1) Prediction Equations

Author	Date	Sex	Ages	Regression Equation	SEE
Adults					
Knudson et al[1]	1976	M	25–90	$0.052H(cm) - 0.027A - 4.203$	0.541
		F	20–90	$0.027H(cm) - 0.021A - 0.794$	0.434
Morris et al[2]	1971	M	20–84	$0.092H(in) - 0.032A - 1.260$	0.55
		F	20–84	$0.089H(in) - 0.025A - 1.932$	0.47
Lapp et al[3]	1974	M/B[a]	35 ± 12	$0.090H(in) - 0.025A - 1.54$	0.23
Schmidt et al[4]	1973	M	20–65	$0.085H(in) - 0.31A - 0.897$	0.393
		F	20–65	$0.067H(in) - 0.027A - 0.525$	0.291
Cherniack & Raber[6]	1972	M	15–79	$0.09107H(in) - 0.02320A - 1.50723$	
		F	15–79	$0.06029H(in) - 0.01936A - 0.18693$	
Ferris et al[8]	1965	M	25–74	$0.036H(cm) - 0.027A - 1.65$	0.49
		F	25–74	$0.025H(cm) - 0.022A - 0.62$	0.40
Berglund et al[9]	1963	M	7–70	$0.0344H(cm) - 0.033A - 1.00$	0.50
		F	7–70	$0.0267H(cm) - 0.027A - 0.54$	0.36
Kory et al[20]	1961	M	20–65	$0.0370H(cm) - 0.028A - 1.59$	0.52
Children and Adolescents					
Weng & Levison[10]	1969	M,F	4–18	$0.04H(cm) - 3.99$	2.04%
Knudson et al[1]	1976	M	8–24	$0.046H(cm) + 0.045A - 4.808$	0.523
		F	8–19	$0.027H(cm) + 0.085A - 2.703$	0.422
Hsu et al[11]	1979	M/MA[a]	7–20	$1.73 \times 10^{-6}H(cm)^{2.85}$	13%
		M/W	7–20	$7.74 \times 10^{-7}H(cm)^{3.00}$	13%
		M/B	7–20	$1.03 \times 10^{-6}H(cm)^{2.92}$	17%
		F/MA	7–20	$1.61 \times 10^{-6}H(cm)^{2.85}$	14%
		F/W	7–18	$3.79 \times 10^{-6}H(cm)^{2.68}$	14%
		F/B	7–20	$1.14 \times 10^{-6}H(cm)^{2.89}$	15%
Dickman et al[13]	1971	M	5–11	$0.085H(in) - 2.855$	0.159
		M	12–18	$0.143H(in) + 0.121A - 7.864$	0.303
		F	5–11	$0.074H(in) - 2.482$	0.166
		F	12–18	$0.100H(in) + 0.085A - 4.939$	0.290
Polgar & Promadhat[12]	1971	M,F	—[b]	$2.10 \times 10^{-6}H(cm)^{2.799}$	—[b]

[a] B = black, MA = Mexican American, W = white.
[b] Composite data from several studies.

Table B-8 Forced Expired Volume in 2 Seconds (FEV$_2$) Prediction Equations

Author	Date	Sex	Ages	Regression Equation	SEE
Adults					
Knudson et al[1]	1976	M	25–90	$0.061H(cm) - 0.032A - 5.021$	0.566
		F	25–90	$0.033H(cm) - 0.023A - 1.433$	0.474
Children and Adolescents					
Knudson et al[1]	1976	M	8–24	$0.056H(cm) + 0.056A - 5.484$	0.577
		F	8–19	$0.033H(cm) + 0.081A - 3.369$	0.485

Table B-9 Forced Expired Volume in 3 Seconds (FEV$_3$) Prediction Equations

Author	Date	Sex	Ages	Regression Equation	SEE
Adults					
Knudson et al[1]	1976	M	25–90	$0.063H(cm) - 0.031A - 5.245$	0.575
		F	25–90	$0.035H(cm) - 0.023A - 1.633$	0.496
Children and Adolescents					
Knudson et al[1]	1976	M	8–24	$0.052H(cm) + 0.066A - 5.531$	0.589
		F	8–19	$0.033H(cm) + 0.086A - 3.417$	0.510

Table B-10 Forced Expired Volume in 1 Second to Forced Vital Capacity Ratio (FEV$_1$/FVC) Prediction Equations

Author	Date	Sex	Ages	Regression Equation	SEE
Adults					
Morris et al[21]	1973	M	20–79	$-0.2253A + 84.64$	7.83
		F	20–79	$-0.1789A + 84.23$	6.84
Berglund et al[9]	1963	M	7–70	$-0.373A + 91.79$	7.19
		F	7–70	$-0.261A + 92.11$	5.44
Children and Adolescents					
Weng & Levison[10]	1971	M,F	4–18	85.83[a]	5.98 (SD)
Polgar & Promadhat[12]	1971	M,F	—[b]	86.1[a]	7.0 (SD)
Gandevia[22]	1960	M	5–14	$-0.098H(in) + 87.1$	—
		F	5–14	$-0.561H(in) + 113.9$	—

[a] Regression not significant on any variable.
[b] Composite data from several studies.

Table B-11 Peak Expiratory Flow Rate (PEFR) Prediction Equations

Author	Date	Sex	Ages	Regression Equation	SEE
Children and Adolescents					
Weng & Levison[10]	1969	M,F	4–18	$4.90H(cm) - 379.17$	2.45%
Hsu et al[11]	1979	M/MA[a]	7–20	$7.69 \times 10^{-4}H(cm)^{2.63}$	17%
		M/W	7–20	$3.35 \times 10^{-4}H(cm)^{2.79}$	18%
		M/B	7–20	$1.74 \times 10^{-4}H(cm)^{2.92}$	22%
		F/MA	7–20	$6.97 \times 10^{-4}H(cm)^{2.64}$	18%
		F/W	7–18	$2.58 \times 10^{-3}H(cm)^{2.37}$	18%
		F/B	7–20	$5.51 \times 10^{-4}H(cm)^{2.68}$	20%
Polgar & Promadhat[12]	1971	M,F	—[b]	$5.2428H(cm) - 425.5714$	—[b]
DeMuth et al[14]	1965	M	4–18	$4.796 \times 10^{-4}H(cm)^{2.642}$	—
		F	4–18	$1.415 \times 10^{-4}H(cm)^{2.864}$	—

[a] B = black, MA = Mexican-American, W = white.
[b] Composite data from several studies.

Table B-12 Maximal Forced Expiratory Flow (FEF$_{max}$) Prediction Equations

Author	Date	Sex	Ages	Regression Equation	SEE
Adults					
Knudson et al[1]	1976	M	25–90	$0.094H(cm) - 0.035A - 5.993$	2.078
		F	20–90	$0.049H(cm) - 0.025A - 0.735$	1.605
Bass[5]	1973	M	21–71+	$2.38S - 0.026A + 4.63$	1.48
		F	21–71+	$3.93S - 0.028A - 0.017W(lb) + 2.72$	1.13
Cherniack & Raber[6]	1972	M	15–79	$0.14393H(in) - 0.02403A + 0.22544$	—
		F	15–79	$0.09130H(in) - 0.01776A + 1.13160$	—
Ferris et al[8]	1965	M	25–74	$0.0788H(cm) - 0.0410A - 3.338$	1.51
		F	25–74	$0.0493H(cm) - 0.0285A - 0.6532$	1.15
Children and Adolescents					
Knudson et al[1]	1976	M	8–24	$0.078H(cm) + 0.166A - 8.060$	1.653
		F	8–19	$0.049H(cm) + 0.157A - 3.916$	1.339
Dickman et al[13]	1971	M	5–11	$0.161H(in) - 5.876$	0.451
		M	12–18	$0.181H(in) + 0.205A - 9.538$	0.780
		F	5–11	$0.130H(in) - 4.506$	0.487
		F	12–18	$0.100H(in) + 0.139A - 4.117$	0.798

Table B-13 Forced Expiratory Flow at 25% of the Vital Capacity (FEF$_{25\%}$) Prediction Equations

Author	Date	Sex	Ages	Regression Equation	SEE
Adults					
Knudson et al[1]	1976	M	25–90	$0.088H(cm) - 0.035A - 5.618$	2.012
		F	25–90	$0.043H(cm) - 0.025A - 0.132$	1.53
Bass[5]	1973	M	21–75	$2.88S - 0.031A + 3.38$	1.57
		F	21–75	$0.105H(in) - 0.024A - 0.30$	1.30
Cherniack & Raber[6]	1972	M	15–79	$0.03583H(in) - 0.04142A + 1.98361$	—
		F	15–79	$0.02334H(in) - 0.03450A + 2.21596$	—
Children and Adolescents					
Knudson et al[1]	1976	M	8–24	$0.070H(cm) + 0.147A - 7.054$	1.530
		F	8–19	$0.044H(cm) + 0.144A - 3.365$	1.290

Table B-14 Forced Expiratory Flow at 50% of the Vital Capacity (FEF$_{50\%}$) Prediction Equations

Author	Date	Sex	Ages	Regression Equation	SEE
Adults					
Knudson et al[1]	1976	M	25–90	$0.069H(cm) - 0.015A - 5.400$	1.422
		F	25–90	$0.035H(cm) - 0.013A - 0.444$	1.22
Bass[5]	1973	M	21–75	$2.35S - 0.107H(in) - 0.038A + 9.45$	1.34
		F	21–75	$-0.029A + 5.37$	1.10
Cherniack & Raber[6]	1972	M	15–79	$0.06526H(in) - 0.03049A + 2.40337$	—
		F	15–79	$0.06220H(in) - 0.02344A + 1.42640$	—
Children and Adolescents					
Knudson et al[1]	1976	M	8–24	$0.051H(cm) + 0.081A - 4.975$	1.102
		F	8–19	$0.034H(cm) + 0.120A - 2.531$	1.106

Table B-15 Forced Expiratory Flow at 75% of the Vital Capacity (FEF$_{75\%}$) Prediction Equations

Author	Date	Sex	Ages	Regression Equation	SEE
Adults					
Knudson et al[1]	1976	M	25–90	$0.044H(cm) - 0.012A - 4.143$	1.026
		F	25–90	$-0.014A + 3.042$	.936
Bass[5]	1973	M	21–75	$0.613S - 0.024A + 1.61$	.71
		F	21–75	$-0.023A + 2.59$	.58
Cherniack & Raber[6]	1972	M	15–79	$0.09030H(in) - 0.19870A + 2.72554$	—
		F	15–79	$0.06876H(in) - 0.01926A + 2.14653$	—
Children and Adolescents					
Knudson et al[1]	1976	M	8–24	$0.032H(cm) - 2.455$	.833
		F	8–19	$0.120A + 0.692$	.845

Table B-16 Forced Expiratory Flow from 200 to 1200 ml of the Vital Capacity (FEF$_{200-1200}$) Prediction Equations

Author	Date	Sex	Ages	Regression Equation	SEE
Adults					
Morris et al[2]	1971	M	20–84	$0.109H(\text{in}) - 0.047A + 2.010$	1.66
		F	20–84	$0.145H(\text{in}) - 0.036A - 2.532$	1.19
Schmidt et al[4]	1973	M	20–94	$0.130H(\text{cm}) - 0.068A + 0.940$	1.650
		F	20–94	$0.092H(\text{cm}) - 0.051A + 1.100$	1.024

Table B-17 Forced Mid-Expiratory Flow (FEF$_{25-75\%}$) Prediction Equations

Author	Date	Sex	Ages	Regression Equation	SEE
Adults					
Knudson et al[1]	1976	M	25–90	$0.045H(\text{cm}) - 0.031A - 1.864$	1.159
		F	20–90	$0.021H(\text{cm}) - 0.024A + 1.171$	0.993
Morris et al[2]	1971	M	20–84	$0.047H(\text{in}) - 0.045A + 2.513$	1.12
		F	20–84	$0.060H(\text{in}) - 0.030A + 0.551$	0.80
Schmidt et al[4]	1973	M	20–94	$0.051H(\text{in}) - 0.046A + 2.954$	0.844
		F	20–94	$0.043H(\text{in}) - 0.037A + 2.243$	0.576
Cherniack & Raber[6]	1972	M	15–79	$0.05948H(\text{in}) - 0.03700A + 2.61187$	—
		F	15–79	$0.04931H(\text{in}) - 0.03120A + 2.25610$	—
Birath et al[23]	1963	M	20–65	$-0.0523A + 5.85$	1.00
		F	20–65	$-0.0579A + 5.65$	0.71
Children and Adolescents					
Weng & Levison[10]	1969	M,F	4–18	$0.050H(\text{cm}) - 4.38$	32.9%
Knudson et al[1]	1976	M	8–24	$0.059H(\text{cm}) - 5.334$	0.933
		F	8–19	$0.025H(\text{cm}) + 0.121A - 1.893$	0.860
Hsu et al[11]	1979	M/MA[a]	7–20	$1.52 \times 10^{-5}H(\text{cm})^{2.45}$	25%
		M/W	7–20	$1.33 \times 10^{-5}H(\text{cm})^{2.46}$	26%
		M/B	7–20	$6.02 \times 10^{-6}H(\text{cm})^{2.60}$	36%
		F/MA	7–20	$2.00 \times 10^{-5}H(\text{cm})^{2.40}$	24%
		F/W	7–18	$6.32 \times 10^{-5}H(\text{cm})^{2.16}$	28%
		F/B	7–20	$2.42 \times 10^{-5}H(\text{cm})^{2.34}$	30%
Dickman et al[13]	1971	M	5–11	$0.094H(\text{in}) - 2.614$	0.388
		M	12–18	$0.135H(\text{in}) + 0.126A - 6.498$	0.612
		F	5–11	$0.087H(\text{in}) - 2.389$	0.347
		F	12–18	$0.093H(\text{in}) + 0.083A - 3.499$	0.621
Polgar & Promadhat[12]	1971	M,F	—[b]	$0.043H(\text{cm}) - 3.43$	—[b]
Cherniack[15]	1962	M	3–16	$0.0279H(\text{cm}) + 0.0259A - 1.75$	—
		F	3–16	$0.0198H(\text{cm}) + 0.0647A - 1.08$	—

[a] B = black, MA = Mexican American, W = white.
[b] Composite data from several studies.

Table B-18 Forced End-Expiratory Flow (FEF$_{75-85\%}$) Prediction Equations

Author	Date	Sex	Ages	Regression Equation	SEE
Adults					
Morris et al[24]	1975	M	20–85	$0.013H(\text{in}) - 0.023A + 1.210$	0.48
		F	20–85	$0.025H(\text{in}) - 0.021A + 0.321$	0.45

Table B-19 Maximum Voluntary Ventilation (MVV) Prediction Equations

Author	Date	Sex	Ages	Regression Equation	SEE
Adults					
Bass[5]	1973	M	21–75	$3.65H(in) - 0.814A - 76.78$	25.2
		F	21–75	$-0.692A + 127.43$	16.5
Cherniack & Raber[6]	1972	M	15–79	$3.02915H(in) - 0.81621A - 37.94893$	—
		F	15–79	$2.13844H(in) - 0.68503A - 4.86957$	—
Birath et al[23a]	1963	M	20–65	$-0.1288A + 180.5$	16.6
		F	20–65	$-0.618A + 113.1$	15.1
Kory et al[20]	1961	M	20–65	$1.34H(cm) - 1.26A - 21.4$	29
Children and Adolescents					
Weng & Levison[10]	1969	M,F	4–18	$1.50H(cm) - 134.61$	26.5%
Polgar & Promadhat[12]	1971	M,F	—[b]	$1.276H(cm) - 99.507$	—[b]
Cherniak[15]	1962	M	3–16	$1.075H(cm) + 2.165A - 89.66$	—
		F	3–16	$0.772H(cm) + 2.725A - 57.84$	—

[a] MVV fixed at frequency of 40/min.
[b] Composite data from several studies.

Table B-20 Specific Airway Conductance (Gaw/VL) Prediction Equations

Author	Date	Sex	Ages	Regression Equation	Range
Adults					
Doershuk et al[25]	1974	M,F	19–54	0.25	0.15–0.91
Skoogh[26]	1973	M,F	20–64	0.407	0.223–0.738
Briscoe & Dubois[27]	1958	M,F	4–87	0.24	0.13–0.35
Children and Adolescents					
Weng & Levison[10]	1969	M,F	4–18	$0.227 - 0.041/V_{TG}$	
Doershuk et al[25]	1974	M,F	1–5	0.23	0.15–0.63
		M,F	5–18	0.23	0.14–0.67
Zapletal et al[28]	1969	M,F	6–18	$0.17074 + 0.0025/V_{TG}$	—

Table B-21 Respiratory System Resistance (Rrs) Prediction Equations

Author	Date	Sex	Ages	Regression Equation	SEE
Adults					
Jiemsripong et al[29]	1976	M	21–64	$8.9/V_{TG}$	—
		F	21–64	$1/V_{TG}(0.562 - 0.00263H(cm))$	—
Fisher et al[30]	1968	M,F	18–79	$7.1/V_{TG}$	—
Children and Adolescents					
Mansell et al[31]	1972	M,F	3–17	$10^{(1.877-0.0089H(cm))}$	—
Williams et al[32]	1979	M,F	3–5	$11.02 - 0.0529H(cm)$	—

Table B-22 Static Expiratory Lung Compliance (CLst) Prediction Equations

Author	Date	Sex	Ages	Regression Equation	SEE
Adults					
Begin et al[33]	1975	M	20–82	$0.0131H(cm) + 0.0024A - 0.667$	0.066
		F		$0.0099H(cm) + 0.0019A - 0.471$	0.045
Frank et al[34]	1956	M,F	18–39	$0.00343H(cm) - 0.425$	0.035
Children and Adolescents					
Polgar & Promadhat[12]	1971	M,F	—[b]	$17.09 + 0.0459FRC$	—[b]
Kamel et al[35]	1969	M,F	7–23	$2.49 \times 10^{-8}H(cm)^{3.03}$	—
		M,F	7–23	$0.063FRC^{0.836}$	—

[a] Values measured at FRC
[b] Composite data from several studies

Table B-23 Maximal Respiratory Pressures (MIP and MEP) Prediction Equations

Author SEE	Date	Sex	Ages	Regression Equation[a]	
Adults					
Black & Hyatt[36]	1969	M	20–80	MIP $-0.55A + 143$	16
				MEP $-1.03A + 268$	37
		F	20–80	MIP $-0.51A + 104$	13
				MEP $-0.53A + 170$	20

[a] MIP: Maximal inspiratory pressure, measured at RV; MEP: Maximal expiratory pressure, measured at TLC.

Table B-24 Volume of Isoflow, Percent Vital Capacity ($V_{iso}\dot{v}$/VC%) Prediction Equations

Author	Date	Sex	Ages	Regression Equation	SEE
Adults					
Dosman et al[37]	1975	M,F	24–67	$0.291A + 4.917$	6.88
Gelb et al[38]	1975	M,F	42 ± 13.7	$0.450A + 4.69$	5.27

Table B-25 Change in $\dot{V}$max at 50 Percent of the Vital Capacity ($\Delta\dot{V}$max$_{50\%}$) Prediction Equations

Author	Date	Sex	Ages	Regression Equation	SEE
Adults					
Dosman et al[37]	1975	M,F	24–67	$-0.245A + 57.64$[a]	13.56
		M,F	24–67	47.3	27.4 (SD)

[a] No significant regression was noted on age, therefore the constant predicted value is given as a separate equation.

Table B-26 Closing Volume to Vital Capacity Ratio, Percent (CV/VC%) Prediction Equations

Author	Date	Sex	Ages	Regression Equation	SEE
Adults					
Buist et al[39]	1979	M	25–54	$0.40A - 1.89$	4.56
		F	25–54	$0.40A - 2.90$	4.56
Knudson et al[40]	1977	M,F	25–54	$0.269A - 0.882$	—
Gelb et al[38]	1975	M,F	42 ± 13.7	$0.3A - 0.1H(in) + 6.9$	5.00
Buist & Ross[41]	1973	M	16–83	$0.357A + 0.562$	4.15
		F	16–85	$0.293A + 2.812$	4.90
Children and Adolescents					
Mansell et al[42]	1972	M,F	6–18	$-1.25A + 26.12$	—

Table B-27 Closing Capacity to Total Lung Capacity Ratio, Percent (CC/TLC%) Prediction Equations

Author	Date	Sex	Ages	Regression Equation	SEE
Adults					
Buist et al[39]	1979	M	25–54	$0.53A + 13.25$	4.00
		F	25–54	$0.53A + 15.70$	4.00
Knudson et al[40]	1977	M,F	25–54	$0.471A - 11.492$	—
Gelb et al[38]	1975	M,F	42 ± 13.7	$0.58A + 16.485$	6.44
Buist & Ross[41]	1973	M	16–83	$0.496A + 14.878$	4.09
		F	16–85	$0.536A + 14.420$	4.43

Table B-28 Single Breath Nitrogen Phase III Slope ($\Delta N_2\%/L$) Prediction Equations

Author	Date	Sex	Ages	Regression Equation	SEE
Adults					
Buist et al[39]	1979	M	25–54	$0.001A + 0.81$	0.59
		F	25–54	$0.001A + 1.07$	0.59
Knudson et al[40]	1977	M,F	20–54	$-0.018H(\text{in}) - 0.0002A + 1.717$	—
			54+	$-0.036H(\text{in}) + 0.026A + 1.599$	—
Buist & Ross[43]	1973	M	16–83	$0.010A + 0.710$	0.43
		F	16–60	$0.009A + 1.036$	0.57
		F	61–85	$0.058A - 1.777$	1.30
Children and Adolescents					
Knudson et al[40]	1977	M,F	8–19	$-0.018H(\text{in}) + 1.771$	—

Table B-29 Carbon Monoxide Diffusing Capacity (DL_{CO}) Prediction Equations

Author	Date	Sex	Ages	Regression Equation	SEE
Adults					
			SINGLE BREATH METHOD		
Van Ganse et al[44]	1972	M	25–79	$0.212H(\text{cm}) - 0.246A + 0.572$	4.89
		F	24–76	$0.171H(\text{cm}) - 0.152A - 1.567$	3.72
Miller et al[45]	1983	M	41 ± 17	$0.418H(\text{cm}) - 0.229A + 12.91$	4.84
		F	45 ± 16	$0.407H(\text{cm}) - 0.111A + 2.238$	3.95
Crapo & Morris[46]	1981	M	15–91	$0.416H(\text{cm}) - 0.219A - 22.34$	4.83
		F	17–84	$0.256H(\text{cm}) - 0.144A - 8.36$	3.57
Frans et al[47]	1975	M	38 ± 12	$0.285H(\text{cm}) - 0.14A - 10.3$	4.2
Children and Adolescents					
			SINGLE BREATH METHOD		
Giammona & Daly[48]	1965	M,F	4–13	$0.0059\text{TLC} + 1.7$	—
		M,F	4–13	$21S - 4$	—
Bucci* et al[49]	1961	M,F		$0.384\text{TLC} + 5.5$	—
		M,F		$10^{(0.00656H(\text{cm})+0.308)}$	—
		M,F		$10^{(0.362S+0.806)}$	—
			STEADY STATE METHOD		
Weng & Levison[10]	1969	M,F	4–18	$0.228H(\text{cm}) - 17.56$	30.0%
		M,F	4–18	$14.4S - 2.63$	16.9%
			REBREATHING METHOD		
Demuth et al[14]	1965	M	4–18	$5.504 \times 10^{-6}H(\text{cm})^{2.767}$	—
		F	4–18	$4.969 \times 10^{-6}H(\text{cm})^{2.724}$	—

[a] Included 16 adults in sample of 59.

Table B-30 Specific Carbon Monoxide Diffusing Capacity (DL_{CO}/V_A) Prediction Equations

Author	Date	Sex	Ages	Regression Equation	SEE
Adults					
			SINGLE BREATH METHOD		
Van Ganse et al[44]	1972	M	25–79	$-0.0327A + 6.646$	1.150
		F	24–76	$-0.0098A + 5.869$	1.024
Crapo & Morris[46]	1981	M	15–91	$-0.034A + 7.08$	0.84
		F	17–84	$-0.025A + 6.58$	0.78
Frans et al[47]	1975	M	38 ± 12	$0.000157A^2 - 0.0296A + 6.18$	0.73

Table B-31 Membrane and Intracapillary Diffusing Capacity for Carbon Monoxide (DM_{CO}, θQc, and Qc^a) Prediction Equations

Author	Date	Sex	Ages		Regression Equation	SEE
Adults						
Frans et al[47]	1975	M	38 ± 12	(DM)	$0.56H(cm) - 0.29A - 31.3$	9.4
		M	38 ± 12	(Qc)	93.4	17.9 (SD)
Children and Adolescents						
Giammona & Daly[48]	1965	M,F	4–13	(DM)	$0.0126TLC + 5.9$	—
		M,F	4–13	(DM)	$0.042S + 42$	—
		M,F	4–13	(Qc)	$0.0124TLC + 24$	—
		M,F	4–13	(Qc)	$4.2S + 52$	—
Bucci[b] et al[49]	1961	M,F	7–40	(DM)	$1.1TLC + 3$	—
		M,F	7–40	(DM)	$10^{(0.00855H(cm)+0.333)}$	—
		M,F	7–40	(DM)	$10^{(0.448S+1.033)}$	—
		M,F	7–40	(Qc)	$9.3TLC + 16.5$	—
		M,F	7–40	(Qc)	$10^{(0.00684H(cm)+0.674)}$	—
		M,F	7–40	(Qc)	$10^{(0.359S+1.220)}$	—

[a] Commonly abbreviated Vc.
[b] Included 16 adults in sample of 59.

Table B-32 Specific Membrane and Intracapillary Diffusing Capacity for Carbon Monoxide (DM_{CO}/VA and $\theta Qc/VA$) Prediction Equations

Author	Date	Sex	Ages		Regression Equation	SEE
Adults						
Frans et al[47]	1975	M	38 ± 12	(DM/VA)	$0.000688A^2 - 0.0936A - 11.06$	1.39
		M	38 ± 12	($\theta Qc/VA$)	14.52	3.21 (SD)

ANNOTATED REFERENCES

1. Knudson, RJ, Slatin, RC, Lebowitz, MD, Burrows, B: The maximal expiratory flow-volume curve. Normal standards, variability, and effects of age. Am Rev Respir Dis 113:587, 1976.
   Flow-volume loops were obtained from 746 asymptomatic nonsmoking white subjects randomly selected in Tucson, Arizona. The recording device was a portable pneumotachometer that was tested against Stead-Wells spirometers for accuracy. The best two of five curves were averaged and corrected to BTPS.

2. Morris, JF, Koski, A, Johnson, LC: Spirometric standards for healthy nonsmoking adults. Am Rev Respir Dis 103:57, 1971
   This study used a sample of 988 nonsmoking asymptomatic adults from an area of Oregon free of air pollution at an altitude less than 500 feet above sea level. Most (79 percent) were church members. Stead-Wells spirometers were used to obtain at least two tracings from subjects in the standing position. Calculations, reported in BTPS, were based on the method of Kory et al[20]

3. Lapp, NL, Amandus, HE, Hall, R, Morgan, WKC: Lung volumes and flow rates in black and white subjects. Thorax 29:185, 1974.
   A study of more than 9000 coal miners from which 66 blacks and 66 matched whites were used to develop prediction equations. Smokers were accepted but all were asymptomatic with normal chest radiographs.

4. Schmidt, CD, Dickman, ML, Gardner, RM, Brough, FK: Spirometric standards for healthy elderly men and women. Am Rev Respir Dis 108:933, 1973
   Spirometric measurements from 532 elderly subjects were combined with those from a sample of younger subjects for a total of 1177 volunteer smoking and nonsmoking

asymptomatic subjects from Salt Lake City, Utah (820 males and 357 females). A computerized 13.5 liter Collins spirometer was used to obtain at least three spirograms on each subject.

5. Bass, H: The flow volume loop: Normal standards and abnormalities in chronic obstructive pulmonary disease. Chest 63:171, 1973
    A sample of 247 asymptomatic nonsmoking adults, presumably from the Boston area, were tested with a wedge spirometer. Two loops were obtained from each subject.

6. Cherniack, RM, Raber, MB: Normal standards for ventilatory function using an automated wedge spirometer. Am Rev Respir Dis 106:38, 1972
    Prediction standards were obtained from a sample of 879 male and 452 female healthy nonsmokers residing in Manitoba, Canada, a pollution-free area. A wedge spirometer was used to obtain at least three tracings from each subject in the standing position.

7. Abramowitz, S, Leiner, GC, Lewis, WA, Small, MJ: Vital capacity in the Negro. Am Rev Respir Dis 92:287, 1965.
    Spirometry was performed by 161 black and white males and females who were hospital employees and physicians in East Orange, New Jersey. All were asymptomatic with negative chest radiographs. A Gaensler-Collins timed vitalometer was used for measurements and reported in BTPS. The method of Kory et al[20] was used for calculations. Prediction equations were reported for FVC. No difference between blacks and whites was found for the forced expired volumes and peak flow.

8. Ferris, BG, Anderson, DO, Zickmantel, R: Prediction values for screening tests of pulmonary function. Am Rev Respir Dis 91:252, 1965
    A random sample was drawn from a town register of Berlin, New Hampshire. A total of 1227 asymptomatic adults were studied, and separate equations for the 156 male and 433 female nonsmokers were derived. Five tracings from each subject were recorded on a 6 liter Collins vitalometer (corrected to BTPS), and peak flow was obtained with a Wright peak flowmeter. The mean of the last three measurements was used as the true value. Timing was by back-extrapolation.

9. Berglund, E, Birath, G, Bjure, J et al: Spirometric studies in normal subjects. Part I. Forced expirograms in subjects between 7 and 70 years of age. Acta Med Scand 173:185, 1963
    Two hundred ninety-six male and 201 female residents of Sweden were studied and equations were derived for those above age 20. A Plexiglas bell water seal spirometer was used, with subjects in the sitting position. Values were reported in ATPS. Three to five tracings were recorded. The starting point was defined as the point where the first deflection occurred.

10. Weng, T, Levison, H: Standards of pulmonary function in children. Am Rev Respir Dis 99:879, 1969
    Complete pulmonary function studies were performed on 62 boys and 77 girls. Most were children of relatives of physicians. Lung volumes were obtained with a 9 liter spirometer using the closed circuit method. Forced expiratory measurements were obtained with the same instrument. Diffusing capacity was measured using the steady state method. Airway resistance was obtained with a 600 liter plethysmograph.

11. Hsu, KHK, Jenkins, DE, Hsi, BP et al: Ventilatory functions of normal children and young adults-Mexican-American, white, and black. Part I. Spirometry. J Ped 95:14, 1979
    This study was designed to study spirometry in asymptomatic nonsmoking Mexican-American and black children as well as white children. The children were selected from several schools in the area of Houston, Texas with various pollution levels. A dry seal spirometer was used to record spirograms in the standing position until two satisfactory tracings were obtained. All volumes were corrected to BTPS.

12. Polgar, G, Promadhat, V: Pulmonary Function Testing in Children: Techniques and Standards. WB Saunders Co, Philadelphia, 1971
    A textbook that presents twelve studies by other authors and derives equations which are a composite of these studies.

13. Dickman, ML, Schmidt, CD, Gardner, RM: Spirometric standards for normal children and adolescents (ages 5 years through 18 years). Am Rev Respir Dis 104:680, 1971
    A 13.5 liter Collins water seal spirometer was used to obtain spirograms on 482 healthy boys and 468 healthy girls in the area of Salt Lake City, Utah.
14. Demuth, GR, Howatt, WF, Hill, BM: The growth of lung function. Pediatrics 35(suppl):159, 1965
    A study of a comprehensive battery of tests in 147 school children in Ann Arbor, Michigan.
15. Cherniack, RM: Ventilatory function in normal children. Can Med Assoc J 87:80, 1962
    Two hundred sixty boys and 261 girls from the wards and outpatient clinics in Winnepeg, Manitoba were studied with a 9 liter Collins water seal spirometer. All were free of cardiopulmonary disease.
16. Boren, HG, Kory, RC, Syner, JC: The Veterans Administration-Army cooperative study of pulmonary function. Part II. The lung volume and its subdivisions in normal men. Am J Med 41:96, 1966.
    A total of 422 male subjects selected from hospital employees, military personnel, medical students, physicians, and patients, from 15 hospitals were studied with helium dilution and nitrogen washout methods.
17. Grimby, G, & Soderholm, B.: Spirometric studies in normal subjects. Part III. Static lung volumes and maximum voluntary ventilation in adults with a note on physical fitness. Acta Med Scand 173:199, 1963
    The study consisted of 152 men and 58 women from Sweden in whom lung volumes were determined.
18. Goldman, HI, Becklake, MR: Respiratory function tests. Normal values at median altitudes and the prediction of normal results. Am Rev Respir Dis 79:457, 1959
    Forty four male and 50 female asymptomatic subjects were tested. The subjects were medical and clerical workers and relatives living at an altitude of 5760 feet. Spirometry was performed in the sitting position with a Knipping-type spirometer. FRC was measured by the closed circuit method using hydrogen as the test gas. All volumes were adjusted to BTPS.
19. Needham, CD, Rogan, MC, McDonald, I: Normal standards for lung volumes, intrapulmonary gas mixing, and maximum breathing capacity. Thorax 9:313, 1954.
    Two age groups, 11 to 19 and 20 to 70 years, consisting of 105 men, 69 women, and 150 children were studied at sea level. All were asymptomatic, but smokers were included. Closed circuit helium dilution was used for lung volumes.
20. Kory, RC, Callahan, R, Boren, HG, Syner, JC: The Veterans Administration-Army cooperative study of pulmonary function. Part I. Clinical spirometry in normal men. Am J Med 30:243, 1961
    A study of 468 male subjects selected from among hospital employees, patients, medical students, and resident and full-time physicians of 15 cooperating hospitals. All measurements were made on a 13.5 liter Collins spirometer, and repeated until values reached 5 percent agreement. Volumes were converted to BTPS. The starting point for timing was 200 ml below the baseline.
21. Morris, JF, Temple, WP, Koski, A: Normal values for the ratio of one-second forced expiratory volume to forced vital capacity. Am Rev Respir Dis 108:1000, 1973
    Using the same population in Morris et al[2] of 963 healthy nonsmoking adults in Oregon, the FEV$_1$/FVC ratio was calculated.
22. Gandevia, B: Normal standards for single breath tests of ventilatory capacity in children. Arch Dis Child 35:236, 1960.
    Ninety-one boys and 79 girls randomly chosen from among school children in Melbourne, underwent spirometry.
23. Birath, G, Kjellmer, I, Sandqvist, L: Spirometric studies in normal subjects. Part II. Ventilatory capacity tests in adults. Acta Med Scand 173:193, 1963.

A group of 62 male and 58 female asymptomatic students, nurses, factory workers, office workers, and housewives was studied. All had normal chest radiographs, but smokers were included. The equipment used was that of Berglund et al.[9]

24. Morris, JF, Koski, A, Breese, JD: Normal values and evaluation of forced end-expiratory flow. Am Rev Respir Dis 111:755, 1975

The end-expiratory flow was calculated from the spirograms obtained from the 803 of 988 asymptomatic subjects from Oregon reported in a previous study by Morris et al,[2] and used to form prediction equations. For this test, the 75 percent of normal limit was more useful than the −1.65 SEE limit in screening for abnormalities.

25. Doershuk, CF, Fisher, BJ, Matthews, LW: Specific airway resistance from the perinatal period into adulthood. Am Rev Respir Dis 109:452, 1974

Specific airway resistance at FRC was measured in 51 newborns, 35 young children, 103 older children and adolescents, and 74 adults who were healthy and asymptomatic. A minority of adults were smokers, but smoked less than one pack per day. A 120 liter pressure plethysmograh was used for those under age five, and a 620 liter pressure plethysmograph was used for those older than five.

26. Skoogh, B-E: Normal airways conductance at different lung volumes. Scand J Clin Lab Invest 31:429, 1973

Twenty-nine men and 27 women who were free from symptoms, were nonsmokers, and had normal chest radiographs were studied in a volume displacement body plethysmograph. Gaw was calculated at different volumes in each subject, from which a regression line was derived to obtain SGaw. Each conductance line encompassed a range of 50 percent of the vital capacity.

27. Briscoe, WA, DuBois, AB: The relationship between airway resistance, airway conductance, and lung volume in subjects of different age and body size. J Clin Invest 37:1279, 1958

A 600 liter pressure body plethysmograph was used to measure airway resistance at FRC in 8 children, 7 women, and 11 men.

28. Zapletal, A, Motoyama, EK, Van de Woestijne, KP et al: Maximum expiratory flow-volume curves and airway conductance in children and adolescents. J Appl Physiol 26:308, 1969

A group of volunteer subjects, 39 boys and 26 girls, was studied with volume displacement plethysmography for airway conductance and MEFV curves. Equations were derived for Gaw as a function of VTG.

29. Jiemsripong, K, Hyatt, RE, Offord, KP: Total respiratory resistance by forced oscillation in normal subjects. Mayo Clin Proc 51:553, 1976

The method of forced oscillation was used in a study group of 76 asymptomatic nonsmoking women and men. Subjects were tested at a frequency of 3 Hz with forced flow superimposed over tidal breathing.

30. Fisher, AB, DuBois, AB, Hyde, RW: Evaluation of the forced oscillation technique for the determination of resistance to breathing. J Clin Invest 47:2045, 1968

The forced oscillation technique was performed on 25 male and 17 female subjects who had no pulmonary abnormality and who were living in Philadelphia. Some of the subjects were smokers. The variable frequency method was used.

31. Mansell, A, Levison, H, Kruger, K. & Tripp, TL.: Measurement of respiratory resistance in children in forced oscillations. Am Rev Respir Dis 106:710, 1972

The subjects were 79 normal children who were relatives of hospital personnel and patients in Ontario, Canada with nonrespiratory disorders. A fixed frequency of 5 Hz was superimposed over normal tidal breathing.

32. Williams, SP, Fullton, JM, Tsai, MJ et al: Respiratory impedance and derived parameters in young children by forced random noise. J Appl Physiol 47:169, 1979

Sixteen children in a day-care center were studied using forced signals of random frequency, from which respiratory resistance was obtained by methods based on spectral analysis.

33. Begin, R, Renzetti, AD Jr, Bigler, AH & Watanabe, S.: Flow and age dependence of airway closure and dynamic compliance. J Appl Physiol 38:199, 1975
    The single breath nitrogen test, spirometry, and airway resistance and gas dilution volume measurements were performed in 40 male and 26 female asymptomatic subjects with normal chest radiographs, from Salt Lake City, Utah.

34. Frank, NR, Mead, J, Siebens, AA, Storey, CF: Measurements of pulmonary compliance in 70 healthy young adults. J Appl Physiol 9:38, 1956
    Pulmonary compliance was measured by the interrupted breathing method using an esophageal balloon in 38 men and 32 women in St. Albans, New York. Subjects were tested in the seated position.

35. Kamel, M, Weng, TR, Featherby, EA et al: Relationship of mechanics of ventilation to lung volumes in children and young adults. Scand J Respir Dis 50:125, 1969
    Twenty-five boys and 14 girls from Toronto, Canada were studied. Compliance was measured at FRC with an esophageal balloon.

36. Black, LF, Hyatt, RE: Maximal respiratory pressures: normal values and relationship to age and sex. Am Rev Respir Dis 99:696, 1969
    Maximal respiratory pressures were measured in 60 men and 60 women while seated. Subjects were outpatients without respiratory symptoms and with normal chest radiographs who were seen for general physical examinations in Rochester, Minnesota.

37. Dosman, J, Bode, F, Urbanetti, J et al: The use of a helium-oxygen mixture during maximum expiratory flow to demonstrate obstruction in small airways in smokers. J Clin Invest 55:1090, 1975
    The study involved volume of isoflow measurements in 66 nonsmokers without respiratory disease, in Montreal, Canada. FRC was measured by plethysmography and flow-volume by pneumotachometry.

38. Gelb, AF, Molony, PA, Klein, E, Aronstam, PS: Sensitivity of volume of isoflow in the detection of mild airway obstruction. Am Rev Respir Dis 112:401, 1975
    Volume of isoflow was measured in thirty-four male and 9 female asymptomatic volunteers in Long Beach, California using 80 percent helium and 20 percent oxygen, in the sitting position. A waterless spirometer was used for flow-volume and FRC was measured by plethysmography.

39. Buist, AS, Ghezzo, H, Anthonisen, NR et al: Relationship between the single-breath N_2 test and age, sex and smoking habit in three North American cities. Am Rev Respir Dis 120:305, 1979
    This report describes a collaborative study conducted in Portland, Oregon, Montreal, and Winnepeg involving 122 male and 191 female subjects. The single breath nitrogen test and conventional measures of airflow obstruction were performed.

40. Knudson, RJ, Lebowitz, MD, Burton, AP & Knudson, DE: The closing volume test: Evaluation of nitrogen and bolus methods in a random population. Am Rev Respir Dis 115:423, 1977
    Using Fowler's single breath nitrogen method and a bolus helium method, 1900 random white subjects from Tucson, Arizona were studied. A dry rolling seal spirometer-mass spectrometer system was used.

41. Buist, AS, Ross, BB: Predicted values for closing volumes using a modified single breath N_2 test. Am Rev Respir Dis 107:744, 1973
    The researchers selected 132 male and 152 female asymptomatic nonsmokers of Portland, Oregon who were employees of the University of Oregon Medical School and screenees of an emphysema screening center, and studied them using Fowler's single breath method. A Stead-Wells spirometer and a rapid response nitrogen meter were used.

42. Mansell, A, Bryan, C, Levison, H: Airway closure in children. J Appl Physiol 33:711, 1972

*Fowler's single breath nitrogen test was used in 62 normal children of Toronto,
Canada to measure closing volume with a wedge spirometer and rapid response
nitrogen meter.*

43. Buist, AS, Ross, BB: Quantitative analysis of the alveolar plateau in the diagnosis of
early airway obstruction. Am Rev Respir Dis 108:1078, 1973
    *The slope of phase III from single breath N₂ tests of 134 males and 203 females from
    the population sample in the reference 41 is studied.*
44. Van Ganse, WF, Ferris, BG, Cotes, JE: Cigarette smoking and pulmonary diffusing
capacity (transfer factor). Am Rev Respir Dis 105:30, 1972
    *The study included 142 normal adult subjects (70 male and 72 female) from Berlin,
    New Hampshire in which the single breath diffusing capacity was measured by
    Forster's modification of the Krogh technique as standardized by Ogilvie et al. (see refs
    1, 3, and 4 in Chap. 9).*
45. Miller, A, Thornton, JC, Warshaw, R et al: Single breath diffusing capacity in a
representative sample of the population of Michigan, a large industrial state. Predicted values, lower limits of normal, and frequencies of abnormality by smoking
history. Am Rev Respir Dis 127:270, 1983
    *Seventy-four male and 130 female nonsmokers obtained by a random sample of
    households throughout Michigan were tested with the single breath diffusion test.*
46. Crapo, RO, Morris, AH: Standardized single breath normal values for carbon monoxide diffusing capacity. Am Rev Respir Dis 123:185, 1981
    *The Intermountain Thoracic Society technique was used to measure diffusing capac-
    ity in 122 male and 123 female nonsmoking members of the Church of Jesus Christ of
    Latter-Day Saints in Salt Lake City, Utah, at an altitude of 1400 meters.*
47. Frans, A, Stanescu, DC, Veriter, C et al: Smoking and pulmonary diffusing capacity.
Scand J Respir Dis 56:165, 1975
    *The study involved 64 asymptomatic nonsmoking medical and paramedical personnel
    in Belgium and used the method of Ogilvie et al (see refs 1, 3, and 4 in Chap. 9), to
    measure the single breath diffusing capacity. In 14 subjects membrane diffusion and
    capillary volume were measured.*
48. Giammona, STJ, Daly, WJ: Pulmonary diffusing capacity in normal children, ages 4 to
13. Am J Dis Child 110:144, 1965
    *Twenty children of physicians in Indiana were studied. Diffusing capacity was
    measured by the Forster/Ogilvie modification of the Krogh method, and membrane
    diffusion and capillary volume by the method of Roughton and Forster (see refs 1, 3,
    and 4 in Chap. 9).*
49. Bucci, G, Cook, CO, Barrie, H: Studies of respiratory physiology in children. Part V.
Total lung diffusing, diffusing capacity of pulmonary membrane, and pulmonary
capillary blood volume in normal subjects from 7 to 40 years. J Ped 58:820, 1961.
    *Fifty-nine normal subjects from Boston, Massachusetts, of which 16 were adults and
    43 were children, were tested for diffusion capacity by the Ogilvie modification of the
    Krogh method. Membrane diffusion and capillary volume were determined by the
    method of Roughton and Forster (see Ref. 10 in Chap. 9).*

Appendix C

Derivation of Equations Used in Pulmonary Function Testing

Steven A. Conrad, M.D.

This appendix describes the derivations of many of the equations used in the testing of pulmonary function and presented in this book. The final equations are developed from simple starting assumptions in a step-by-step fashion. For those with a deeper interest in methods, this appendix provides an in-depth analysis of the physiologic basis of certain pulmonary function tests. The appendix is organized into functional categories in a fashion similar to Section II of the book, and most of the derivations require only a knowledge of basic algebra.

GAS DILUTION VOLUME METHODS

The underlying principle in gas dilution determinations is that mass is conserved in a closed system despite changes in its volume. This is expressed in equation form as

$$M_i = M_f$$

where M_i is the initial mass within the system and M_f is the mass after a change in the system volume. Since the mass of a gas at a constant pressure is directly proportional to its volume, then we can substitute gas volume for mass, where gas volume is equal to its fractional concentration (F) times the system volume (V).

$$V_i F_i = V_f F_f$$

This basic principle is applied to volume determination by rearranging to give

$$V_f = V_i(F_i/F_f) \qquad \text{(Eq. C-1)}$$

If we know the initial volume V_i of the system and the fractional concentration of the gas prior to a change in system volume F_i, and we measure the fractional concentration after the change in system volume F_f, then we can calculate the new system volume V_f. The method involves an important assumption—that the gas within the system is well mixed and its concentration is the same throughout the system.

Equation C-1 can be modified to suit the configuration of a particular method. Some of the most common methods are described below.

Helium Equilibrium Method (Constant Volume)

In this method, helium in a spirometer system of volume Vs at initial concentration F_iHe distributes into a new volume consisting of the spirometer plus the FRC of the subject (Vs + FRC) with a final concentration F_fHe. The equation is

$$(Vs + FRC)F_f He = Vs(F_i He) \qquad \text{(Eq. C-2)}$$

which rearranges to

$$FRC(F_f He) = Vs(F_i He) - Vs(F_f He)$$

or

$$FRC = Vs \frac{F_i He - F_f He}{F_f He} \qquad \text{(Eq. C-3)}$$

The spirometer system volume Vs typically includes the volume under the bell or within the housing and all dead space produced by conduits and connections.

Helium Equilibration Method (Decreasing Volume)

In this method the spirometer system is filled with helium to a volume designated VHe. The initial spirometer system volume then consists of the helium volume. The concentration is unity prior to adding oxygen. Since the added oxygen is consumed by the end of the procedure, the *effective* initial concentration is still unity ($F_i He = 1$).

The final volume consists of the FRC, system dead space DS, and the volume of He added. The final system He concentration is designated F_fHe. The equation is

$$(FRC + VHe + DS)F_f He = VHe(F_i He) = VHe \qquad \text{(Eq. C-4)}$$

or

$$FRC(F_f He) + (VHe + DS)F_f He = VHe$$

which rearranges to

$$FRC = \frac{V_{He} - (V_{He} + DS)F_f He}{F_f He}$$

or

$$FRC = (V_{He}/F_f He) - (V_{He} + DS) \qquad \text{(Eq. C-5)}$$

Nitrogen Equilibration Method

The nitrogen contained in the FRC is distributed into a new volume consisting of the FRC plus the spirometer

$$FRC(F_i N_2) = (FRC + V_S)F_f N_2 \qquad \text{(Eq. C-6)}$$

which is similar to the equation for the helium method. Since nitrogen diffuses more readily than helium, the volume of gas in the spirometer has a contribution from the volume of nitrogen that diffused from the blood and tissues ($V_t N_2$), which must be subtracted:

$$FRC(F_i N_2) = (FRC + V_S)F_f N_2 - V_t N_2 \qquad \text{(Eq. C-7)}$$

which rearranges to

$$FRC(F_i N_2 - F_f N_2) = V_S(F_f N_2) - V_t N_2$$

or

$$FRC = \frac{V_S(F_f N_2) - V_t N_2}{(F_i N_2 - F_f N_2)} \qquad \text{(Eq. C-8)}$$

Multibreath Nitrogen Washout Method

In this method there is incomplete equilibrium between the alveolar nitrogen concentration and the nitrogen concentration in the mixed expired gas. This calculation is approached in a slightly different manner:

$$N_2 \text{ volume lost from lungs} = N_2 \text{ volume gained by reservoir} \quad \text{(Eq. C-9)}$$

where:

$$N_2 \text{ volume lost} = FRC(F_i N_2 - F_f N_2) + V_t N_2$$

and

$$N_2 \text{ volume gained} = V_E(F_e He)$$

Thus Equation C becomes:

$$FRC(F_iN_2 - F_fN_2) + V_tN_2 = V_E(F_eN_2)$$

or

$$FRC = \frac{V_E(F_eN_2) - V_tN_2}{F_iN_2 - F_fN_2} \qquad \text{(Eq. C-10)}$$

which is the equation for the reservoir method. If the open analyzer method is used, the equipment reports the volume of nitrogen exhaled (V_eN_2) as opposed to the nitrogen concentration and volume of exhaled volume. Equation C-10 then becomes

$$FRC = \frac{V_eN_2 - V_tN_2}{F_iN_2 - F_fN_2} \qquad \text{(Eq. C-11)}$$

Single Breath Nitrogen Method

In the single breath test the nitrogen present in the residual volume is distributed into a new volume (the TLC) following the inhalation of oxygen. Since TLC = VC + RV, we have the following balance equation:

$$RV(F_iN_2) = (RV + VC)F_eN_2 \qquad \text{(Eq. C-12)}$$

where F_iN_2 is the initial alveolar nitrogen concentration, usually estimated as 0.81 instead of measured, and F_eN_2 is the average concentration of nitrogen in the exhaled gas, measured by the method described in Chapter 6. The above equation rearranges to:

$$RV(F_iN_2 - F_eN_2) = VC(F_eN_2)$$

or

$$RV = VC \frac{F_eN_2}{F_iN_2 - F_eN_2} \qquad \text{(Eq. C-13)}$$

If the volume of interest is TLC instead of RV, Equation C-12 can be rewritten:

$$(TLC - VC)F_iN_2 = TLC(F_eN_2)$$

which rearranges to

$$TLC(F_iN_2 - F_eN_2) = VC(F_iN_2)$$

or

$$TLC = VC \frac{F_iN_2}{F_iN_2 - F_eN_2} \qquad \text{(Eq. C-14)}$$

BODY PLETHYSMOGRAPHY

Thoracic Gas Volume

The physical behavior of ideal gases is described by the general gas law

$$PV = nRT \qquad \text{(Eq. C-15)}$$

where P is absolute pressure, V is volume, n is the molar fraction (number of moles of gas), R is a constant, and T is the absolute temperature. The value of R depends upon the units of measurement used.

Boyle's law is a simplification of the general gas law in which temperature is held constant, so that the value nRT may be expressed as a constant (k):

$$PV = k$$

with the result that pressure is inversely proportional to volume. If we increase the volume of a given mass of gas by a small fraction ΔV, to $V + \Delta V$, the pressure will decrease by the small value ΔP, to $P - \Delta P$. Since the product is the constant k, we have:

$$PV = (V + \Delta V)(P - \Delta P) \qquad \text{(Eq. C-16)}$$

By expansion of the product on the right:

$$PV = V(P - \Delta P) + (P - \Delta P)\Delta V$$
$$= PV - V\Delta P + (P - \Delta P)\Delta V$$

This rearranges to

$$V\Delta P = (P - \Delta P)\Delta V$$

or

$$V = (P - \Delta P)(\Delta V/\Delta P)$$

Since ΔP is a small fraction of P, the value $(P - \Delta P)$ may be approximated by the value P with little loss of accuracy, leading to:

$$V = P(\Delta V/\Delta P) \qquad \text{(Eq. C-17)}$$

where V represents the absolute gas volume (of the thoracic cavity, V_{TG}), P the absolute pressure (atmospheric), and ΔP the small change in intrathoracic pressure resulting from changing the intrathoracic volume by the small quantity ΔV. This is the plethysmographic equation for V_{TG}.

In a volume plethysmograph the values for ΔV and ΔP can be directly measured. The use of a pressure plethysmograph, however, requires that box pressure be used to estimate the change in intrathoracic volume. To do this, the pressure-volume relationship of the box must be determined at a frequency corresponding to the panting frequency by measuring the pressure response to a cyclically injected volume. This is nearly linear for small volume, and defined by:

$$C_{box} = \Delta V_{box}/\Delta P_{box} \qquad \text{(Eq. C-18)}$$

Since, by rearranging:

$$\Delta V_{box} = C_{box}(\Delta P_{box})$$

we can substitute:

$$V_{TG} = P_B(\Delta P_{box}/\Delta P_{ao})C_{box} \qquad \text{(Eq. C-19)}$$

where V_{TG} is the thoracic gas volume, P_B is the barometric pressure, P_{ao} and P_{box} are airway and box pressures, respectively, and C_{box} is the box compliance as determined above. This is the plethysmographic V_{TG} equation for the pressure plethysmograph.

DISTRIBUTION OF VENTILATION AND PERFUSION

Alveolar Gas Equation

The alveolar gas equation, commonly used in clinical practice, was derived by Gray for the study of the oxygen requirements and the use of inspired carbon dioxide at altitude.[1,2] His derivation is summarized here.

The alveolar respiratory quotient (RQ) is defined as the volume of CO_2 (V_{CO_2}) eliminated by the lungs, divided by the volume of O_2 absorbed from the lungs (V_{O_2}). In the steady state this is equal to the minute CO_2 production ($\dot{V}_{CO_2}$) divided by the minute O_2 consumption ($\dot{V}_{O_2}$):

$$RQ = \frac{V_{CO_2}}{V_{O_2}} = \frac{\dot{V}_{CO_2}}{\dot{V}_{O_2}} \text{ (steady state)} \qquad \text{(Eq. C-20)}$$

The volume of CO_2 transferred to the alveoli during a breath is the difference in the total alveolar volume of CO_2 before and after gas exchange during a single breath. The volume is calculated from the total alveolar volume before (V_{A_i}) and after (V_{A_f}), as well as the fractional concentrations of CO_2 before ($F_iA_{CO_2}$) and after ($F_fA_{CO_2}$) gas exchange:

$$\begin{aligned}
V_{CO_2} &= V_f A_{CO_2} - V_i A_{CO_2} \\
&= F_f A_{CO_2}(V_{A_f}) - F_i A_{CO_2}(V_{A_i}) \\
&= \frac{P_{A_{CO_2}}}{P_B} V_{A_f} - \frac{P_B - P_{H_2O}}{P_B} F_{I_{CO_2}}(V_{A_f})
\end{aligned} \qquad \text{(Eq. C-21)}$$

$P_{A_{CO_2}}$ is the alveolar CO_2 tension after gas exchange, P_B is the barometric pressure, and P_{H_2O} is the water vapor pressure. $F_{I_{CO_2}}$ is the inspired CO_2 fractional concentration. The factor $(P_B - P_{H_2O})/P_B$ is the dilution factor resulting from humidification of inspired gas.

Similarly, the volume of oxygen transferred from the alveoli to the pulmonary blood is the difference in the total alveolar volume of O_2 before and after gas exchange:

$$\begin{aligned}
V_{O_2} &= V_i A_{O_2} - V_f A_{O_2} \\
&= F_i A_{O_2}(V_{A_i}) - F_f A_{O_2}(V_{A_f}) \\
&= \frac{P_B - P_{H_2O}}{P_B} F_{I_{O_2}}(V_{A_i}) - (P_{A_{O_2}}/P_B)V_{A_f}
\end{aligned} \qquad \text{(Eq. C-22)}$$

Substituting Equations C-21 and C-22 into C-20, then rearranging the resulting equation to solve for V_{A_i}, we obtain

$$V_{A_i} = \frac{P_{A_{CO_2}} + RQ(P_{A_{O_2}})}{(P_B - P_{H_2O})(RQ(F_{I_{O_2}}) + F_{I_{CO_2}})} \cdot V_{A_f} \qquad \text{(Eq. C-23)}$$

We now examine nitrogen balance. The volume of N_2 at the beginning of gas exchange is:

$$V_i N_2 = \frac{P_B - P_{H_2O}}{P_B} F_{I_{N_2}}(V_{A_f}) \qquad \text{(Eq. C-24)}$$

where $F_{I_{N_2}}$ is the fractional concentration of N_2 in dry inspired air and V_{A_i} is the alveolar volume at the beginning of gas exchange. After gas exchange, the N_2 concentration has changed as a result of exchange of O_2 for CO_2:

$$V_f N_2 = (P_{A_{N_2}}/P_B)V_{A_f} \qquad \text{(Eq. C-25)}$$

where $P_{A_{N_2}}$ is the alveolar partial pressure of N_2 after gas exchange has taken place.

Since N_2 does not readily cross the alveolar-capillary membrane, the volume of N_2 does not change (only its concentration changes), so that

$$V_f N_2 = V_i N_2 \qquad \text{(Eq. C-26)}$$

Substituting Equations C-24 and C-25 into C-26 and rearranging for $P_{A_{N_2}}$ yields

$$P_{A_{N_2}} = (P_B - P_{H_2O})F_{I_{N_2}}(V_{A_i}/V_{A_f}) \qquad \text{(Eq. C-27)}$$

Substituting Equation C-23 into C-27 yields

$$P_{A_{N_2}} = \frac{P_{A_{CO_2}} + RQ(P_{A_{O_2}})}{F_{I_{CO_2}} + RQ(F_{I_{O_2}})} F_{I_{N_2}} \qquad \text{(Eq. C-28)}$$

The partial pressures of N_2, O_2, CO_2 and H_2O sum to give P_B (other gases exist in insignificant concentrations):

$$P_B = P_{A_{N_2}} + P_{A_{O_2}} + P_{A_{CO_2}} + P_{H_2O} \qquad \text{(Eq. C-29)}$$

Substituting Equation C-28 into C-29 and rearranging for $P_{A_{O_2}}$ yields

$$P_{A_{O_2}} = \frac{(P_B - P_{H_2O} - P_{A_{CO_2}})(F_{I_{CO_2}} + RQ(F_{I_{O_2}})) - F_{I_{N_2}}(P_{A_{CO_2}})}{RQ(F_{I_{N_2}} + F_{I_{O_2}}) + F_{I_{CO_2}}}$$

By substituting $(1 - F_{I_{CO_2}})$ for $(F_{I_{N_2}} + F_{I_{CO_2}})$ and $(1 - F_{I_{O_2}} - F_{I_{CO_2}})$ for $F_{I_{N_2}}$, we obtain

$$P_{A_{O_2}} = \frac{(P_B - P_{H_2O})(RQ(F_{I_{O_2}}) + F_{I_{CO_2}}) - P_{A_{CO_2}}(1 - F_{I_{O_2}}(1 - RQ))}{RQ + F_{I_{CO_2}}(1 - RQ)} \qquad \text{(Eq. C-30)}$$

which is the *general form* of the alveolar gas equation.

When $F_{I_{CO_2}}$ is zero, as occurs when rebreathing does not occur, Eq. C-30 reduces to a simpler form

$$P_{A_{O_2}} = (P_B - P_{H_2O})F_{I_{O_2}} - P_{A_{CO_2}}(F_{I_{O_2}} - (1 - F_{I_{O_2}})/RQ) \qquad \text{(Eq. C-31)}$$

which is the form used in clinical practice. For ease of computation, Equation C-31 is often reduced to

$$P_{A_{O_2}} = (P_B - P_{H_2O})F_{I_{O_2}} - P_{A_{CO_2}}/RQ \qquad \text{(Eq. C-32)}$$

but this form ignores the effect of $F_{A_{N_2}}$, and may err by as much as 10 torr. For most clinical decisions, however, this accuracy is usually adequate.

Physiologic Dead Space Fraction

The physiologic dead space fraction as measured by the Bohr technique, is based on a gas dilution principle. The simple model for this technique assumes two alveolar compartments in parallel, one functioning (V_A) and one dead space ($V_{D_{alv}}$). The anatomic dead space ($V_{D_{an}}$) is represented by a third compartment which connects the two. The sum of the two dead space compartments is equal to the physiologic dead space (V_D).

Expired tidal gas (V_T) receives contributions from all three compartments. Only the alveolar compartment (V_A) contributes CO_2 from the blood, while V_D is free of CO_2. The volume of CO_2 in the functioning alveolar compartment is diluted into the larger (CO_2-free) V_T, according to the following relation, where $P_{E_{CO_2}}$ is the mixed expired gas in the expired tidal volume:

$$V_T(P_{E_{CO_2}}) = V_A(P_{A_{CO_2}}) \qquad \text{(Eq. C-33)}$$

The value V_A is equal to $V_T - V_D$:

$$V_T(P_{E_{CO_2}}) = (V_T - V_D)P_{A_{CO_2}}$$
$$= V_T(P_{A_{CO_2}}) - V_D(P_{A_{CO_2}})$$

rearranging:

$$V_D(P_{A_{CO_2}}) = V_T(P_{A_{CO_2}}) - V_T(P_{E_{CO_2}})$$
$$= V_T(P_{A_{CO_2}} - P_{E_{CO_2}})$$

or

$$V_D/V_T = (P_{A_{CO_2}} - P_{E_{CO_2}})/P_{A_{CO_2}} \qquad \text{(Eq. C-34)}$$

Physiologic Shunt Fraction

The determination of the physiologic shunt fraction is based on the simple model consisting of blood flow dividing into two parallel compartments which then rejoin. One portion is in contact with a functioning alveolus ($\dot{Q}_A$) and the second is shunt portion ($\dot{Q}_S$) that delivers venous blood to mix with arterial blood.

Oxygen delivery is the product of blood flow and oxygen content ($\dot{Q}C$). The total oxygen delivered out of the lungs ($\dot{Q}_TC_a$) is the sum of the oxygen delivered from the functioning capillary bed containing end-capillary blood ($\dot{Q}_AC_{c'}$) and from the shunt capillary bed containing mixed venous blood ($\dot{Q}_S C\bar{v}$):

$$\dot{Q}_T Ca = \dot{Q}_A Cc' + \dot{Q}_S C\bar{v} \qquad \text{(Eq. C-35)}$$

Since total flow is the sum of the alveolar and shunt fractions, we can substitute $\dot{Q}_T - \dot{Q}_S$ for $\dot{Q}_A$:

$$\dot{Q}_T Ca = (\dot{Q}_T - \dot{Q}_S)Cc' + \dot{Q}_S C\bar{v}$$

or

$$\dot{Q}_T Ca = \dot{Q}_T Cc' - \dot{Q}_S Cc' + \dot{Q}_S C\bar{v}$$

Rearranging:

$$\dot{Q}_S Cc' - \dot{Q}_S C\bar{v} = \dot{Q}_T Cc' - \dot{Q}_T Ca$$

or

$$\dot{Q}_S(Cc' - C\bar{v}) = \dot{Q}_T(Cc' - Ca)$$

which becomes:

$$\frac{\dot{Q}_S}{\dot{Q}_T} = \frac{Cc' - Ca}{Cc' - C\bar{v}} \qquad \text{(Eq. C-36)}$$

which is the physiologic shunt fraction.

Anatomic Shunt Fraction

   If a subject were to breathe oxygen ($F_{I_{O_2}} = 1.00$) for several minutes to washout the nitrogen in his alveoli, then even slowly ventilating spaces (comprising the relative shunt) will contain high concentrations of oxygen, and end-capillary blood will be completely saturated with oxygen. The only remaining venous admixture is then the anatomic shunt. There are two considerations under the above condition:
   1) Both end-capillary and arterial blood hemoglobin are fully saturated, such that $Sc' = Sa$, and therefore $C_{hgb}c' = C_{hgb}a$.
   2) the contribution of physically dissolved oxygen is significant at higher partial pressures, therefore whole blood oxygen content must be expressed as the sum of hemoglobin content and the content of physically dissolved oxygen ($C_{hgb} + 0.0031P_{O_2}$).
   Therefore, Eq. C-36 above is replaced by

$$\frac{\dot{Q}_{S_{an}}}{\dot{Q}_T} = \frac{(C_{hgb}a + 0.0031P_{A_{O_2}}) - (C_{hgb}a\ a\ 0.0031P_{a_{O_2}})}{(C_{hgb}a + 0.0031P_{A_{O_2}}) - (C_{hgb}\bar{v} + 0.0031P\bar{v}_{O_2})}$$

or

$$\frac{\dot{Q}_{S_{an}}}{\dot{Q}_T} = \frac{0.0031P_{(A\text{-}a)_{O_2}}}{(C_{hgb}a + 0.0031P_{A_{O_2}}) - (C_{hgb}\bar{v} + 0.0031P\bar{v}_{O_2})}$$

By adding and subtracting Pa_{O_2} to the denominator we have:

$$\frac{\dot{Q}s_{an}}{\dot{Q}_T} = \frac{0.0031P(A\text{-}a)_{O_2}}{(C_{hgb}a + 0.0031Pa_{O_2}) - (C_{hgb}\bar{v} + 0.0031P\bar{v}_{O_2}) + 0.0031(P_{A_{O_2}} - Pa_{O_2})}$$

which reduces to:

$$\frac{\dot{Q}s_{an}}{\dot{Q}_t} = \frac{0.0031P(A\text{-}a)_{O_2}}{c(a\text{-}\bar{v})_{O_2} + 0.0031P(A\text{-}a)_{O_2}} \qquad \text{(Eq. C-37)}$$

which is the anatomic shunt fraction.

GAS DIFFUSION

Single Breath Diffusing Capacity

The $D_{L_{CO}sb}$ involves the introduction of a foreign gas into the alveolar volume and recording the volume of gas transferred during a single breath. As opposed to steady state methods in which the alveolar concentration of CO is maintained nearly constant by continuous inhalation of test gas, the single breath method involves a decline in CO concentration as gas is transferred.

The model for $D_{L_{CO}}$ consists of a single alveolar compartment and a single capillary compartment (Fig. 9-1). The process is described by a form of the Fick equation:

$$\dot{V}_{CO} = D_L(P_{A_{CO}}) \qquad \text{(Eq. C-38)}$$

which assumes a Pa_{CO} of zero (a reasonable assumption in the nonsmoker). Using the equalities

$$\dot{V}_{CO} = F_{A_{CO}}(V_A)$$

and:

$$P_{A_{CO}} = F_{A_{CO}}(P_B - P_{H_2O})$$

we can express Eq. C-38 in terms of $F_{A_{CO_2}}$. Representing $\dot{V}_{CO}$ in terms of derivatives we have

$$V_A \frac{dF_{A_{CO}}}{dt} = -D_L(P_B - P_{H_2O})F_{A_{CO}} \qquad \text{(Eq. C-39)}$$

where the negative sign is intended only to indicate that $F_{A_{CO}}$ decreases with time. The derivative $d\,F_{A_{CO}}/dt$ may be thought of as the instantaneous rate of change of $F_{A_{CO}}$ with time. Rearranging to

$$\frac{d\,F_{A_{CO}}}{F_{A_{CO}}} = -D_L \frac{(P_B - P_{H_2O})}{V_A}\,dt$$

Integrating this equation, we obtain

$$\ln F_{A_{CO}} = -D_L \frac{(P_B - P_{H_2O})}{V_A} t + C \qquad \text{(Eq. C-40)}$$

The constant of integration (C) of is found by setting $t = 0$, representing the start of the test, when $F_{A_{CO}} = F_{i A_{CO}}$, the initial value of $F_{A_{CO}}$. We then have:

$$C = \ln F_{A_{CO}} \text{ (at } t = 0) = \ln F_{i A_{CO}}$$

thus Eq. C-40 can be arranged to:

$$D_L = \frac{V_A}{P_B - P_{H_2O}} (1/t)(\ln F_{i A_{CO}} - \ln F_{A_{CO}}) \qquad \text{(Eq. C-41)}$$

or

$$D_L = \frac{-V_A}{t(P_B - P_{H_2O})} \ln \frac{F_{i A_{CO}}}{F_{A_{CO}}} \qquad \text{(Eq. C-42)}$$

which is the diffusion equation for the single breath method. The negative sign indicates that the alveolar CO concentration decreases with time, but this may be ignored for clinical purposes.

To understand the behavior of $F_{A_{CO}}$ during the test, Eq. C-41 can be arranged to

$$\ln F_{A_{CO}} = \ln F_{i A_{CO}} - (D_L/V_A)(P_B - P_{H_2O})t$$

which by taking the exponential function of each side becomes

$$F_{A_{CO}} = F_{i A_{CO}} e^{-D_L/V_A(P_B - P_{H_2O})t} \qquad \text{(Eq. C-43)}$$

This indicates that $F_{A_{CO}}$ declines exponentially from an initial value of $F_{i A_{CO}}$. The rate of decline is dependent upon the diffusing capacity, the alveolar volume, and the barometric pressure.

REFERENCES

1. Gray, JS: The derivation and certain uses of an equation relating alveolar composition to altitude. AAF Sch Aviat Med Proj 131, Report 1, 1943
2. Gray, JS: Concerning the use of carbon dioxide to counteract anoxia. AAF Sch Aviat Med Proj 310, Report 1, 1944

Index

Page numbers followed by f represent figures; those followed by t represent tables.